# The Lessons
## and
# The Legacy
## of the
# Pew Health
# Policy
# Program

# The Lessons
# and
# The Legacy
# of the
# Pew Health
# Policy
# Program

Jon A. Chilingerian
Corinne M. Kay

**INSTITUTE OF MEDICINE**

SPONSORED BY THE PEW CHARITABLE TRUSTS

**NATIONAL ACADEMY PRESS** ✳ 2101 Constitution Avenue, N.W. ✳ Washington, D.C. 20418

The Institute of Medicine was chartered in 1970 by the National Academy of Sciences to enlist distinguished members of the appropriate professions in the examination of policy matters pertaining to the health of the public. In this, the Institute acts under both the Academy's 1863 congressional charter responsibility to be an adviser to the federal government and its own initiative in identifying issues of medical care, research, and education. Dr. Kenneth I. Shine is president of the Institute of Medicine.

Support for this project was provided by The Pew Charitable Trusts, Philadelphia, Pennsylvania.

Additional copies of this report are available from the National Academy Press, 2101 Constitution Avenue, N.W., Box 285, Washington, D.C. 20055. Call 800-624-6242 or 202-334-3313 (in the Washington Metropolitan Area). **http://www/nap.edu.**

# Foreword

This document describes the creation, evolution, and future opportunities in health policy training that have emanated from The Pew Charitable Trusts' 15-year support of the Pew Health Policy Fellows Program. It is intended to help stimulate and strengthen health policy training programs at a time when rich and diverse approaches are so crucial to preparing leaders to deal successfully with the many compelling health care delivery and financing issues that we face as a nation. The document portrays the strategic approaches taken over the life of the program, as well as their strengths and weaknesses, conveys a sense of optimism about how much can be achieved by creating an environment in which talented people can learn new skills to use in analyzing problems and devising improved policies for addressing them.

In 1982, the Pew Charitable Trusts initiated the Health Policy Fellows Program, with a grant of $11.85 million. The program was based on a premise that the challenges that lay ahead in health care would require a cadre of people with finely honed skills to analyze issues and to translate those analyses into public policy. The program was also an attempt to bridge the gap between policy research and policy-making, and to infuse a variety of perspectives into the search for ways to improve access to and the quality of health care while controlling its cost. At that time, there were few places where this kind of multidisciplinary environment flourished. Instead, people interested in pursuing health policy research usually defaulted to discipline-specific academic departments and, if they were highly motivated, sought perspectives from other fields and disciplines. The Pew program was an attempt to break down barriers, to stimulate the creation of a multidisciplinary training environment, and to promote an interchange among policymakers, academic faculty, and students. It was also designed to apply rigorous methodological approaches to applied health policy research. These goals and changes were fundamental to the program's success, and achieving them required the dedication, commitment, and foresight of project directors and faculty in each of the participating sites.

In the early years of the Program, four sites were funded, each of which is described in the pages that follow. The University of Michigan program offered people working full time, often in government, the opportunity to pursue a doctorate through weekend sessions and through work on a dissertation topic related to their job. Boston University and Brandeis jointly offered a 2-year doctoral "corporate fellows" program for high-level executives in the health care field, and an "associates" program to provide technical assistance to select cities. The University of California San Francisco (UCSF) program offered a 2-year predoctoral fellowship and postdoctoral opportunities for health care professionals. Last, the RAND/University of California Los Angeles (UCLA) program offered a 2-year doctoral degree and a 1-year (nondegree) midcareer fellowship designed primarily for academic health care professionals. The four programs ran the gamut in terms of enabling people at any stage of their career—whether at a predoctoral, postdoctoral, or corporate continuing education level—to develop the skills needed to become leaders in health policy research and policy-making.

Funding for a central administrative office was provided initially to the American Enterprise Institute and later to the Institute of Medicine, to support Marion Ein Lewin's leadership and direction of the program. From the beginning, she worked tirelessly to guide the implementation of the program by its leaders at the four sites: Richard Egdahl and Stuart Altman at Boston University/Brandeis; Albert Williams at RAND/UCLA; Philip Lee and Carroll Estes at UCSF; and John Griffith and Leon Wyszewianski at Michigan. Early Fellows were guided through their studies by the likes of Steve Crane at Boston University, Kate Korman at RAND/UCLA, and David Perlman at Michigan. Early advisory committee members who helped critique and refine the program included Bruce Vladeck (chair), Bob Blendon, Walter McNerney, Judy Miller-Jones, Bill Richardson and Gail Warden. Following Dr. Richardson's thoughtful evaluation of the program in 1985, the Trusts renewed their commitment with an $8.1 million grant. The advisory committee added new experts as well, including Diane Rowland (chair), Richard Curtis, David Kindig, Faith Mitchell, and

Helen Smits. The sites continued to modify and refine their efforts based on the advisory committee's recommendations, and in 1991 the grant was renewed one last time for $5.7 million. This time, however, the funding supported three distinct models: the UCSF postdoctoral program, directed by Hal Luft and Carroll Estes; the Brandeis University doctoral program codirected by Stan Wallack and Jon Chilingerian; and the continuation of the Michigan nonresidential program for full-time workers, directed by Bill Weissert.

Several common themes transcended the different program structure. For instance, Fellows and faculty alike flourished thanks to the commitment of the faculty in fusing a direct link between theory and practice. Most faculty moved easily between policy research and policy-making, thus demonstrating for students that this divide was an artificial construct that could be traversed effectively. Second, all of the programs were sharply focused. It is easy in a multidisciplinary environment to become vague and fuzzy. Instead, the programs required strategic thinking on explicit topics. The topics could be synthetic (i.e., systems approaches) rather than reductionist, but underlying the topical framework was a third shared characteristic: methodological rigor. Fourth, the Fellows learned from one another as well as from their faculty mentors, and this created a strong network of leaders who soon became mentors in their own right.

Throughout the program's 15-year history, the sites incorporated the lessons they learned as they worked to reconcile the tensions that naturally arose between conflicting demands. For example, there is always a tension between breadth or depth in multidisciplinary studies, and each program took its own road in defining the appropriate balance. Moreover, applied research methodologies inherently call for trade-offs between pragmatic constraints and research design needs. Finally, all programs entered into the final several years of funding recognizing that the Trusts' support was coming to an end, and that the their future viability would depend on finding other sources of support. Their continued viability also would require a willingness by the sponsoring universities to "institutionalize" this multidisciplinary approach and to legitimize health policy research as an academic discipline. Recognizing that its support could facilitate only a handful of models, and appreciating how much these models have to contribute to the field, the Trusts requested that the project leaders develop the present document so other institutions could benefit from the programs' experiences—both their successes and their problems—and might develop their own health policy training programs to expand the available options for interested students.

The network of Fellows is now more than 300 strong. Many of the alumni play leading roles in policy-making positions in both the public and private sectors as well as in academia throughout the country. We owe the early faculty and Fellows a great debt of gratitude for taking the risk of entering into a new type of program and for establishing ties with and mentoring new Fellows. We are grateful to the Fellows of the early 1980's for strengthening the programs through their candid feedback and critiques. We owe the current Fellows special thanks for enrolling in the program during this time of transitional funding, when they and their faculty have had to rely on creative means of generating additional support. We are greatly indebted to the faculty for their unflagging commitment to the program, and for their devotion to making it better year after year. We are enormously grateful to Marion Ein Lewin who has directed the program for 15 years, has facilitated its refinement and evolution, and has served as its enthusiastic advocate and emissary. Finally, we owe a tremendous debt of thanks to the sites, advisors, Fellows, and alumni for their candor in sharing their experiences and thoughts in this document, and to Jon Chilingerian and Corinne Kay for pulling all of this material together to create what we hope will be a useful resource for years to come. Of course, the good works of the over 300 Fellows and alumni are a legacy of their own.

**Carolyn H. Asbury, PhD**
Director, Health and Human Services
The Pew Charitable Trusts
Philadelphia, Pennsylvania
April 24, 1997

# Acknowledgments

Books are rarely creations of their authors alone; rather they synthesize and build on the ideas, opinions, and work of many. This "legacy" is an example of that fact. We have relied on archival materials, program evaluations, and interviews with dozens of Pew Fellows, program staff and faculty, and Institute of Medicine staff. Grateful acknowledgment is made to those who allowed us to carry forward their knowledge and ideas, especially those who were part of the focus groups (Washington meetings in November 1995 and December 1996 and Atlanta meeting in June 1995) and to the BU/Brandeis Pew Fellows who were in Jon's Pew Seminar.

We are happy to thank all those many friends who shared and helped us, especially the interviewees who not only gave of their time to discuss their Pew experiences but then meticulously read through sections of the document and provided helpful comments. They are (in alphabetical order): Stuart Altman, Dennis Beatrice, Lisa Bero, Sarita Bhalotra, Patricia Butler, Steve Crane, Joan DaVanzo, Carroll Estes, Kathleen Eyre, John Griffith, Terry Hammons, Jonathan Howland, Kate Korman, Leighton Ku, Mark Legnini, Marion Ein Lewin, Hal Luft, John McDonough, Pamela Paul-Shaheen, Dan Rubin, Stan Wallack, Linda Simoni-Wastilla, Bill Weissert, Al Williams, and Leon Wyszewianski. Furthermore, there were several Pew alumni who were not interviewed but who graciously reviewed sections of the document and provided suggestions: Nora Maloy (Michigan), Debbie Ward (BU), Linda Bergthold (UCSF), Ruth Malone (UCSF), and Faith Mitchell (UCSF). Their criticism guided us. If, in places, we did not take their advice, we alone are to blame. We would also like to express our gratitude to Kevin Dombkowski, a current Michigan Pew Fellow, for his valuable assistance with graphics.

We are deeply indebted to Marion Ein Lewin for all her help in the construction of this book. Our gratitude also goes to Shirley Stewart for her assistance in getting the project started and locating some interesting archives, Carolyn Asbury for writing the preface, and Stan Wallack and Steve Crane for their stimulating comments on the manuscript. Special thanks to Valerie Tate Jopeck for her great patience and exceptional organizational skills and to Nancy Marley and Kathleen Keck for their most expert assistance in preparing the manuscript. We thank Michael Hayes for his help in editing this book, and to Linda Humphrey for her inspired design work. We are grateful to Dean Jack Shonkoff for his kindness in providing us with a haven to do this work.

Thank you Dianne, Christine, Johnny, and Chris (with love). Last but not least, we would like to thank each other for the pleasure of working together to complete this project. It was fun.

Finally, we dedicate this book to the Pew Fellows, in recognition of their sacrifice, interest, criticism, and deep concern for the future of our health care system.

# Contents

## List of Tables

## List of Figures

# Part I.

## *Introduction*

he idea of writing about the legacy and experiences of the Pew Health Policy Fellowship Programs was first articulated several years ago by the Pew Health Policy Program Advisory Board. Under the direction of Marion Ein Lewin, the Program Office began negotiating with outside consultants and writers. Logistical difficulties postponed the production for several years, and it was not until August 1995 that the project took off. It was at that time that the process of gathering information about the various Pew Health Policy Fellowship Programs began.

Over the next year, 25 telephone and focused, in-depth, face-to-face interviews with key individuals were conducted to enlarge the range of perspectives (see Appendix A), round-table discussions and focus groups were held at a November 1995 Pew Networking Dinner at the institute of Medicine in Washington, D.C. and at the Association for Health Services Research (AHSR) annual meeting in Atlanta in June 1996, and the manuscript was circulated among several program directors and alumni for feedback. Detailed archival information, including three program evaluations conducted by outside consultants, case studies, directories, and minutes, were collected, synthesized, and summarized. Ultimately, these many and varied sources of information came together to tell a most provoking and stimulating story.

The Program Office, in consultation with the program directors, envisioned—and ultimately produced—a report that would capture some of the history of the Pew Health Policy Fellowship Programs, include the curriculum from each of the program sites, and report on interviews with program directors regarding specific issues. Questions included the following: How had the programs evolved over time? What lessons and insights have been learned? How were the program directors able to make an innovative and often unconventional training program work within the traditional academic environment? The report was also to include

> Archival information, including three program evaluations conducted by outside consultants, case studies, directories, and minutes, were collected, synthesized, and summarized. These many and varied sources of information came together to tell a most provoking and stimulating story.

interviews with fellows and alumni sharing their experiences in pursuing midcareer, fast-track doctorate and postdoctorate education. In describing the field, the report would illustrate the importance of health services and health policy research and the role that the Pew Health Policy Program (PHPP) has played in this arena, as well as in the areas of leadership training and health policy development. Finally, the report was to describe the next generation of such programs and how and where they might be developed and funded. A report such as this was deemed important because the PHPP experience was an especially rich one due to the various formats of graduate training in health policy that the program helped to develop. The original thinkers hypothesized that differentiating between these programs would help guide future programs and identify aspects that were replicable and transferable.

## THE BIRTH OF THE PEW HEALTH POLICY PROGRAM

By 1994, the Pew Charitable Trusts had eight signature scholarship programs. The Pew Health Policy Program (PHPP) was the oldest of the eight programs and the first with a national scope.[1]  In many ways PHPP, which was established in 1982 and which selected its first fellows in 1983, was a crucial experiment for the Pew Charitable Trusts, because, until the establishment of PHPP,  Pew grants had predominantly been distributed in Pennsylvania.

When PHPP was designed, the operating philosophy of the Pew Charitable Trusts was strikingly different from what it had been during the development of earlier signature fellowship programs. PHPP was the first Trusts-initiated program, and it represented Pew's desire to play a more active role in the programs that it sponsored. The Pew Charitable Trusts developed their own programmatic initiatives and, together with the institutions selected to run the programs, helped to shape the process (Hamilton, 1995).

Traditionally, the Pew Charitable Trusts had focused on supporting the "bricks and mortar" endeavors in health and education. Rapid growth, however, in both the assets and the interests of the Pew Charitable Trusts during the 1970s, combined with significant changes in the nation's health care delivery, research, and funding systems, influenced the Pew Charitable Trusts to change their focus toward program building and human development. With the establishment of PHPP, Pew aimed to enrich the content of a subject area that was suffering from limited academic recognition and

[1] *The seven other signature scholarship programs were: The Pew Scholars Program in the Biomedical Sciences/ Latin American Fellows; Pew Fellowships in the Arts; Pew National Arts Journalism Program; Pew Economic Freedom Fellowships; Pew Global Security Initiative; Pew Evangelical Scholars; and Pew Scholars in Conservation and the Environment.*

student interest. PHPP was created to stimulate the development of the nation's health policy through the development of multidisciplinary educational programs that would prepare fellows for leadership roles in health policy.

The Pew Charitable Trusts invited a Health Advisory Group of nine experts in health care to assist them in developing their programmatic initiatives. Eight members of this advisory group were academicians, and the ninth person was a physician representing the foundation community (see Table 1). The Health Advisory Group recommended that Pew sponsor one to three programs in health policy and suggested the incorporation of several different educational models (i.e., master's degree programs, doctoral programs, and combined on-job/on-campus doctoral programs). The development strategy included assembling several consultants who would be charged with designing a request for proposal (RFP), selecting the appropriate institutions to receive the RFP, reviewing the responses and recommending the best institutions proposing the best programs, and developing a strategy to evaluate the programs (Hamilton, 1995).

> PHPP was created to stimulate the development of the nation's health policy through the development of multidisciplinary educational programs that would prepare fellows for leadership roles in health policy.

## Table 1.
### Health Advisory Group Membership, The Pew Charitable Trusts, 1980

**Robert W. Berliner, M.D.**
Yale University School of Medicine
New Haven, Connecticut

**Hilary Koprowski, M.D.**
Director
Wistar Institute of Anatomy and Biology
Philadelphia, Pennsylvania

**Thomas W. Langfitt, M.D.**
Vice President of Health Affairs
University of Pennsylvania
Philadelphia, Pennsylvania

**Irving M. London, M.D.**
Harvard–MIT Program for Health Science and Technology
Cambridge, Massachusetts

**Vernon B. Mountcastle, M.D.**
Director
Department of Physiology
Johns Hopkins University School of Medicine
Baltimore, Maryland

**Ray D. Owen, Ph.D.**
Vice President, Student Affairs and
Dean of Students
Division of Biology
California Institute of Technology
Pasadena, California

**Frederick C. Robbins, M.D.**
Office of the Dean
School of Medicine
Case Western Reserve University
Cleveland, Ohio

**Timothy R. Talbot, Jr., M.D.**
President
Fox Chase Cancer Center
Philadelphia, Pennsylvania

**Kerr L. White, M.D.**
Deputy Director
Director of Health Sciences
The Rockefeller Foundation
New York, New York

Ultimately, 15 academic institutions with health centers and four nonacademic health centers that were conducting high-quality programs in health policy-related areas were selected to receive the RFP. All 19 organizations sent proposals. Four university programs, each of which proposed a unique educational model, and one nonacademic center-based site providing independent programming and support services to the university sites received funding. The proposals from the institutions selected to receive funding are briefly described here.

### RAND Corporation/University of California at Los Angeles (RAND/UCLA)

**Four university programs, each of which proposed a unique educational model, and one nonacademic center-based site providing independent programming and support services to the university sites received funding.**

RAND and UCLA proposed a joint venture in the Los Angeles area. The proposal contained three components: the Health Policy Fellowship Program, a 3-year interdisciplinary program leading to a PhD in policy analysis at RAND or the PhD in health policy at UCLA; the Policy Career Development Program, a 1-year nondegree program aimed at improving the individual's ability to critically evaluate health policy studies and to collaborate knowledgeably with professionals from varied disciplines; and the Medical Student Policy Seminar, a 10-session lecture and discussion series designed to introduce medical students to health policy issues early in their training.

### Boston University/Brandeis University (BU/Brandeis)

Boston University and Brandeis also proposed a joint venture. The proposal contained three specific elements: the Pew Scholars Program, an intensive 2-year, post-master's, multidisciplinary program leading to a PhD in health policy, offered at both universities; the Pew Fellows Program, which included a 2-year seminar program to raise the level of health resource management skills of upper-level corporate and government managers (called senior fellows), and a 2- to 3-year commitment of selected midcareer-level corporate staff to focus on improving access to health care services through the implementation of cost-containment strategies within selected communities (called mid-level fellows).

### University of California San Francisco (UCSF)

UCSF proposed a two-component program designed to meet needs at various levels. The first component was the

Pew Health Policy Research Program, which offered two distinct programs: a 2-year postdoctoral fellowship aimed at augmenting research skills, particularly methodological and statistical skills, and improving the fellows' ability to work effectively in both large and small interdisciplinary research studies requiring significant cooperation, and a 2-year predoctoral fellowship providing broader exposure to health policy issues in a multidisciplinary environment and encouraging research on health policy-related topics that would result in a dissertation. The second component was the Pew Health Policy Management Program, offering a 2-year term of diverse management experiences in hospitals, the School of Medicine, and other UCSF professional schools and participation in the Health Policy Research Seminar.

### University of Michigan

The University of Michigan proposed a 2- to 3-year, non-residential on-job/on-campus doctoral program providing 20 4-day sessions and two 4-week sessions for health services policy makers and administrators and offering doctoral-level training without requiring fellows to leave their current employment for extended periods of time. The program was to be housed in the School of Public Health, and those participants who completed the program received a doctorate in public health.

### American Enterprise Institute (AEI)

The American Enterprise Institute provided a two-component effort designed to support the basic aims of PHPP: (1) a program for state officials offering nine seminars over a 2-year period focusing on new cost-containment strategies for state and local governments and (2) semiannual 3-day seminars for fellows and faculty from the four university-based programs to expose fellows to policy leaders on national and regional levels.

**Over time, various changes took place.**

### Changes to the Programs

The programs are described as they were originally designed during the period of initial funding. Over time, various changes took place. For example, one entire program (RAND/UCLA) was not refunded after the program's first 11 years; however, fellows matriculating in the Fall of 1990 were funded through July 1993. (As will be discussed further,

*Three evaluations contracted out first in 1985, then in 1990, and finally in 1995 guided the evolution of PHPP.*

the RAND program continued to thrive past the termination of Pew funding.) Boston University, one of the partner institutions at the BU/Brandeis site dropped out at the same point. The site and administration of the program office also changed after 5 years. Finally, some programmatic elements at each site were either dropped or became self-financed.[2]

## VAGUE GOALS THAT ALLOWED FOR REFLECTIVE ORGANIZATIONAL LEARNING

The purpose of PHPP was clear:

> *To stimulate the development of multidisciplinary health policy education programs that will equip a cadre of leaders with the required skills to deal effectively with the nation's complex current and future health policy issues.*

In spite of this clear purpose, a review of the available archives and discussion records reveals an absence of performance measures or benchmarks to gauge the progress or success of PHPP.

Although the goals and objectives were not explicit, three evaluations contracted out first in 1985, then in 1990, and finally in 1995 guided the evolution of PHPP. The data obtained from the comprehensive and instructive evaluations by William Richardson (1985, 1990) and Ed Hamilton (1995) formed the foundation for this report. Eight performance indicators used in those evaluations greatly influenced the progress and development of the individual programs:

1. The interdisciplinary strength of the curricula
2. The richness of the health policy-related research and policy analysis environments accessible to fellows
3. The existence of a nurturing orientation and structured mentoring function and the quality of the fellows
4. The impact of the program on local, state, and national scenes
5. The degree to which Pew funding has had a capacity-building influence within the universities housing the programs
6. The ability of the fellows to routinely secure appointment to appropriate health professional positions having a significant health policy content
7. The impact of the fellowship experience on the fellow's career paths
8. The degree to which grantees' programs complement rather than duplicate each other

[2] *The evolution of the programs will be described in further detail in Part II.*

To decipher the legacy of PHPP, the programs will be examined on each of these levels. A few other factors found to play critical roles in the successful growth and development of these programs are also described.

## HISTORY AND ORIGINS OF DEVELOPMENT

PHPP was established in response to several challenging environmental needs. First, the nation's health care system was becoming increasingly competitive, complex, customer focused, and community oriented, generating the need for an ever larger pool of highly qualified health policy professionals. Second, Pew realized that the key players at the forefront of resolving and reshaping the future of the U.S. health care system would need to represent a spectrum of disciplines and perspectives.

The objective of the program was to develop and support a unique program of advanced training and education in health policy that would attract talented young and mid-career professionals interested in preparing for leadership roles in policy development at the highest levels of government and industry. The program envisioned that these future health policy leaders would come from a variety of disciplines—including medicine, public health, other health professions, law, management, social sciences, economics, and political science—but that all would benefit from multidisciplinary training in policy research and analysis, hands-on-experience, and management. Multidisciplinary learning would ideally enable the Pew fellows to function in the world of health policy with an ability to work not only with each other but with professionals from many fields.

It was further envisioned that these programs should be formulated in a way that would support and supplement the advanced health policy training and education activities that were being undertaken at various universities and institutes, building on existing efforts at a few selected institutions of excellence.

The request for proposals was not prescriptive regarding the type of educational experience to be provided or its format, content, length, or cost. It did, however, indicate that programs should draw from the perspectives of a variety of disciplines. As Stuart Altman of Brandeis University recalled:

> *If you go back to the very beginning, one of the things that was very impressive and very unique about the original solicitation, that I have never seen before and have never seen since, was the fact that a small group of advisers to Pew said that there are*

Pew realized that the key players at the forefront of resolving and reshaping the future of the U.S. health care system would need to represent a spectrum of disciplines and perspectives.

*important issues that are likely to develop in health care over the next few years, rather than the foundation saying what they are. Therefore, the small group of institutions that were selected to train people were allowed to (a) indicate what they believe[d] [were]going to be some of the major health care problems that this country would face over the next decade and (b) how they could design a training program to help individuals meet those needs.*

Granting the individual universities the creative freedom to create programs that best fit their institutions and their perspectives resulted in several very different kinds of training centers and a rich diversity of health policy professionals. The program evaluations were subsequently used to tighten and improve the programs. Today, PHPP fellows have been able to take leadership positions throughout the health care system at strategic levels and locations. The incredibly broad scope of PHPP fellows has elevated their influence, impact, and effectiveness as policy engineers and change agents.

## PROGRAM DESCRIPTIONS
### University of California at San Francisco

**Granting the individual universities the creative freedom to create programs that best fit their institutions and their perspectives resulted in several very different kinds of training centers and a rich diversity of health policy professionals.**

The UCSF program, jointly sponsored by the university's Institute for Health Policy Studies in the School of Medicine and the Institute for Health and Aging in the School of Nursing, initially offered three types of 2-year fellowships: predoctoral, postdoctoral, and management. Following the first 5-year funding cycle, however, predoctoral and management fellowships were discontinued in favor of strengthening the postdoctoral program. At the same time, the postdoctoral program was expanded to include some midcareer fellows, people who entered the program from an employment setting as opposed to postdoctoral fellows who entered the program directly from a graduate degree program or residency. The program was made more flexible so that 1-year and part-time fellowships could also be offered. Part-time fellowships were typically for 20 to 40 percent of a full-time fellowship for a period of 2 years.

The program offers multidisciplinary training in applied collaborative health services and health policy research through apprenticeship models. Fellows learn to think broadly and work collaboratively with people from a variety of disciplines and then develop a base of skills that can be applied to health policy issues at various levels of government and in the private sector. The faculty from the two institutes serve as teachers, mentors, and research preceptors to the fellows. Additional faculty are drawn from other departments and units at UCSF.

From its inception, the UCSF Pew fellowship program has been unique in that it is housed in and cosponsored by organized research units (ORUs) of the university rather than departments: the Institute for Health Policy Studies and the Institute for Health and Aging. The ORUs are designed to facilitate cross-departmental and cross-school research, but they do not have formal teaching responsibilities or sponsor degree programs. Furthermore, the majority of the faculty in these two ORUs are supported entirely by outside grants and contracts. The two Institutes have more than 65 faculty, and fellows have the opportunity to work directly with policy analysts and researchers from a wide range of disciplines and interests on a large number of important projects. The interdisciplinary nature of these institutes also makes their position unique. Both settings draw upon faculty from a wide range of disciplines, including sociology, economics, psychology, political science, medicine, nursing, pharmacy, dentistry, law, public health, and bioscience.

The role of key people in the development and evolution of the UCSF postdoctoral program cannot be overstated. In particular, the role of its founder, Phil Lee, as program champion is widely acknowledged, as cited by Hal Luft:

> *Phil Lee's commitment to training, to doing health policy and health policy research, and incorporating a wide range of people with different backgrounds and expertise was crucial [to the development of the UCSF program]. . . . Many of the faculty come out of a multidisciplinary background and believe that good integrative health policy research and policy analysis is something that is valued and good to do, and this gave us an opportunity, in a sense, to reproduce.*

The development of the UCSF doctoral program was based on a strongly held belief that excellent health services research can often be better accomplished through a team effort involving people of different backgrounds who understand each other's assumptions and perspectives on the world. Thus, the program was designed as a model in which social scientists would learn to work with health professionals and health professionals would learn to work with social scientists. If physicians or other health professionals really wanted extensive research skills, they were encouraged to enroll in a master's of public health or doctoral program.

At UCSF, there was no preexisting set of courses to serve as a basis for the program. There were excellent, but

The incredibly broad scope of PHPP fellows has elevated their influence, impact, and effectiveness as policy engineers and change agents.

small, programs in sociology, medical anthropology, and health psychology, but there was little institutional support for a new PhD program in health policy on this campus, nor did the faculty think that such a program should be developed. Instead, they supported a "learning by doing" model, widely used in both the medical and nursing schools at UCSF, that enabled the fellows to gain facility with the methodology needed to conduct sound, policy-relevant research. The course work and hands-on research experience resulted in the development of an effective network for fellows that included academicians, health professionals, and policy makers (UCSF Report, 1994).

In an effort to make the Pew Health Policy Program at UCSF self-sufficient, its faculty implemented major steps toward institutionalizing the training approach. A series of new formal courses has been developed, and the curriculum has been greatly enriched. The issues surrounding the difficulties of institutionalizing the fellowship program without financial support will be discussed later. However, UCSF has made a commitment to exploring new avenues of funding. Faculty have worked collaboratively to identify new funding sources and have been quite successful (UCSF Report, 1994).

> At UCSF, there was no preexisting set of courses to serve as a basis for the program. Instead, they supported a "learning by doing" model, widely used in both the medical and nursing schools at UCSF.

### University of Michigan

At the University of Michigan, another new and innovative advanced training model emerged. A nontraditional, nonresidential Pew health policy doctoral (DrPH) program was created. The program has been sponsored by the Department of Health Services Management and Policy in the School of Public Health at the University of Michigan. Every 2 years, the program selects approximately 10 to 15 health policy makers from across the nation. These Pew fellows hold graduate degrees or the equivalent in public health, medicine, law, or business and have at least 5 years of experience in health policy positions.

The PHPP at Michigan was designed for individuals who were seeking doctoral-level education to enhance their ability to function in the health policy arena. The program is offered in an on-job/on-campus (OJ/OC) format, which allows the doctoral students to continue working full time while pursuing their degree. The OJ/OC format was initiated at the University of Michigan in the early 1970s and has been extremely successful. It began as a single master's program in health services administration and has evolved into a total of seven different graduate-level programs at the

School of Public Health (Michigan Report, 1994). John Griffith stated that although Michigan had experimented with this type of nonresidential training before PHPP, the real challenge was transferring it to the doctoral level.

Bill Weissert explains how Michigan met and continues to meet the challenge:

> We had an innovation here that dates back 25 years, which is this midcareer weekend program where people come in and take 2 years of the same courses. That was a proven idea that worked and cranked a huge number of people out into the health management community. So, we extended that to the health policy community with this [doctoral] program. And, I think it's a good idea. And, it gets better every year. That's how it developed. It was basically an incremental change over a proven program that was and is unique in the country. It was innovative at the time and continues to be innovative.

Participants meet once each month for a 4-day weekend session in Ann Arbor. The weekend comprises 30 hours of classroom work, and the fellows are expected to spend an additional 20 to 25 hours on independent work between monthly sessions. During the third year of the program the students meet for three weekend sessions, scheduled several months apart, as part of a series of activities and services designed to support their work on the dissertation.

**The work experiences brought to the classroom by the students provide a unique opportunity to integrate both the theoretical and practical sides of policy.**

Added to the responsibilities of a full-time job, the Michigan full-time doctoral program offers an intense experience that only very carefully selected students are able to sustain for the full 2 years of course work plus 2 to 3 years spent on the dissertation. At the same time, however, the work experiences brought to the classroom by the students provide a unique opportunity to integrate both the theoretical and practical sides of policy. The OJ/OC format complements the DrPH's practitioner orientation quite well. It does not require students to leave the world of practice and action to acquire skills that are ultimately meant for that world. This contrasts with the traditional PhD programs, whose principal aim is to prepare future teachers and researchers and whose students therefore benefit from being immersed full time in the academic and research environment for which they are being prepared (Michigan Report, 1994).

## RAND/University of California at Los Angeles

The RAND/UCLA program evolved out of a long-term relationship between the University of California at Los Angeles and the RAND Graduate School of Policy Studies.

As explained by faculty members Al Williams and Kate Korman, however, this relationship was not formalized until the joint proposal submission to the Pew Charitable Trusts. Kate Korman reflected that the preexisting loose ties between the UCLA Department of Medicine, the UCLA School of Public Health, and RAND greatly facilitated the creation of a joint program:

> *Those loose ties were individual faculty at UCLA who also had appointments in the RAND Health Sciences Program. It must have seemed a natural progression to create programs which formally built on the strengths of each institution. RAND already had the RAND Graduate School of Policy Studies, which offered just a PhD, but no real emphasis on health, and UCLA had programs in health services, community health, and epidemiology, but no stated emphasis on policy.*

Like for the other programs, the commitment and dedication on the part of the faculty were crucial to the success of the RAND/UCLA program. Faculty members like Bob Brook and Bob Kane who were at UCLA but who had appointments at RAND were "groundbreakers," says Kate Korman, in that they worked tirelessly to bridge the different cultures of UCLA and RAND.

The RAND/UCLA doctoral program prescribed a 3-year enrollment period of study during which time students completed the requirements of either the RAND Graduate School of Policy Studies or the appropriate division of the UCLA School of Public Health. In addition, fellows participated in health policy workshops, completed a course in research methodology, and worked approximately half time as staff on health policy research projects at one of the two institutions. Doctoral (and midcareer fellows) were required to work 16 to 20 hours a week, and this project work was held with the same importance as the courses. It was this on-the-job training (OJT) that many of the fellows and faculty considered the most innovative aspect of the training program. The research projects and mentor relationships that were developed during the OJT enabled the students to align themselves with the dissertation process (or the research process for midcareer fellows) from the outset of their training.

RAND/UCLA also offered a 1-year (nondegree) fellowship for midcareer professionals involved in a variety of backgrounds, such as policy formulation, health care administration, the health professions, law, and management. There was a deliberate emphasis on providing real world applications in the midcareer workshops and research pro-

At RAND/UCLA, fellows worked approximately half time as staff on health policy research projects at one of the two institutions. It was this on-the-job training (OJT) that many of the fellows and faculty considered the most innovative aspect of the training program.

jects. Fellows developed skills and tools that could easily be transferred back into the health policy field.

Although the midcareer fellows left the field for a year of study, they spent much of their RAND program back in the field focused on health care-related problems. Like the RAND doctoral students, the midcareer fellows were required to align themselves with an OJT research project early on. The fellows that we interviewed, discussed projects that involved them working with the U.S. Department of Health and Human Services, the National Institutes of Health, and the Health Care Financing Administration and in many other exciting health policy environments. During their year of study many midcareer fellows worked on projects that resulted in publications and new career opportunities.

At the point of the second renewal of the program in 1991, additional objectives were added to the operating design of PHPP, which recommended that none of the basic models represented by the program sites be duplicative (Hamilton, 1995). This resulted in the discontinuance of Pew funding for the RAND/UCLA doctoral and midcareer programs. Nonetheless, the residential doctoral program continued after the Pew funds were discontinued, and it remains a vibrant program today, with the courses created for the Pew program fully institutionalized at both universities. Without outside funding, however, the midcareer program was unable to continue.[3]

> The RAND/UCLA residential doctoral program continued after the Pew funds were discontinued, and it remains a vibrant program today, with the courses created for the Pew program fully institutionalized at both universities.

## Boston University/Brandeis University (BU/Brandeis)

Established in 1983 as a joint program with Boston University, the Pew Doctoral Program at Brandeis has undergone two distinct phases. Phase One of the program (1983 to 1991) was offered jointly by Boston University and Brandeis University. Phase Two of the program (1991 to 1995) has been directed by Brandeis alone.

Phase One was built on the successful relationships that had been established between Boston University and Brandeis University faculty and research staff through the Institute for Health Policy at Brandeis University. The major objective of the program was to train a cadre of health policy leaders in health policy formulation, research, and education. The program focused on providing doctoral training in health policy to six students per year (three from each school). It was an individualized advanced program of study offering doctoral-level training in health policy to a diverse

---

[3] *The issues surrounding program institutionalization will be discussed later in this report.*

group of midcareer-level individuals. The curriculum focused on ensuring that students received a thorough grounding in the underlying disciplines while becoming quickly involved in the more divergent aspects of policy research and decision making. An important part of the training and education involved developing strong research skills with a policy research attitude. This attitude would incorporate, for example, a willingness to make policy decisions under conditions of high risk and an ability to inspire confidence in areas of uncertainty (Raskin, Chilingerian and Wallack, 1992).

Steve Crane discussed how the merging of the two institutions and their philosophies created programs that aimed at involving the business community in the health policy world:

> *The particular center at BU that was involved was the Center for Industry and Health Care. . . . [T]he Pew Corporate Fellows Program at BU brought together major industry leaders who were involved in health care issues, brought them to Boston twice a year, and created a network in the business community, the results of which are still being seen today in terms of the corporate coalitions that have been created and the analyses that continue to be done on health outcomes. I think these are things that are attributable to the types of discussions that took place, not just at BU, but I think we were a catalyst for a lot of that. It was a very important part of our total program. Likewise, Bruce Spitz's Community Program at Brandeis was very important. The notion was that we needed to create change, not just at the intellectual level but at the institutional level as well. Bruce's effort to try to get communities to move, to link together business and public sectors was highly innovative and a precursor to the coalitions of today and the more population-based research being employed today.*

**An important part of the training and education involved developing strong research skills with a policy research attitude.**

Phase Two of the program (1991 to 1995) developed out of a recognition that there had been considerable growth in health policy information over the previous decade, particularly in areas dealing with the identification of social problems in health care and the changing nature of delivery systems. To address these trends, Brandeis believed that policy makers needed to be prepared to draw on a broad range of disciplines and conduct action-oriented policy research.

The major change in the program from Phase One to Phase Two was structural. At Brandeis the program was administered through the Institute for Health Policy and had a social policy focus. At Boston University the program was offered either through the University Professors Program or through other university departments, and the primary focus of the program was cost-containment. However, as time went on, the combined program of Boston University and Brandeis University evolved from having a primary focus on cost-containment to having a concern for broader social welfare goals and health policy reform. This evolution induced curriculum, program design, and faculty changes. Due to the uncertainty of the renewal of funding and the lack of an organizational structure to sustain the health policy focus of the Pew program, Boston University changed its role to that of an affiliated institution responsible for providing several core courses. Brandeis had the potential to provide a strong organizational component through the Heller Graduate School and the Institute for Health Policy and wanted to continue the program. The Heller School had the support of the faculty and the Dean and of the Institute for Health Policy, which was located within the school.

To better integrate the Pew fellows into the Heller School's existing doctoral program, a traditional academic Heller School faculty member codirected the Pew program with a research faculty member from the Institute for Health Policy. The codirectors were then able to link the Heller School faculty and the institute research faculty in a close and substantive way (Raskin et al., 1992). The affiliation with the institute was a real strength for the Brandeis Pew program. Established in 1978, the institute is one of the largest academically based health policy research groups in the country. It provides an excellent working laboratory for Pew fellows interested in conducting and pursuing careers in health policy research.

Boston University's Health Policy Institute and the Institute for Health Policy at Brandeis University's Heller School initially offered three distinct programs: The Pew Corporate Fellows Program, the Pew Associates Program, and the Pew Doctoral Program. The Pew Corporate Fellows Program was a thematically oriented executive conference and publication program established to help some of the nation's businesspeople deal more effectively with their internal efforts to provide cost-effective and quality health services for their employees. It accepted cohorts of 30 to 40 corporate managers every 2 years to collaborate with each other and to attend two conferences per year in an effort to give the involved corporations a broader view of their responsibilities with respect to health policy issues. With the end of Pew funding, a self-funding continuation of the program was developed, with nine major international corporations becoming charter members of the new structure.

> As time went on, the combined program of Boston University and Brandeis University evolved from having a primary focus on cost-containment to having a concern for broader social welfare goals and health policy reform.

The Pew Associates Program was intended to bring technical assistance and related collaborative project work to selected cities or to programmatic activities within cities. It focused its efforts in three locations—Cleveland, Denver, and Tampa—using university staff guidance and support to help strengthen public-private collaboration in achieving community goals with respect to cost-containment and access to health care. Funding discontinued at the end of the second year of the second cycle of funding, but the Institute for Health Policy obtained a successor 4-year grant from the W. K. Kellogg Foundation to establish a center on local health policy issues in conjunction with the National Association of Counties, based in Washington, D.C. The Kellogg Foundation project provided technical assistance and policy analysis to county officials in selected sites.

**Boston University's Health Policy Institute and the Institute for Health Policy at Brandeis University's Heller School initially offered three distinct programs: The Pew Corporate Fellows Program, the Pew Associates Program, and the Pew Doctoral Program.**

The Pew Doctoral Program provided a 2-year educational and research base for training future health policy leaders. It was envisioned that these health policy leaders might work in either the public or the private sector or might assume academic or nonacademic roles in policy formulation, research, and education. With the withdrawal of Boston University as a joint sponsor of the training program, the Heller School's complement of fellows increased from 6 to 12, and an effort was made to better integrate the Pew program into the Heller School's existing doctoral program in social policy.

Research at the Institute for Health Policy is concentrated around nine areas: national health policy; state health policy; substance abuse services research; health care management; long-term care for elderly and disabled people; finance, reimbursement, and organization; managed care; community health models; and vulnerable populations. Under the direction of Stanley Wallack, the codirector of the Pew Fellows Program, the institute has been committed to developing a health policy curriculum that integrates both the theory and the practice of applied health research. Research staff have been involved in the educational process, and the fellows have been involved in the research activities of the institute.

The implications of current trends have led to a third phase that will make important changes in the curriculum and learning process as well as organizational changes within the program (Wallack and Chilingerian, 1994). During this third phase, highly experienced health care professionals such as physicians, nurses, and top health care managers have been targeted.

## THE ROLE OF THE IOM

As mentioned earlier, the Pew Charitable Trusts awarded a separate grant for administering the Pew Health Policy Program, including the planning of national conferences for fellows, faculty, and the advisory committee. For the first 5 years (1982 to 1987), this role was assumed by the American Enterprise Institute (AEI), but in 1987, the responsibility was transferred to the Institute of Medicine (IOM) of the National Academy of Sciences.

The IOM Office of Health Policy Programs and Fellowships directs and coordinates the joint activities of PHPP, including convening conferences and producing various related publications. The Program Office also cultivates linkages among Pew fellows, the program of studies at IOM and the health policy community in Washington, D.C.

The 1990 Richardson Evaluation Report commended the IOM Program Office for its effective work in helping to link those involved with separate scholarly training efforts into a "community of scholars with a special identity and national recognition." Bill Richardson praised the Program Office for its success in helping Pew fellows gain important exposure to the Washington policy environment. This sentiment can be found throughout the interviews with faculty and alumni (see Appendix A) and will be explored further in Part III.

In an article written for the commemoration of IOM's 25th anniversary, Marion Ein Lewin, Director of the Office of Health Policy Programs and Fellowships, discussed the relationship between IOM and its fellowship programs. Lewin states that over the years, the Pew Health Policy fellows have developed a close relationship with IOM, even though most fellows only formally interact with IOM twice during their Pew program training. A meeting conducted each fall in Washington, D.C., provides first-year fellows with a national perspective on the health care scene. As part of the agenda, fellows meet in small groups with leading congressional and executive branch staff who are working on issues of particular interest to program participants. The fall meetings also provide an opportunity for Pew fellows to become better acquainted with the mission of PHPP and the three distinct models that are used to train the future leaders in health policy. The fellows use this time to network among themselves and to become familiar with the IOM's other programs.

An annual conference is held each spring. The conference is designed to bring all current Pew fellows, faculty, and some alumni together. Leading public policy themes are addressed in

**The IOM Office of Health Policy Programs and Fellowships directs and coordinates the joint activities of PHPP, including convening conferences and producing various related publications.**

depth from a number of different perspectives. Each of the funded sites takes a turn playing the lead role in developing the program agenda. Occasionally, background papers have been commissioned, and proceedings of some of the meetings have been published. These annual meetings provided opportunities for fellows to meet in small groups as part of skills workshops, to hear presentations on research or career activities, to network, and to discuss issues related to their dissertations.

In addition to its convening responsibilities, the Program Office produces *Pew Fellow News,* a semiannual newsletter and a fellow and alumni directory with current addresses, positions, and academic status for all Pew fellows and alumni. Each year a number of other networking and program enhancement activities are conducted as well.

The joint activities of PHPP have achieved a high level of success in developing educational forums, networking opportunities, and dissemination vehicles that complement the more formal doctoral and postdoctoral work conducted at the individual sites. The regular convening and dissemination activities have given the overall effort broadened visibility and recognition among the nation's health policy leaders (IOM Narrative Report, 1993). Knowledge about IOM and interest in its program activities are further provided by the program directors at each of the sites, many of whom are IOM members (Lewin, 1995).

Marion Ein Lewin indicated that in preparation for her report, the Office of Health Policy Programs and Fellowships conducted an informal mail survey "to get a better sense of the degree to which Pew alumni have been involved in IOM activities." Forty percent of Pew alumni responded to the survey, and of that group approximately 20 percent reported participation in an IOM activity. One Pew alumnus is an IOM member, 6 percent of respondents have served on IOM committees, and 11 percent would like to be involved with IOM but have not been asked to do so. Lewin acknowledges that although these numbers appear to be quite low, they are impressive given that the Pew fellows tend to be younger and at less senior stages in their careers than fellows in other programs that may have greater rates of interaction with IOM (e.g., Robert Wood Johnson Foundation Health Policy Fellows).

Steven A. Schroeder, President of The Robert Wood Johnson Foundation, prepared an article responding to Lewin's review (Schroeder, 1995). Schroeder reflects on the historical role of IOM, best known for its "honorific membership and scholarly reports." He states that operating ongoing programs is an unusual activity for IOM, whose

> The joint activities of PHPP have achieved a high level of success in developing educational forums, networking opportunities, and dissemination vehicles that complement the more formal doctoral and postdoctoral work conducted at the individual sites.

work usually centers around historical accomplishments or focuses on the condition of the current knowledge base. "By contrast, fellowship programs are an investment in the future, and health policy fellowships focus on the health policy process rather than on discrete knowledge base" (Schroeder, 1995, p. 161).

Schroeder reinforces Lewin's conclusion that limited ongoing participation of the Pew fellows with IOM is related to the ages of the Pew alumni. He compares the differences in age between the fellows and IOM members, emphasizing the different challenges and responsibilities these age chasms introduce.

Schroeder recognizes that during the life of the Pew program (and more so since the initiation of the Robert Wood Johnson Health Policy Fellowships Program), health policy has become an increasingly dominant focus of national attention. He suggests that as a result, IOM's interests and programs have become more closely aligned with the activities of the fellowship programs. "The Pew program provides formal linkages to top academic health policy institutions and their faculties. This intellectual linkage should expand the knowledge and the network of the IOM and thereby benefit its formal projects" (Schroeder, 1995, p. 162).

Schroeder gives an insightful analysis of the impact of fellowship programs on sponsoring institutions. He addresses the issues that have made fellowship programs unpopular among foundations: cost and the "invisibility" of fellowship program payoffs to foundation staff and trustees. The impact of fellowship programs is more difficult to assess than the quality of research and demonstration programs. This awareness leads Schroeder to commend the Pew Charitable Trusts and the Robert Wood Johnson Foundation for continuing their fellowships in light of these impediments. He praises the Pew Charitable Trusts and the Robert Wood Johnson Foundation for their commitment to investing in the future through long-range projects. Schroeder concludes with admiration for Marion Ein Lewin's "wise and comforting counsel" and success in performing the critical role of providing the "personal glue that holds together" these fellowship programs.

*The Pew program provides formal linkages to top academic health policy institutions and their faculties.*

## NOTES ON PROGRAM STRENGTHS AND WEAKNESSES
### University of Michigan
The highly innovative model of OJ/OC nonresidential doctoral training at the University of Michigan has enabled

many talented professionals to enrich and expand their knowledge base without losing their influence or positions in the field. Fellows are immediately able to use their newly acquired skills into the workplace, making this approach of great value to both the fellow and health policy. Fellows working in the field also bring real-world issues into the classroom, which further enriches the curriculum and training process. The uniqueness of the OJ/OC design is cited as one of the greatest strengths of the Michigan Pew program.

Pamela Paul-Shaheen, a Michigan doctoral alumna, explained that she would not have gone for her doctorate if not for Michigan's nonresidential approach. The other two Michigan fellows who were interviewed, Patricia Butler and Dan Rubin, agreed that it was the opportunity offered at Michigan that brought them back to the classroom. In that way, the structure of the program enabled many high-powered professionals to go back and get the additional training needed to more effectively influence health policy. Pamela Paul-Shaheen discussed the benefits of this type of training approach:

> *I would hope and encourage other institutions to look at these kinds of projects, both from the standpoint that if you go after individuals who are in mid- or upper-level career positions, bring them into a university setting, and have in the class a diversity of interest, expertise, and ability, it creates an incredibly diverse and interesting learning environment. Secondly, when you combine that, as the Michigan program did, with people who are actively engaged in activities at work, a symbiotic relationship occurs between problems from work and techniques learned from class, adding an interesting dynamic into the program. The program empowered these individuals in their own workplaces.*

**The structure of the Michigan program enabled many high-powered professionals to go back and get the additional training needed to more effectively influence health policy.**

Leon Wyszewianski remarked that the University of Michigan continues to corner the market for this type of doctoral training and that it still has no competition. However, many believe that Michigan's success with the Pew health policy nonresidential doctoral program in health policy will inspire other institutions to follow suit. Stan Wallack views the Michigan model as "state of the art" and "highly effective" and is sure that other universities will adopt this training approach.

Although Michigan's nonresidential nature was one of its greatest strengths, it simultaneously represented one of the biggest challenges that the Michigan program faced. Nonresidential programs have the potential to be disjointed and fragmented, and fellows have the potential to feel extremely isolated. In an effort to combat these potential dangers, Michigan fellows and faculty were linked through a sophisticated computer conferencing system. This highly effective method of communication enabled the fellows to simulate the closeness and intensity of a residential doctoral program. Leon Wyszewianski describes this state-of-the-art method of communication as an invaluable component of faculty-fellow and fellow-fellow interaction:

> *Computer conferencing that all the fellows participate in . . . has been a unifying element [at Michigan]. There is a lot of conversation going back and forth among the scholars and the faculty. . . . The fellows also have their own encoded conference that the faculty can't participate in. It's very important for the fellows to have this opportunity. The only people that understand the kind of hell they're going through are the people going through it with them. They support each other, and we foster that.*

Patricia Butler, a Michigan doctoral alumna, also spoke about the uniqueness of the Michigan program in terms of fellow-fellow and fellow-faculty interaction. She found that although the computer conferencing kept the faculty and fellows in touch, it could not compensate entirely for the non-residential structure. Butler explained that because the program was nonresidential, approximately 30 hours of classes were held during one long weekend each month. This intensity would have been even more beneficial, she says, if there had been an opportunity to process all that was learned with fellow classmates. Although the group did usually venture out together one evening during the weekend, they were often too exhausted from the intense course sessions to actually discuss the material. Traditional doctoral programs allow for that peer group processing, an activity that Patricia Butler and others believe is very important to any program at this level.

Bill Weissert discussed another concern related to nonresidential doctoral programs. He stated that a program like that at Michigan is particularly vulnerable because it is not training people to go into academia; rather it is training them to go into the health policy field. One can only hope that that is where they will stay or where they will go. The Michigan program was not trying to train people to become ivory tower academics; rather, it was training them to become policy activists, that is, health policy analysts and change agents:

> *There is a real risk when you give a degree without requiring residence. You wind up giving a degree to people who are not really academics, but are now qualified to teach. That's the downside of our program and something we are constantly vigilant on.*

**Michigan fellows and faculty were linked through a sophisticated computer conferencing system.**

Although the program at Michigan has been highly successful, it, like the other programs, has had its share of trials and tribulations. Fellows needed to learn not only how to be students all over again but also how to balance their student lives with their professional lives. The faculty had to learn how best to teach nontraditional students in this nontraditional setting.

Although the program at Michigan has been highly successful, it, like the other programs, has had its share of trials and tribulations. For the first two program cohorts, the competing demands of work and study resulted in a problem with fellows' completion of program requirements. Over the course of the 2 years of required classes, fellows were accumulating large numbers of incompletes in their courses because of unfinished papers (Richardson, 1990). This problem was largely resolved in the latter half of the program through a combination of adjustments in faculty expectations, revised and increased curriculum structure, and the recruitment of students who were stronger in their academic preparation and ability. Leon Wyszewianski discussed one way that the program went about changing the curriculum structure without sacrificing depth so that the fellows were better able to meet the requirements:

> *What we did was to discourage very strongly the faculty from having a major paper due at the end of the course. You just can't do that with this population. Instead, we encouraged the faculty to have the term paper develop in pieces over the course of the term. The students had deliverables that by the end of the course would add up to the product they were looking for. This worked far better than waiting for it to somehow magically appear in the last flurry of the term. The rate of incompletes dropped dramatically.*

The Michigan program directors recognized that many of their fellows had been in the career mode for a while and needed to be readjusted to the school mode. Fellows needed to learn not only how to be students all over again but also how to balance their student lives with their professional lives. The faculty also had a lot to learn. They needed to learn how best to teach nontraditional students in this nontraditional setting. Leon Wyszewianski reflects on the early years:

> *We initially thought that we would bring in all these bright, successful people who would have no problem writing a dissertation because they would just thirst for learning, when, even with their thirst for learning, they needed structure due to the heavy demands of their full-time careers. They were too busy. These were people who were working 50-60 hours a week and trying to go to school full-time. We should have realized the need for structure. We had a lot of experience with this type of student. We somehow forgot that at the beginning of the Pew program, but we soon remembered and then set up the program much as we had done for our master's-level program. This worked much better. We concentrated on the dissertation early on rather than just assuming the students would know how to find a topic, how to find a committee, and how to move along the path. Lesson learned.*

Another challenging issue for a program structured like the Michigan program is getting good faculty to commit to teaching in an intensive mode of one weekend a month. When asked what advice he would give to another university attempting to organize a similar program, Bill Weissert stated that getting the best faculty to commit to the unusual teaching requirements was key to the success of the program. He further stressed that this commitment needs to be established up front, because many faculty do not realize that they will be teaching at least 5 of the 7 or 7 of the 9 months on weekends, both Saturdays and Sundays.

According to the alumni who were interviewed, Michigan's challenge of finding the best faculty to commit to the training program resulted in an exceptionally strong faculty base. Because most of the fellows were in senior-level positions with some level of influence within the health care world, external faculty were brought in when necessary to ensure that the appropriate policy relevance was incorporated into the courses. Fellows also appreciated the very small student-to-faculty ratio (8:1) and the intense commitment of the faculty to the fellows. All four Michigan fellows interviewed mentioned the benefits of having in the classroom students with a rich diversity of backgrounds. Bringing together professionals from many different sectors of the health care community added dimension to the educational experience.

> Getting the best faculty to commit to the unusual teaching requirements was key to the success of the program. The RAND/UCLA curriculum had a strong analytical orientation with a heavy emphasis on methodological skills.

## RAND/University of California at Los Angeles

The RAND/UCLA curriculum had a strong analytical orientation with a heavy emphasis on methodological skills. Doctoral-level workshops covered the necessary core of knowledge for all fellows and provided cohesion and joint exposure to faculty and content for doctoral students from both RAND and UCLA (Richardson, 1990). The fellows considered program content to be a strength, because of the seminars, research opportunities, and courses that allowed them to develop their analytical skills and that showed the link between analysis and policy. Moreover, the fellows also considered the faculty to be a great strength (Richardson, 1990). Faculty member and Program Director Al Williams described the workshops and seminars as one the most innovative aspects of the RAND/UCLA program design:

> [W]e have workshops or seminars on broad policy domains with a set of modules dealing with particular things. For example, there is one on technology, regulation, innovation, and diffu-

One of the major challenges faced by the RAND/UCLA program, like most multidisciplinary programs, was how not to include the whole world of health policy in the curriculum.

*sion, and we deal with everything from the NIH process of awarding grants to drug regulation. The one on health care has modules that deal with the hospital side and now the managed care side. That has worked well. Another thing that was unique (and one never knows just how unique one's own program is, as you only hear about the others) was that the exercises were in the form of short policy exercises: a short policy memo, a presentation, etc., all oriented toward current problems which captures the fellows. . . . The workshop model was a modification of part of the curriculum at the RAND Graduate School. It's oriented toward health and has become more stylized. That basic model was there, and what we tried to do was to apply it to health policy programs.*

Student integration at RAND was strong, and Al Williams attributed this in part to the fact that the workshops were open to people outside the Pew program. Integrating Pew and non-Pew fellows in the workshops led to a more diverse student body that enriched class discussions. Al Williams attributes much of the success in bringing students together to the integrated seminars and the small size of the RAND program.

One of the major challenges faced by the RAND/UCLA program, like most multidisciplinary programs, was how not to include the whole world of health policy in the curriculum. Kate Korman elaborated on this point:

*Initially, the curriculum was pretty enthusiastic, far-reaching, even overreaching. One course was eliminated after 2 years because it was just too much. The students couldn't learn everything. This was challenging, because as parts of courses or whole courses were cut out or restructured, some faculty found their role changed. However, the program design was much too ambitious in the beginning.*

Yet, RAND continued to try and reach the whole multifaceted world of health policy by bringing in guest speakers for regular colloquia. This way the students were able to get some exposure to all areas of health policy. This technique was used, in various ways, by all of the PHPP and was cited as a great strength.

According to the Richardson (1990) evaluation, the UCLA program was weakened over time because of the loss of several senior faculty. This point, however, did not come out in the recent interviews (see Appendix A). Richardson (1990) reported that despite the rich mix of research projects at RAND and UCLA, students expressed concern about their inability to gain access to a research project that was compatible with their own interests and professional goals, and complaints about the lack of access to faculty mentors grew over time. In Richardson's (1990) evaluation, fragmentation was listed as a major weakness, existing as a result of the difficulty of matching a diverse mix of students with faculty or projects that reflected each fellow's interests. On the contrary, Kate Korman rated the relationships between faculty and students as one of the long-run strengths of the program, and explained that the collaborative student-faculty research projects led to close relationships:

> Over time very strong bonds were created between faculty and students, since the students were not just faces in the classroom but integral members of research teams with faculty team leaders. . . .There was a lot of camaraderie, and our faculty showed up for every award ceremony or whatever. . . . Lots of support.

Furthermore, Joan DaVanzo, a RAND/UCLA doctoral alumna who started out at RAND and then graduated from UCLA, cited the work project requirements as a bonding experience between the fellows and the faculty:

> Working on the projects allows you to get to know the professors in a different way. As a student you know a professor is a professor and you are both locked into that role, then you're thrown on a project with a professor and all of a sudden they are more collegial. You're not just one of the graduate students anymore. You have access to them in a different way. Being able to switch the role is very important when you are a student.

Like Joan DaVanzo, several other RAND doctoral fellows started out at one of the two jointly sponsored institutions and then switched over to the other institution to complete the degree. This flexibility was cited as one of the most innovative and unique aspects of the program. DaVanzo described RAND as supplying the necessary depth in quantitative skills and economics, with UCLA providing the equally necessary breadth in health, epidemiology, and public health: "The combination was invaluable," she said.

Terry Hammons, a RAND alumnus considered the work projects a great strength of the midcareer program for another reason: the reality focus. This concept comes up again and again with the Pew fellows, whether they are doctoral, postdoctoral or midcareer fellows. To most, PHPP was fully representative of the health policy world, with health policy leaders teaching in a relevant, timely, and applicable manner. Hammons explained that the workshops and seminars were always structured in the context of real-world application:

> The second part of our program was working on real projects, and I thought in contrast to my experience in graduate school, for example, these workshops and seminars were more effective

RAND supplied the necessary depth in quantitative skills and economics and UCLA provided the equally necessary breadth in health, epidemiology, and public health: The combination was invaluable.

*than traditional graduate education (I did economics at MIT [Massachusetts Institute of Technology]). Most important were the projects. I was fortunate enough to be involved in four and a half really wonderful projects during the year I was there. They were real projects, such as helping DHHS [U.S. Department of Health and Human Services] understand what academic medical centers were going through and how to make policy that related to graduate medical education, research and training, and so forth and that was appropriate for the nation's goals but that took into account what academic medical centers could do and were doing.*

Kathleen Eyre, another RAND midcareer alumna, underscored Hammons' emphasis on the value of being able to apply newly learned skills to specific on-the-job projects. She also considered the work projects to be a great strength of the RAND midcareer program. However, she would have liked to have seen more general discussions of the big-picture health policy issues. She explains that there was a lack of regular, organized, high-level discussions on, for instance, health reform, which was the hot topic of the time:

*We just didn't have opportunities to take cuts at the big picture. That's the major criticism I would have of the midcareer program. I don't know if it was because of time constraints. I think some of it was that and some of it was that the focus was one giving you your basic skills. That was the most useful part of the program. I think being able to put that in context would have been useful as well.*

The tension between breadth and depth is not uncommon in fast-paced multidisciplinary programs, and because it was cited by most PHPP directors and fellows, this tension is probed further, later in the report.

### University of California at San Francisco

The tension between breadth and depth is not uncommon in fast-paced multidisciplinary programs.

The UCSF program's shift to a postdoctoral focus was based on a desire to take advantage of the interaction among several groups of advanced doctoral and postdoctoral students (Pew fellows and others) at UCSF and to contribute to that interaction (Richardson, 1990). This fellow-fellow and fellow-faculty interaction was nurtured throughout the fellowship and was considered a great strength of the program. Hal Luft discussed how the process of integrating Pew fellows among all students was facilitated by the flexibility of Pew funding. He stressed the importance of treating all fellows (Pew fellows and others) equally. Equality among the students fostered integration and collaboration, whereas separation would have led to a divisive elitism.

> *[There was] a conscious strategy of using Pew funds to supple-*
> *ment other fellowship funds so we [had] people who were fully*
> *funded by Pew and others who basically got $1,000 all mixed*
> *together in the same classes. We did not . . . establish a pecking*
> *order. We set a standard for fellowship applicants and said this*
> *is what all our applicants have to meet, and then once they*
> *were in that acceptable pool, who we give what kinds of dollars*
> *to out of what pot will partly depend on the constraints of the*
> *pot. . . .Everybody is on equal footing. That integration worked*
> *very well.*

The program typically enrolled five postdoctoral fellows per
year, drawing from a national pool of applicants to create a
mix of medical and nonmedical doctorates. Physicians came
primarily from preventive medicine and primary care specialties, with the PhDs typically drawn from among individuals
with social science backgrounds. The Pew program at UCSF
also took advantage of the opportunity of bringing together
clinicians and PhDs already committed to health policy and
health services research with physicians completing their
clinical fellowship. Integrating these two groups served a
dual purpose. The Pew fellows' experiences were further
enriched by exposure to other key players in the health policy world, and the purely clinical fellows' experience was
broadened and enriched with policy-relevant training. Hal
Luft discussed this unique interaction:

> *The clinicians attend the Pew seminars, get involved with a fac-*
> *ulty member's research project, and are basically integrated into*
> *the fellowship program, although paid by someone else. These are*
> *people who might have otherwise been doing bench research on*
> *pulmonary function. They are now doing work on risk adjust-*
> *ment models and health care costs of AIDS, etc., exactly the*
> *kinds of things Pew fellows do.*

This kind of cross-fertilization of individuals who had
worked in the policy arena and other health care professionals is what the Pew Charitable Trusts hoped to accomplish
with PHPP. Collaboration and communication between
various players in the health policy arena can lead to more
effective and appropriate policies. Carroll Estes considered
the aspect of mixing physicians with social scientists as one of
the greatest challenges and one of the greatest rewards of the
UCSF program.

The commitment of UCSF faculty has been maintained
throughout the program, and many fellows cited this as the
greatest strength of the UCSF program. Fellows were
pleased that the faculty had top-level policy influence and
real-world perspectives, were committed to teaching and
being supportive, and treated the fellows as peers (Richard-

> Cross-fertilization of
> individuals who had
> worked in the policy
> arena and other health
> care professionals is
> what the Pew
> Charitable Trusts hoped
> to accomplish with
> PHPP. The aspect of
> mixing physicians with
> social scientists was one
> of the greatest
> challenges and one of
> the greatest rewards of
> the UCSF program.

son, 1990). Hal Luft and Carroll Estes both underscored this sentiment, stating that most of the faculty treated and truly believed that the fellows were more like colleagues than students. Outside evaluators cited UCSF's research and policy environment as a "tremendous" strength of the program. Richardson (1990) stated that all faculty were intricately involved in a range of activities at the local, state, and national levels, including high-priority areas such as AIDS policy, physician reimbursement, and policies related to aging.

The UCSF program believed that its goal was not merely to train competent researchers and practitioners but to ensure that graduates be effective and relevant participants in the health policy process, and so it considered supervised field placements in public- and private-sector organizations a valuable "learning-by-doing" part of the fellowship program, especially for midcareer fellows (UCSF Annual Report, 1992). Mark Legnini, a postdoctoral alumnus, recalled the benefits of the learning-by-doing educational model:

> *[The most innovative aspect of the Pew program is] the emphasis on networking and getting involved in the politics and the art of doing things rather than just plugging people into existing research projects and making sure they have a job.*

For alumna Lisa Bero, the field placements were a vital part of her training and posttraining placement:

> *[The program] positioned me for doing a lot of international work. I had my first contact with the World Health Organization while I was a Pew fellow. That rocketed me into doing international health policy work which was great. I got a real jump start on that through the fellowship.*

Early on the lack of physical space for fellows was a problem and precluded some valuable interaction between faculty and fellows and among fellows. Close proximity to peers and mentors, a seemingly simple logistical issue, is one of the strongest integrative and bonding forces. Hal Luft describes the situation at UCSF:

> *In general, one of the biggest challenges early on was space. When we were located in our old site, on the main campus, there wasn't even enough room for faculty. So there was no place for the postdocs. They were hanging out in weird and bizarre places. They were often off site in office space that had been provided, but this hindered interaction. When we moved 5 years ago, we provided real office space for all the fellows as part of the unit. They were integrated with the faculty, with the unit. [It] works a lot better.*

The UCSF program believed that its goal was not merely to train competent researchers and practitioners but to ensure that graduates be effective and relevant participants in the health policy process.

Like fellows from the other program sites, the UCSF postdoctoral fellows discussed at length the tension between depth and breadth. However, unlike the RAND fellows, at UCSF the feeling was that depth was often sacrificed for breadth (Richardson, 1990). Fellows also cited the lack of structure and guidance in establishing fellow-mentor relationships early in the program, although this situation was said to improve over time. As the program evolved, the fellow-mentor relationships and career planning services became more formalized (see Appendix C for specifics on the Fellow-Mentor Relationship Guidelines at UCSF). UCSF program directors concluded that the optimal amount of structure depends on the needs of individual fellows. Whereas an appropriate core curriculum is necessary, a health policy training program must also be flexible enough to allow it to adapt to the unique needs of individual fellows (UCSF Annual Report, 1992). In a multidisciplinary program such as the PHPP, where fellows come into the program with many different perspectives and experiences, faculty really need to have the capacity and commitment to cater to each fellow. Lisa Bero stated that the UCSF faculty mastered this approach, and she cited this ability as one of UCSF's greatest strengths:

> The most unique aspect [of the UCSF program] was that it was very tailored to the individual fellow. Every fellow came into the program with different experiences. We had some core courses, but most were tailored to the individual and the faculty spent a lot of time talking to each fellow to find out what specifically were our needs at the beginning. It was a needs assessment. We were asked: where do you want to go? And what do you need to do that? And then efforts were made to give the fellows what they needed to get where they wanted to be. This individual attention was by far the strongest point.

## Boston University/Brandeis University

Raskin and colleagues (1992) discuss the BU/Brandeis program's greatest challenge: the idea of a 2-year accelerated doctoral program. This concept was new to Brandeis and Boston universities, and required a different pedagogical approach. Some of the faculty believed that the best way to produce good policy makers in health policy was to get researchers to learn skills quickly and get them "out there" doing policy research. Many believed that candidates with a master's degree could attain the necessary research skills that could be used on an applied research dissertation within a 2-

**Whereas an appropriate core curriculum is necessary, a health policy training program must also be flexible enough to allow it to adapt to the unique needs of individual fellows.**

to 3-year period. Stan Wallack discussed the way that the Heller School at Brandeis University approached the 2-year curriculum challenge:

> *[One] thing that was key in terms of our 2-year curriculum and our very high success rate was the focus on problem solving and learning how to get to an answer. The seminar led by Jon Chilingerian was very critical in getting people to work together and to see studies of successes. How does someone who is in political science move ahead on an entire project and complete it? How does an economist go ahead and do it? Our educational process or approach was pragmatic, using the procedures as any business or person would adopt in solving a problem. Being exposed to this process from the beginning of the program to the end is very important. It is very difficult but very important for students to see at the outset how they get from where they are starting to the end. This road map became a backdrop for students, one they could put hooks into as they moved along.*

For those students who were very focused and self-directed, the 2-year time frame was found to be manageable. Jonathan Howland, in the unique position of having been a Pew fellow at BU and then subsequently a program director, reflected on his doctoral experience and how the time pressures worked to his benefit:

> *I thought it was great that we could essentially design our own curriculum and decide what tools we wanted to get. One of the reasons I thought that was so great was that the program enabled me to study epidemiology, which is what I wanted to do, and I was free from taking a whole lot of required courses and able to pursue the courses that were really of interest to me. That was really nice. The other thing that was really nice was that I was able to . . . [do] my course work and dissertation at the same time. There are very few programs that would have allowed me to do that. It was a fast-track program.*

Jonathan Howland and Steve Crane discussed not only the benefits of a fast-track, flexible program but also the potentially negative aspects. For instance, people fall through the cracks and get their doctorate without having acquired the necessary tools. The lack of structure associated with the BU program worked for some but not for others, which meant that students needed to be self-motivated. For those students who did not identify a dissertation topic early on in the process and preferred to be exposed to broad social policy perspectives, it was very difficult for them to complete the requirements in the 2-year time frame. Steve Crane explained how determining program structure was a learning experience for the program directors as well as the fellows:

*The [BU] program wasn't as assertive with the students in say-*
*ing you must take this and this. We weren't sure what the "musts"*
*should be. As we went along in the program and we saw what*
*students did, we saw then what we needed to do and towards the*
*end we probably had a much better sense of what we needed to do*
*in terms of requirements than we had in the beginning.*

Jonathan Howland recommends that future fast-track,
loosely structured programs develop some sort of mechanism to ensure that people get the necessary skills without
taking away all sense of control. A minimum skill set requirement was one example that he offered. This issue will be
addressed further later in this report.

Another issue found to have a substantial impact on the
completion rate was the lack of funding for the third year.
This meant that the fellows had to secure other sources of
funding for the additional time required to complete the dissertation. When funding ceased, many students had to take
jobs, which distracted them from their dissertation work. A
Brandeis survey found that many students complained that
after the 2 years they were no longer linked with the program and felt isolated. Following the 2-year funding period,
students would have liked to have been able to keep in touch
with faculty and other students for dissertation support.

Raskin and colleagues (1992) found that some students
saw the Pew program as creating rigidity in the pacing of the
curriculum. Since the Pew fellows were expected to complete their dissertations within 2 years, they were forced to
think about their proposals prior to the Qualifying Examination, which is administered in January of the second year.
The delay of the Qualifying Examinations until students had
been in residence for a year and a half was viewed as a significant hurdle by the Pew fellows. Their schedule required
them to assemble a dissertation committee early on in the
process and conduct a literature review prior to taking the
exams. This fast track obligated students to make decisions
about how they used their time. They often missed the special seminars and colloquiums offered at the school and felt
disconnected from some excellent learning opportunities at
the Heller School. In addition, networking with other students, a valuable resource, was limited.

Boston University faculty and fellows alike cited the
involvement and dedication of several faculty and program
directors as a major strength of the program. Steve Crane
described how several key people, Diana Chapman Walsh,
Sol Levine, and Dick Egdahl, worked to build and define the
BU Pew Health Policy Fellowship Program. The whole BU

> The greatest strength
> reported by the
> Brandeis fellows was
> the support of the well-
> known and highly
> respected faculty.

program was modeled on Diana Chapman Walsh's program in the University Professors Program (UPP), where she ultimately became a mentor. According to Steve Crane, "UPP was the educational home for the BU Pew Doctoral Program, and Diana was the intellectual inspiration." Sol Levine was the academic director at BU and a leading national expert on medical sociology. He was the faculty member who bridged the gap between students, UPP, and BU. Steve stated that it was Sol who "made it happen at the academic level" by focusing on the importance of change and emphasizing values, policy, and "the quest to do what was right and good. Sol was always there for the students at BU and Brandeis, and they loved him." Debbie Ward, a BU alumna, reflected upon her memories of Diana Chapman Walsh and Sol Levine:

> Diana Walsh constructed several important bridges at the Health Policy Institute at BU. One was to the business community, where she had done extensive work and where her understanding of business imperatives was quite a bit more sophisticated than that of we run-of-the-mill capitalist scorners. The second bridge built by Diana was specifically for the women in the program. Diana had a feminist core which exhibited itself in her humor as well as her intellectual and personal pursuits. All the women at Pew in my day were grateful for that. . . .Sol Levine was a grand facilitator. He used his rolodex and his prodigious memory to send us to the vast resources of Boston and beyond. In my case, he sent me to the great urban historian, Sam Bass Warner and to Mike Miller whose course in sociology of poverty led me to the text I still have students use: Beeghley's Living Poorly in America. Sol made us remember that we were in a great university setting, not only budding policy wonks ("wonk," as I recall it, was not a word in use during my Pew days).

At Brandeis, fellows are trained to focus on critiquing, understanding, and finding solutions to problems through integrated problem-solving techniques.

Similarly, the greatest strength reported by the Brandeis fellows in Richardson's 1990 evaluation and during the interviews was the support of the well-known and highly respected faculty. The Institute for Health Policy was in a unique position as a leading health care and research center; thus, key faculty and research staff were available to assist Pew doctoral students in the pursuit of their PhDs (Raskin et al., 1992).

The multidisciplinary training approach was another strength of the Brandeis program cited by alumni. Health policy issues are often approached from several different paradigms: economics, political science, and sociology. At Brandeis, on the other hand, fellows are trained to focus on critiquing, understanding, and finding solutions to problems through integrated problem-solving techniques. The multidisciplinary approach was not unique to Brandeis; rather, it was a cornerstone of the PHPP vision. Approaching health policy from a variety of disciplines brings about a deeper understanding of the related issues and consequences of policy. This style of advanced graduate training is relatively unique and will be discussed further later in this report.

## COMMON THEMES

The strengths and weaknesses discussed above in no way encompass an exhaustive list. Rather, those issues highlighted above were those mentioned most often during the interviews. However, several common themes emerged from the interviews, themes that transcended the different program structures. First, most fellows and faculty emphasized the importance of having a strong, well-known, committed faculty. As will be discussed later in the report, excellent faculty may be one of the greatest recruitment tools that a university can employ. Even beyond that, however, the use of a strong and dedicated teaching faculty with one foot in the world of academia and research and the other foot in the world of health policy making and development is the best way a university can ensure a successful program and produce future leaders. The Pew programs were able to offer as faculty leaders in the field of health policy.

A second common theme that emerged from the interviews is the "reality focus" of the Pew programs. Almost all of the fellows commented on how the programs were applicable to the real world and how the research and work projects were focused on current health care issues and problems. All of the programs except the Michigan program, whose fellows were already engaged in full-time employment in the health field, required their fellows to become involved with ongoing research projects either internally or outside the university. Many of these work projects or internships led to publications or job placements for the fellows. For the Michigan fellows and the RAND midcareer fellows, the educational experience was easily translated into immediate on-the-job applications. This feature of PHPP situated the programs in a class by themselves, and the fellows and faculty considered this feature a great strength.

The multidisciplinary nature of the PHPP curricula will be discussed in Part II, however, it should be noted that every person interviewed emphasized that this aspect of the Pew program was one of its greatest strengths. Incorporating many disciplines and perspectives into health policy cur-

> The programs were applicable to the real world and the research and work projects were focused on current health care issues and problems.

*There is a strong consensus that the multidisciplinary approach remains the most effective way to train health policy professionals.*

ricula acknowledges that health care problems are not unidimensional and that effective change cannot be achieved without a thorough understanding of the multiple aspects of a given issue. The Pew Health Policy Program trained fellows to view health care problems through many different lenses. The ultimate strength of PHPP can thus be described as a training approach that gave future health policy leaders the ability to understand and speak fluently in the many languages of health policy development.

Although the PHPPs had common strengths, no weaknesses were common to all programs. There was frequent discussion about the tension between breadth and depth inherent in a multidisciplinary curriculum; however, some programs focused more on giving the fellows a broad training in health policy, whereas other programs zeroed in on certain perspectives or disciplines and rarely looked at the big picture. In both cases, fellows and faculty mentioned the gaps and weaknesses in the approach. Nonetheless, there was a strong consensus that the multidisciplinary approach remains the most effective way to train health policy professionals.

# Part II.
## Successes and Failures

## CRITICAL SUCCESS FACTORS

ne of the goals of this report is to reveal some of the factors that appear to have made the Pew Health Policy Programs (PHPPs) a success. In so doing, it is hoped that the constraints as well as the lessons learned by the programs can be identified and ultimately that the legacy or legacies can be uncovered. It is hoped that incipient health policy and graduate programs can learn from these experiences and use this narrative to guide them through the process of planning, implementing, and developing innovative and effective programs.

This section focuses on what has been termed the *critical success factors* of PHPP, as a whole. Critical success factors are a "limited number of areas in which results, if they are satisfactory, will ensure successful performance" (Rockhart, 1978). These factors, identified by the 25 interviewees, through discussions held at the Pew meetings, and by sifting through archival information, form the foundation of the Pew Health Policy Fellowship Program.[4] These performance areas represent program activities that are interdependent, that work in unison to generate success, and that should therefore receive attention. They are (in no particular order) recruitment, mentoring, building a community of scholars, an early focus on the dissertation, networking, leadership, and multidisciplinary education and training. As a result of different service concepts, different operating strategies, and other variables, each program emphasizes different sets of success factors at different points in time.

## RECRUITMENT

Kate Korman stated that "a variety of needs . . . exist in the potential student population: postdoctoral, doctoral (both

[4] *Hal Luft noted that these factors are derived from people closely involved in the program and do not reflect the type of formal assessment one could derive from a study of many programs, some of which are successful and some of which are not.*

35

residential and nonresidential), and midcareer; and no one program can fulfill all these requirements." With this in mind, the Pew programs pioneered a joint recruitment effort, both implicitly and explicitly, to supplement their individual efforts. Understanding that each program had a unique approach to health policy education and training, those involved in recruitment from all four sites worked together to guide potential fellows toward the program that best met their individual needs and expectations. As a team, Steve Crane (Boston University [BU]/Brandeis University), Kate Korman (RAND/University of California at Los Angeles [UCLA]), Ted Benjamin (University of California at San Francisco [UCSF]), and David Perlman (University of Michigan) searched for potential recruits who would be appropriate and beneficial for the program as a whole and who would also fit well into a particular program site. Steve Crane and Kate Korman explained that students more interested in a traditional academic career were steered toward RAND/UCLA. People more business or problem oriented were directed toward the BU/Brandeis program. For those who could not or did not want to leave their careers or their homes for an extended period of time, the on-job/on-campus Michigan program was recommended. For students looking for postdoctoral education, UCSF was most appropriate, and for professionals without doctorates, seeking additional training in an intensive 1-year midcareer program, RAND/UCLA was suggested. "We all had something to contribute," says Steve Crane, "we were competitive only in that we all wanted to be seen to do well by Pew and to stand in the best light." The four program sites were related in that they all shared the same vision and mission. Their commonality enabled them to work together in team recruitment efforts, and their diversity enabled them to capture the best students from all levels and areas of health care and health policy.

> Even though each program had a unique approach to health policy education and training, the four program sites worked together in team recruitment efforts, and their diversity enabled them to capture the best students from all levels and areas of health care and health policy.

## Profiles and Targets

The 1994 Michigan Proposal Narrative states that a program "lives or dies by the quality of [the] student applications." Therefore, Michigan, like the other programs, engaged in major public outreach efforts. Targeted for the Michigan program were highly successful, often high-profile, midcareer professionals who were public sector representatives engaged in health policy formulation as either policy makers, policy analysts, or influential participants in the policy process, such as people in state legislatures and consulting

firms. However, Michigan learned early on that other vital-
ly important aspects beyond professional position and influence are included in an applicant's profile. Leon Wyszewianski commented on the appropriate measures for recruiting
fellows for the Michigan program and how this process
changed over time:

> *[Michigan] is an academic program. [It] is not another job.
> When all is said and done we offer pretty standard, straightfor-
> ward doctoral-level courses. The students had to have the acade-
> mic know-how to make it through these courses no matter what
> their other qualities were or accomplishments may be. We may
> have lost sight of that in the beginning. We tried to take in peo-
> ple who were very accomplished in the field but who were not nec-
> essarily great achievers in the academic realm. It was a disaster.
> They just couldn't cope with all this. If you're going to work full-
> time and go to school, you have to be very good at the "school"
> business. You have to already have mastered the craft of being a
> student. . . . We learned to pay a lot more attention to grades,
> past academic accomplishments, as well as GREs. We began to
> look for people who have shown that they can handle work and
> school at the same time. That is a good predictor of success. This
> was another lesson learned: no matter how applied this was, and
> even though we were not looking to create scholars, ultimately
> they can't take full advantage of what we have to offer if they
> are not good students.*

Brandeis wanted to
participate in PHPP was
so that the university
could use the prestige
and stipend to propel it
into a more attractive
position and recruit
students of the highest
quality.

## Program Champions

The BU/Brandeis faculty and administration underscored
Michigan's emphasis on the value of public communication
and outreach in the recruitment process. Stan Wallack
explained that one of the reasons that Brandeis wanted to
participate in PHPP was so that the university could use the
prestige and stipend to propel it into a more attractive position and recruit students of the highest quality. He conced-
ed that although Brandeis was doing much state-of-the-art
work in health policy that was being recognized and that was
highly regarded, "students weren't just naturally coming to
Brandeis." Stan Wallack stressed the need for active recruitment and the importance of having "program champions,"
people deeply committed to maintaining a high-quality student body:

> *We found ourselves still needing to get out there and do a lot of
> recruitment. . . . Steve Crane really took this program on as his
> mission. He was a key force. . . . You need a champion. Steve
> Crane was a champion in terms of recruitment. . . . The success
> of the program had a lot to do with Steve running this program,
> going out there, really identifying, working hard, writing to
> people, and going to the right kinds of meetings.*

Joan DaVanzo stated that having a "point person" functioning inside the program with the fellows was also critical to the success of the fellows and the program. At RAND/UCLA Kate Korman functioned as the program champion. According to DaVanzo:

*Kate Korman was very nurturing and supportive of us—it was like a little family, with her as the "mother hen." She looked after us, made sure we all knew what was going on. . . . She made us feel connected to the institution and "on the inside," even though we were just these new, somewhat wet-behind-the-ears fellows.*

A "point person" functioning inside the program with the fellows is critical to the success of the fellows and the program.

Joan DaVanzo discussed the difficulty of uprooting one's life to go back to school full-time, and in some cases even switch fields completely. Kate Korman made this potentially rocky midcareer transition smoother for the Pew fellows. Furthermore, DaVanzo indicated that Marion Ein Lewin, director of the Program Office, and her staff were always responsive to and supportive of the Pew fellows. Together, these experiences fostered a defined identity for the fellows and the Pew program.

At BU/Brandeis, the doctoral applicant pool almost always included people who had been thinking about the need for more systematic and rigorous training in health policy analysis as a result of their professional activities (Richardson, 1990). Stuart Altman commented on Brandeis' recruitment goals:

*We were trying to recruit, and we did recruit, people who had worked for governments either at the state or federal level, but who had started out without a lot of formal training and needed a deeper understanding. We did attract a number of individuals who had been working in the health policy arena at the government level, but who had come in as pretty junior people. We added a conceptual framework to what they were doing. Then they reinserted themselves back into the policy process, often at higher levels.*

Proven academic ability and independent, organizational skills were major determinants for admission to the BU/Brandeis Pew program because of its accelerated nature. Steve Crane explained that recruiting for fast-track programs is different than recruiting for traditional graduate-level programs, and this difference must be taken into consideration:

*We wanted to create a doctoral program that would get you in and out within 2 years through a challenging process. We wanted to give students a great degree of flexibility in the courses they chose so that they would waste the least amount of time taking*

*courses that someone thought were important but weren't direct-
ly relevant. We wanted to take in students who already had an
advanced degree and substantial experience and didn't have to
learn what they wanted to do with their lives. We tried to identify and choose people who knew exactly what they wanted to do,
and who could find what they were looking for here at BU and
in that way get them in and out very quickly.*

Although this type of program is not made for everyone,
Stan Wallack stated that for many fellows, the fast-paced curriculum was the primary attraction, and thus an effective
recruitment tool:

> *There are people out there who, when we first started the pro-
> gram, were ideally suited, who were seasoned people, who were
> out there in the real world a long time, and who didn't want to
> spend a lot of time in graduate school. . . .They just wanted to
> pick up some tools. The 2-year program was appealing to some
> students, even if they struggled a little when they got here. . . .We
> expected them to be done with their course work in 2 years and
> have a dissertation subject and be pretty well along when they
> leave. They could be expected to finish their dissertation within
> the third year. We wanted to make it a very fast-paced program
> that would distinguish us.*

**Finding the Best and Brightest**

The postdoctoral PHPP at UCSF emphasized the importance of recruiting the very best among the highly qualified
pool of potential applicants. The collective mission of the
Pew programs is to train the future leaders of the health policy field; therefore, only the best and most promising applicants are selected. According to Carroll Estes, to achieve
this level of applicants, the institution and faculty must also
represent the best: "The excellence of our faculty and their
reputations were the single most important attraction in
recruitment. . . .You need a sterling faculty and a sterling
institution for recruitment."

The UCSF program typically enrolled five postdoctoral
fellows each year, drawing on a very high quality national
pool of applicants. Each year, there was a mix of medical and
nonmedical doctorates, with the physicians drawn from preventive medicine and primary care specialties and the PhDs
typically drawn from largely social science backgrounds.
Placing fellows on research projects with the faculty is the
most important aspect. "Identifying a good match is one of
the key things that needs to be done," says Hal Luft. The
process of identification begins during recruitment and
entails not only matching people to the project with regard
to energy levels and similarities of interests but also finding

> Recruiting for fast-track
> programs is different
> than recruiting for
> traditional graduate-
> level programs, and this
> difference must be
> taken into
> consideration.

someone who fits well into the program and who will fit well with the faculty and in ongoing projects. Like UCSF, the RAND/UCLA program incorporated hands-on research projects into the curriculum; thus, the importance of matching student profiles with faculty research projects and interests was an essential part of its recruitment process as well.

Al Williams discussed the interrelatedness of targeting recruitment to the highest-quality students and of creating a thriving, high-quality program, since you cannot do either one well without mastering the other:

> [F]rom the beginning we tried to [skim the] cream. We intentionally made it a rich program because we wanted to get the best students. . . .We were looking for people who had already done work that required, in the case of the PhD students, their commitment to health and in the case of the midcareer folks, we basically took in people that had convinced us that they were committed. . . .[Most] had demonstrated substantial capability in a domain other than policy.

**Without Pew funds, "skimming the cream" would not have been possible.**

However, Al Williams noted that without Pew funds, "skimming the cream" would not have been possible and laments that today RAND is unable to recruit health policy fellows in the same way. Another factor that enabled RAND/UCLA to succeed in attracting high-quality students was the relationship between the two institutions and the availability of cross-registration. He provided the example that although the RAND Graduate School did not teach epidemiology, fellows had access to multitude epidemiology courses at UCLA. Thus, many students were going back and forth between RAND and UCLA, an opportunity that allowed for the development of a rich and comprehensive program. The joining of forces between BU and Brandeis also allowed for these cross-registration and program enrichment opportunities.

Steve Crane expressed the commonly held belief that one of the great strengths of the program as a whole was the individual faculty members who were committed to Pew's mission and who were accessible to the fellows:

> Can you imagine sitting down in a room with Phil Lee, Stu Altman, Stan Wallack, Dick Egdahl, Al Williams, Bob Brook, and . . . I could go on and list dozens of names . . . and be able to go up to them and talk with them and think and discuss for a day or two [at the conferences] and then go back to your institutions and do that on an ongoing basis or if you want call someone up in another institution? Phil Lee, Assistant Secretary of Health; Stu Altman, Chairman of ProPAC [Prospective Payment Assessment Commission]; Joe Newhouse at Harvard, to speak with the people who are writing the articles, who are changing the world? Incredible. It was just incredible. . . .The Pew HPP

*was just unbelievably rich, and the commitment that the senior people had to this group of students was just extraordinary. That is something that can be replicated by another program. There is still a strong need to get people from different institutions together. That phrase "inter" is really so important. Not "intra," as doctoral programs traditionally are. They only look within themselves. This was "inter" in every respect of the word.*

Marion Ein Lewin has the unique perspective of having been the overseer of PHPP as a whole and having been closely involved in the evolution of each program. From her perspective, there have been tremendous improvements in terms of the recruitment process. Over time, the targeted market changed from highly intelligent people vying for a predoctoral, postdoctoral, or midcareer program to highly intelligent people with the same wants in terms of getting a degree or higher-level training, but who also had unique motivation, discipline, and organizational skills. The task imposed upon the Pew fellows was exceedingly demanding not only because of the complexity and unstable health care environment (the basis of the curriculum) but also because of the fast-paced nature of the program. In her words:

*The schools learned to recruit people who had the initiative and the discipline and the interest to pursue this kind of program, and who had what it would take to be a successful Pew fellow once they completed the program. My feeling is that the recruitment really was very much improved to ensure the success of the alumni.*

Jonathan Howland agrees with Lewin's conclusion that the recruitment process needs to include screening for motivation, but he adds the dimension of screening for completion. He stated that with regard to the doctoral programs, it should be made clear from the start that there is an expectation that comes along with being accepted into the program and that is, that the fellow will complete the program. This topic will be revisited later in the report.

Hal Luft discussed some unique recruitment issues that come up in postdoctoral-level programs. People applying for postdoctoral fellowships are often applying for tenure-track positions simultaneously. Thus, if the postdoctoral application process ends before most institutions notify their new faculty recruits, the fellowship may lose some of the very best because they will be holding out to hear about faculty positions. This may seem like a simple logistical matter; however, competing external factors like this could have long-term effects on the quality of the student body and must therefore be addressed.

> Over time, the targeted market changed from highly intelligent people vying for a predoctoral, postdoctoral, or midcareer program to highly intelligent people with the same wants in terms of getting a degree or higher-level training, but who also had unique motivation, discipline, and organizational skills.

This section has elaborated mostly on the comments of the program directors, those with firsthand knowledge of the recruitment process. However, Dan Rubin noted that it would be interesting to look at how the fellows actually came to choose a particular program or even how they came to be interested in seeking the kinds of degrees and programs offered by PHPP. Although this was not one of the questions specifically asked of the alumni who were interviewed, the information gathered showed a clear consensus that going back for more rigorous training in health policy was the best way that the fellows imagined that they could either empower themselves in their current positions or have greater influence on policy making and change in the future.

## MENTORING

During an advisory meeting in 1993, Phil Lee stated, "A good fellow-mentor relationship is one of the single most important determinants of a successful health policy fellowship." The importance of mentoring was clearly understood by all the programs, as evidenced by their emphasis on supplementing the classroom experience with various research projects that stimulated faculty and fellow interaction and that taught students how to apply theories and techniques to answer real-life problems.

*A good fellow-mentor relationship is one of the single most important determinants of a successful health policy fellowship.*

The Institute of Health Policy, a leading health care and research center at Brandeis University, expanded its mission to include educational training. This enabled the Pew fellows to have access to key faculty and research staff. All research professors from the institute were held responsible for teaching and mentoring students. The Heller School and the institute firmly believed that a program in health policy would fall short if it relied only on traditional academics to teach policy research and analysis, so research practitioners were integrated into the core faculty (Raskin et al., 1992).

### Access to Key People

The fellows from the BU/Brandeis program spoke highly of the mentorship offered by faculty at both BU and Brandeis. Many stated that because of their rich experiences and strong relationships with the faculty, they were not only inspired to provide but also felt appropriately prepared to provide similar mentoring to other colleagues and to their students. Fostering these kinds of relationships between faculty and fellows and between fellows and other fellows, where people are comfortable and even eager to ask questions, give answers, probe issues, and challenge each other, is exactly what the Pew program was hoping to accomplish. These people trained by PHPP to respect, listen to, and learn from peers and colleagues will inform the debate and stimulate effective change. Linda Simoni-Wastila reflected on her experiences in the BU/Brandeis program:

> [O]n a personal level, I felt nurtured through the program by the staff and faculty, particularly Steve Crane, even though he was at BU; we had a joint program then. He was a real "mentor." I also got some good mentoring here, and the way we nurtured each other . . . and sort of developed a need to mentor other people. . . .Now I find myself in a mentoring position for students and even for some colleagues and I am prepared. The Pew program sort of facilitated that. . . .Key faculty were available and eager to mentor the Pews. We had ready access.

## A Hands-on Approach

Although the seminars and course work are vital parts of the UCSF Pew Health Policy Program, for many fellows the most important reason for participating in the program was the opportunity to participate in multidisciplinary health policy and health services research with the faculty of the institutes. This environment is further enriched by faculty-fellow interaction and the mentoring that faculty provide (Lessons Learned, UCSF, 1992-1993). The issues of faculty-fellow interaction and the mentoring and research training overlap to a great extent. Fellows receive detailed orientation to the faculty and their projects. Intensive, individualized programs of counseling, mentoring, and career development have been implemented. Carroll Estes cites the colleagueship and mentoring stimulated through large-scale projects as one of the most innovative methods of program implementation at UCSF. Hal Luft underscored his colleague's emphasis on the value of mentoring:

> The model that we chose worked well, and that's a model where the fellows basically get involved with one or two faculty members and work on some projects and get that hands-on experience. It's more of an apprenticeship model than a classroom model.

Likewise, says Carroll Estes, "The fact that the two institutes at UCSF together have about $20 million in funded research every year and probably 40 faculty investigators who are well known in their area has really contributed to implementing very significant training opportunities."

For many fellows the most important reason for participating in the program was the opportunity to participate in multidisciplinary health policy and health services research with the faculty of the institutes.

The postdoctoral fellows at UCSF had close contact with their assigned advisers and met with them regularly to review progress in research, field placements, publications, course work, and career planning. Faculty monitor and evaluate each fellow's progress, adjust his or her individualized program according to emerging needs, and provide assistance with specific problems. Regular meetings provide an opportunity for informal discussions and for forming the kind of trainee-mentor relationship that is so vital for career development (Lessons Learned, UCSF, 1992-1993).

In an effort to improve faculty-fellow interaction, all UCSF Pew fellows received guidelines listing the expected goals of the Pew fellow-mentor arrangements. This helped them to know what was expected of them and what they could expect from their faculty preceptor. Fellows and faculty were also provided with general guidelines for establishing a productive and enjoyable relationship with a mentor. These simple guidelines helped to clarify the confusion that often surrounds the roles and responsibilities expected of fellows and faculty in academic programs. (See Appendix C for guidelines.)

Pew funding permitted students to offer free assistance to a faculty member in exchange for ongoing mentoring and inclusion in a research project that would meet the individual fellow's training goals. Faculty usually found that the benefits of working with a fellow far exceeded the time of mentoring, provided that the match was a good one in terms of skills, content, timing, and expectations. It was made clear that fellows were "free agents" in their dealings with faculty mentors, and if things were not working out, they were free to seek out another faculty member and research setting. In the experience at UCSF, changing mentors because of irreconcilable conflicts over the research approach was rare, but conflicts over authorship occasionally occurred. This led to encouraging faculty and fellows to discuss issues of authorship order at the beginning of a writing effort.

When asked how the UCSF postdoctoral fellowship approach differed from a traditional postdoctoral fellowship, Carroll Estes responded:

> *This is much more of an interdisciplinary experience and much less of a lone wolf researcher, do it independently on your own and sink or swim on your own. There is much more of a faculty-planned approach and commitment, with annual reviews, mentorship meetings, preceptor meetings, scheduled reviews of students, and group meetings with faculty members on programs of activity in what they've accomplished and what they want to accomplish and getting mentorship and advice on*

**Faculty usually found that the benefits of working with a fellow far exceeded the time of mentoring, provided that the match was a good one in terms of skills, content, timing, and expectations.**

*papers, research proposals, and jobs. I don't think in  most other fellowships there exists this kind of tutelage. There is a real community commitment here.*

Estes attributes the success of the mentorship program to the general support provided by the Pew program for faculty who would not have support for any teaching or mentorship concerns otherwise.

Research collaboration between fellows and faculty does not end at the conclusion of the fellowship period. Fellows who assume academic positions, in particular, are often involved in completing research and publications initiated during the fellowship as well as developing research proposals out of earlier projects. The extent to which postdoctoral fellows who have graduated continue to collaborate with faculty from their programs may be one way to measure the success of the mentorship available during the training period. For example, Joan DaVanzo, who went through a combined doctoral program at RAND and UCLA, emphasized the value of the work projects in fostering close mentoring relationships. In addition to getting on-the-job, real-world experience, the work projects allowed for close contact with the faculty and project directors.

The University at Michigan program is designed to provide active support for doctoral fellows for a 3-year period. There are 2 years of course work and additional support for the completion of the dissertation. The demands of course work and dissertation projects are substantial, competing with full-time professional activities. To deal with this obstacle, faculty began to closely monitor and provide increased academic and psychological support to the fellows. According to Richardson (1990), this approach has been extremely helpful in assisting students in completing of their course work and dissertations.

> Specific steps were taken at all sites to foster a feeling of community among the Pew fellows.

## COMMUNITY OF SCHOLARS

The fellowship is a transition period, with marked uncertainties about the future and a groping for identity as health policy researchers (Lessons Learned, UCSF, 1992-1993).  In addition, fellows are often at similar stages in their nonprofessional lives, and the sharing of experiences is important. Therefore, specific steps were taken at all sites to foster a feeling of community among the Pew fellows through traditional and formal methods such as seminar-style classes, lunchtime colloquia, and conferences.  However, PHPP helped to create a sense of community through other, less formal routes. These include various social activities, the establishment of research project teams, and the logistical issue of placing the fellows in offices close to each other and the faculty because placing fellows in close proximity to one another and to the hub of communication is an important component of creating a community of scholars.

During the early years of PHPP, however, several of the sites did not have the space to place fellows in such strategic locations. Fellows were strewn about, hindering the vital interaction needed to create a community of scholars. Recognizing the dangers of haphazard placement, most of the programs resolved their space-related problems early on. For instance, the RAND/UCLA and the UCSF programs took the issue of proximity very seriously and worked hard to get fellows space together and close to the faculty members' offices. This enabled the fellows to informally discuss research projects, classes, and shared experiences. This exposure allows for the development of crucial critiquing skills because it provides the fellows with the opportunity to receive and provide feedback to their peers.

UCSF (Lessons Learned, UCSF, 1992–1993) points out the fact that too much space or space in some out-of-the-way location can be detrimental to student evolution. Fellows should be clustered near the power center of the organization. Important business is often transacted during chance encounters while picking up mail or getting coffee. These meetings are particularly important in getting fellows to meet and interact with faculty members with whom they are not primarily attached (Lessons Learned, UCSF, 1992–1993).

> *Pew funding for faculty time spent mentoring and interacting with fellows on research teams fostered a secure and close community of scholars.*

## Faculty Generosity

Carroll Estes attributes much of the success of the Pew programs to the commitment to fostering a community of scholars, in large part due to the general support for faculty provided by the Pew Charitable Trusts. Pew funding for faculty time spent mentoring and interacting with fellows on research teams fostered a secure and close community of scholars. Several program directors cited faculty commitment as one reason why the Pew Health Policy Programs are in a league of their own, and this is due in large part to the general support of the Pew Charitable Trusts. Carroll Estes speculates about how the outcomes have differed because of this unique fellowship training approach:

*The outcomes have differed from the traditional fellowship approach dramatically . . . in terms of research and publications. We would stand [our postdoctoral fellows] up against any postdoctoral program and I think they would probably have twice the rate of explicit measures of productivity. It is that nurturing, collectiveness, orientation, network, and support that the fellows offered each other and were offered by the faculty.*

Richardson (1990) found that fellows greatly valued scholarly interaction with their peers. Fellows considered interaction within the student community and with faculty and other health professionals as being vital to their successful evolution as health policy professionals. The fellows also cited Pew-sponsored conferences as contributing to the learning experience and a great opportunity to make additional contacts in the field. The fellows viewed the annual meeting and the meetings in Washington, D.C. very favorably (Richardson, 1990).

Due to the nonresidential nature of the Michigan program, issues related to physical space and working area proximity are not relevant in terms of establishing a community of scholars. Yet, according to Bill Weissert, the intensity of interaction during the weekend sessions create a scholarly atmosphere where fellows can draw upon each other's strengths and experiences:

*[T]he cohort effect, locking people into being part of a group for two years of intensive course work, I think is a terrifically positive effect and leads to a great success and socializes people. They learn from each other like crazy.*

The high-tech computer conferencing, discussed earlier by Leon Wyszewianski as one of the great strengths of the Michigan program, also allowed for the development of a sense of community among the fellows. Pat Butler and the other Michigan fellows who came from all over the country explained that the computer conferencing minimized the potential of feeling of isolated.

The diversity and maturity of the PHPP student body created a situation ripe for community learning. Steve Crane discussed how at BU the weekly seminars would bring together faculty and fellows from various disciplines to work together to solve problems from many different perspectives:

*We proved that there is a place in an academic institution for the mature learner. The discussions we had, the group we had, the experiences we had were just tremendous. That maturity factor was important. We as faculty sat around the table as much as the students, and the students who were there were as much as faculty as we were. It was a true community of learners.*

**Fellows considered interaction within the student community and with faculty and other health professionals as being vital to their successful evolution as health policy professionals.**

Those involved with the other programs had similar experiences, and most of those interviewed discussed the intensity of the Pew learning community. This environment, besides creating stimulating learning experiences, also reflected the real world of health policy, where problems cannot be solved by people sitting in closed offices. Real-life solutions need communities working together toward common goals.

## EARLY FOCUS ON THE DISSERTATION

The dissertation seminar has been crucial to the success of the program. The weekly seminars in the first year primarily focus on research methods and the interplay between data and conceptual thinking at various stages of the research process.

Most students in the BU/Brandeis program were concerned about the accelerated 2-year doctoral program and their chances of completing their dissertations within that time frame. Raskin and colleagues (1992) found that although all students managed to complete their courses and exams within a year and a half, only a few focused fellows finished the dissertation within the 2-year time frame. For those fellows who did manage to finish the dissertation within 2 or 3 years, most had their dissertation topic (and some even had data) before they started the program. The fast-paced nature of the program and the fact that the fellows did not have to collect their own data but could use an existing data set helped them complete the degree quickly. Jonathan Howland, a BU fellow who went on to direct the program for some time, was one of the few fellows who was able to complete the courses and the dissertation quickly. Howland explained how he went about the process:

> I found out in April that I had been accepted into the program and I started looking for data sets then. I knew I was going to have to do a dissertation, and I finally ended up with a dissertation topic in December of my first year. But I had been working on it since April. So I did it in 23 months, but the fact of the matter is I gave myself a long lead time.

However, Jonathan's case was fairly unique. Most students needed slightly more direction. To assist the students with identifying and getting started with a dissertation topic early on, the training directors in the BU/Brandeis program developed a special dissertation seminar for the Pew students. Initially, the dissertation seminar was led by Sol Levine and Stan Wallack, then Steve Crane and Mary Henderson took over, and for the last 5 years of funding (and beyond) the seminar has been taught by Jon Chilingerian. This dissertation seminar has been crucial to the success of the program. The weekly seminars in the first year primarily focus on research methods and the interplay between data and conceptual thinking at various stages of the research process. The emphasis is on managing the throughput and how one draws inferences from social science data. The seminar offers methodological perspectives for the study of health policy to open the way for fellows to begin developing their own areas of professional concentration. By the end of the first-year seminar, fellows are requested to turn their research interests and ideas into viable research topics. Stan Wallack and Jeff Prottas (a Heller School research professor and political scientist) led the seminar in the second year. The second-year seminar was initiated in 1995 and concentrates on lending support and providing peer critiques of topics regarding data sets, problems, and analysis processes relating to the student's individual projects. At each session one student is selected to lead a discussion of a recently written position paper related directly to that student's proposed dissertation research.

### Dissertation Seminars

Linda Simoni-Wastila believes that the dissertation seminars at BU/Brandeis were one of the most innovative and useful aspects of her Pew doctoral program. She explained that the weekly seminars were attended by second- and third-year students so that all were exposed to different processes and different levels of the process:

> We had a very good idea of what to expect before we actually went through the process ourselves. We even had dry runs for people who were defending their entire dissertations, so by the end of my first year, I was no longer afraid of the dissertation. It was no longer that big, huge "D." It was no longer that big black hole that so many students talk about. They don't see that there are steps to it and there is a sequential process and it happens over time. I was able to see very clearly after 1 year what the process was and what the steps were and what sorts of things I should consider.

Bill Weissert explained that early on the Michigan program did not have anybody whose job it was to make sure that students were equipped to do a dissertation. This concept of having one or more faculty members, outside of advisers, help maintain the dissertation momentum was learned over time. Richardson's evaluation (1990) also found that the University of Michigan greatly refined, over time, its orientation to and preparation of students for dissertation work with an early seminar and faculty mentoring. As part of the strategies developed to help students make timely and satisfactory progress toward their dissertations, the Michigan program established as part of the curriculum a formal dissertation seminar. Its purpose is to provide systematically and concisely information on what is known about effective ways to structure and manage the dissertation (Michigan Proposal Narrative, 1994). The seminar serves as a forum for the discussion of general and specific problems related to the dissertation and their solutions, as well as for students to present their progress to fellow classmates for feedback. This has proven to be a very successful exercise (Michigan Proposal Narrative, 1994). During the final portion of the program, each student must sign up with a faculty member of the student's choosing for an independent study course focusing on the dissertation. The usefulness of the dissertation seminar was cited by all four alumni interviewed, and as explained by Dan Rubin, the dissertation process took on new meaning:

> *I think the way that the dissertation seminar was structured was very good. It really focused on producing a draft of a prospectus as the course material. The discipline of doing that step by step was fabulous. Integrating things that we had thought about before while pushing for production . . . the emphasis on getting organized was very helpful. The dissertation was demystified for us.*

To sustain the momentum to completing the dissertation that was begun during the first and second years of the fellowship, the fellows are brought back to Ann Arbor on three separate occasions during the third year. At each of these sessions, students are expected to meet with their dissertation advisers. They also meet as a group at the dissertation seminar, where they report to the group and professor and receive feedback on the progress they have made, the problems they have encountered, and the insights they have gained about the dissertation progress (Michigan Proposal Narrative, 1994).

## On-the-Job Training

Unlike the two other doctoral programs, RAND/UCLA emphasized an early focus on the dissertation from the outset. Kate Korman and Al Williams explained that at RAND/UCLA, the research projects discussed earlier and called on-the-job training were held with the same importance as the course work, because it was the project work that was supposed to lead to a dissertation. Doctoral and midcareer fellows were encouraged from the very beginning to get involved in research projects that had the potential to

At RAND/UCLA, the research projects called on-the-job training were held with the same importance as the course work, because it was the project work that was supposed to lead to a dissertation.

lead to a dissertation or publication, respectively. Fellows spent about half of their time on projects and were evaluated on the basis of progress and performance. Approximately half of the fellows worked on projects that led directly to dissertations. Kate Korman explains the value of the work projects to the early dissertation focus:

> *This effort produced familiarity with research methods and processes "in the lab" to apply what was being learned in the classroom. As a result, our students progressed rapidly toward the degree, where in the case of the midcareer fellows, they often had a publication as a result of work done while in the program.*

## NETWORKING

According to Altman (1995), one of the strongest aspects of the Pew program has been the networking among the fellows in each of the programs, between the fellows in the different programs, and between the fellows and those engaged in the policy process in Washington, D.C. All the fellows interviewed were extremely appreciative for the commitment made by the Pew Charitable Trusts and the Institute of Medicine (IOM) in establishing and maintaining a network that has extended far beyond the training programs. To many, the network has proved invaluable for their careers by providing ready access to a wide array of highly trained professionals working in all sectors of the health policy field. The network fosters collaborative efforts and enhanced communication among members of academia, government, foundations, the service sector, and the corporate world.

PHPP explicitly adopted the objective of implementing a networking system for fellows that included academicians, health professionals, and policy makers. For example, as the UCSF Pew program strengthened its ties with a number of governmental and nongovernmental organizations at the local, state, and national levels, it introduced postdoctoral and midcareer fellows to an extended network of health policy professionals, including those in the Physician Payment Review Commission, the National Academy of Social Insurance, the Centers for Disease Control and Prevention/U.S. Public Health Service, and the San Francisco Department of Public Health.

*One of the strongest aspects of the Pew program has been the networking among the fellows in each of the programs, between the fellows in the different programs, and between the fellows and those engaged in the policy process in Washington, D.C.*

### Shared Interests

The PHPPs were designed with the understanding that to promote effective change, health policy professionals must be trained in the art of communicating with colleagues from all areas and sectors of the health care arena. The network of Pew fellows, alumni, and faculty reflected this underlying premise. Indeed, it is the multidisciplinary nature of the network that Lisa Bero from UCSF most appreciates:

> *[Pew] established a network of highly trained individuals who will stay in touch forever. That will really be important, as it helps people in different agencies and different states as they approach similar problems with different perspectives.*

The PHPPs were designed with the understanding that to promote effective change, health policy professionals must be trained in the art of communicating with colleagues from all areas and sectors of the health care arena.

Steve Crane explained that another great thing about the Pew program was the multitude of opportunities that the fellows had to meet and network with leaders in the field, academia, and the public and private sectors. Establishing these relationships gave the program "weight of influence in the system" and gave the students access to the people who could use their research more quickly. Steve Crane reiterated the value of the multidisciplinary, multisector, real-world Pew network:

> *[The] network of people continue to interact and continue to have important positions in the policy system, both public and private policy. These people understand and know each other and are able to get things done. The policy system does not work through formal authority channels but most often through informal channels and it's not what you know, but who you know that counts; the networking was really important.*

In terms of the BU Corporate Fellows Program, Crane believes that the effects of the Pew network is still reverberating throughout the business community. Likewise, the success of Bruce Spitz's Community Program at Brandeis, he says, was dependent on networking:

> *The notion was that we needed to create change, not just at the intellectual level but at the institutional level as well. Bruce's efforts to try to get communities to move, to link together business and the public sector was highly innovative and a precursor to the coalitions of today and to the more population-based research being employed today.*

### Fellowship Among Fellows

The overwhelming consensus and unbridled enthusiasm that the alumni used to describe both the career value and the social value of the Pew network was remarkable. Pamela Paul-Shaheen from the University of Michigan stated that she draws upon the extensive Pew network regularly through her work. Furthermore, Pamela finds the network to be extremely broad in scope:

*Pew has created . . . incredible networking opportunities. I use many of the people in the Pew network continually, and I am always amazed, as I go through my daily professional life, the people I run into and find out we share the common framework of having gone through the Pew program. . . .The networking that has resulted has offered me an opportunity to link up, work with, and collaborate with a whole range of people across the nation. That has been invaluable.*

Linda Simoni-Wastila, a graduate of the BU/Brandeis program, stated that the emphasis on building and fostering a far-reaching network tied into the policy scene in Washington, D.C., was one of the Pew program's greatest contributions to the field. She explained how the process of network development began early on and how it functioned as a motivating force from the outset:

*Networking began in the first year. [The] first year you go to Washington, D.C. . . . and are introduced right away to the Washington scene and all the hot issues of the moment. The real cutting-edge issues. If you wanted to know about health care reform you got the latest and the greatest right there. It got people really excited, [and] it helped to bridge the programs, to develop that commonality and similar approach to health and health policy. . . . [It] was almost as if you were a cutting-edge person. The conversations were incredibly intellectual, yet practical at the same point. You felt like, wow, we can change the world.*

Mark Legnini, John McDonough, Sarita Bhalotra, Terry Hammons, and Kathleen Eyre all discussed how becoming part of the network was just as important and valuable as the other aspects of the program to their successes as health policy professionals. Bhalotra explained that being part of the Pew network meant interacting with some of the leading minds in the world of health policy. John McDonough explained that the Pew program was about acquiring skills and making unique relationships:

> **Networking is essential to the growth of health policy professionals.**

*[Pew] exposed me to folks in the health policy community who have been very important and helpful and who I wouldn't have otherwise had the opportunity to meet. It exposed me to an excellent network of people.*

Terry Hammons, an alumnus of the RAND midcareer program, found networking with people around the country who were engaged in policy-relevant health services research very valuable. He stated that as a result of relationships established during his year at RAND, he continues to talk regularly with academics from RAND, Brandeis, and Harvard and policy analysts in the Congressional Budget Office and the U.S. Department of Health and Human Services.

Pew may have only 306 fellows and alumni penetrating the health policy field, but with the relationships they have developed among themselves and with non-Pew professionals, their impact and their ability to get things done are enormous.

Kathleen Eyre found the network to be a huge advantage not only for the alumni influencing policy, but also for the field itself. The Pew network has linked the many different sectors of the health care arena, thereby increasing the possibility of effecting change.

Joan DaVanzo, also from RAND, gave a personal anecdote to describe the value and accessibility of the Pew network once she had completed her doctoral degree and was looking for a job out in the field. She also cited the value of the continued effort on the part of IOM to produce the directory, a means of getting in touch with alumni:

*I moved from San Francisco to Washington, D.C. because I said to myself 'if you want to be in health policy, Washington is the place to be.' When I landed in Washington I found this whole community of Pew folks that I had access to. It was like being home. Not only people that you know, even people from the Pew directory, you could just ring them up. Marion and the IOM do a really good job of keeping the network alive with the newsletter, having functions, and updating the Pew directory. I know that takes a lot of time to pull that all together, but that's part of the Pew legacy, part of creating an entity and then calling it the Pew legacy. You have to devote time and space.*

Although it was through Marion Ein Lewin's and IOM's nurturing that the extensive Pew network was formed, it would not have been nearly as successful without the commitment of the faculty and program administrators at the individual program sites. PHPP faculty considered networking to be a vital part of the curriculum. Therefore, they were committed to networking activities, such as the annual or semiannual Pew conferences. Carroll Estes stated that networking is essential to the growth of health policy professionals:

*Networking and socialization to the field, the norms of work, and networking of colleagues have been important parts of the educational process.*

Marion Ein Lewin expressed some concern about the future of the Pew network. Although she stated that the foundation of the network is securely in place and that nearly 300 Pew alumni and many faculty are already tied in with the Washington, D.C. health policy scene, there will no longer be that concerted effort by an organizing body (like IOM) to monitor and foster the networking activities. She hopes that the programs that continue beyond the last funding cycle will continue to recognize the importance of linking fellows from across the country:

*I think one of the really wonderful aspects of the program has been the learning curve at every stage. The evolution of the four programs and the IOM program thinking of themselves as mostly individual fiefdoms, all a little bit in competition with each other, to an evolution where everyone now is working to a common goal. . . . So in the first few years we spent a lot of time just promoting mutual understanding and linkages across the programs, and I think what started off as a challenge became very much a reason for the success of this program. The programs now have common objectives, and there is much more commonality among the fellows . . . they are all working toward mutual goals.*

Integrating health policy fellows is vital to the success of any program, if success is measured by policy influence and communication of health care issues between the sectors. Even if future programs are not financially or academically linked, there would be great value in organizing some networking activities. Such activities not only broaden the scope and extend the reach but also magnify the ultimate products of advanced graduate programs. Pew may have only 306 fellows and alumni penetrating the health policy field, but with the relationships they have developed among themselves and with non-Pew professionals, their impact and their ability to get things done are enormous.

*PHPP fosters a cross-fertilization of different theoretical perspectives, as well as different methodological approaches in solving concrete policy problems.*

## MULTIDISCIPLINARY EDUCATION AND TRAINING

Altman (1995) discussed the changing needs of the U.S. health care system and stated that what was lacking was a sufficient supply of well-trained individuals who could understand and synthesize the clinical, practical, political, and economic implications of the policy process. He stated that the future of the U.S. health care system is dependent on policy decisions that reflect the problem-solving strategies of different disciplines and perspectives. Altman (1995) cites the Robert Wood Johnson Foundation's Health Policy Fellowships and the Pew Charitable Trust's Health Policy Programs as the driving forces behind educating and training health care professionals about policy making and "bringing the synergy of an interdisciplinary approach to problem solving." He described the Pew Health Policy Program as "an effort to bridge the gap between health economists and other disciplines." Furthermore, Altman (1995) stated that PHPP "fosters a cross-fertilization of different theoretical perspectives, as well as different methodological approaches in solving concrete policy problems."

Hamilton's 1995 evaluation states that PHPP "has had from its inception a single stated goal, which was expressed in the RFP: to stimulate the development of multidisciplinary health policy education programs that will equip a cadre of leaders with the required skills to deal effectively with the nation's complex current and future health policy issues." The interdisciplinary strength of the curriculum was cited as a primary success indicator by all three evaluations (Hamilton, 1995; Richardson 1985, 1990) and was underscored by the more recently conducted interviews.

### Agents of Change

Steve Crane stated that the Pew program was all about change. He explained that the programs were not intended to produce policy makers or academic researchers per se but, rather, change makers. Being an agent of change is a subtle and important role, says Dan Rubin, and one that is difficult to observe and measure. Rubin commented that in his career he makes many contributions to change that are invisible outside his organization. Change, says Steve Crane, requires interdisciplinary people who can talk and understand the complex and interdisciplinary nature of the current health care system:

> One of the defining purposes of the Pew HPP, and one that set us apart from other PhD programs was that while we were striving to create people who could produce policy, our emphasis was more so on creating people who could use policy. In essence we were creating change agents. Certainly, BU and Brandeis focused on the intersection of the three worlds of public, private, and academia. We trained people to straddle the fence. Change comes from the interaction of these sectors, and we knew that and we emphasized that. Focusing on that intersection effects lasting change. We are seeing that borne out today in the health care sector.

**The programs were not intended to produce policy makers or academic researchers per se but, rather, change makers.**

Many Pew fellows agreed that their multidisciplinary training enabled them to understand the mechanisms of change and work toward solving problems using a variety of disciplinary approaches and perspectives. However, as the following quote from Lisa Bero so poignantly illustrates, most graduate programs do not realize the value of multidisciplinary training:

> I came from basic science, and I thought I was coming from such a narrow background no one will understand me and I'm not going to understand anybody else. I thought all these sociologists would be much better off than me, but as it turns out we were all in the same boat. I didn't realize that every discipline was so narrow in terms of PhD training. . . . And so we had to learn to understand each other and to really gain an appreciation for all those other disciplines, and I think it was a win-win situation.

Patricia Butler explained that because the Michigan program was housed in the School of Public Health, the curriculum was able to incorporate a fundamental set of disciplines whose influence is often lacking in the national health policy debate:

> *When we talk about health policy we often think of financing and delivery systems, but at the core should be some of the public health disciplines. Michigan offered that interdisciplinary focus, and I think that's unusual at this point among the other programs. I found that very valuable.*

Butler discussed another aspect of a multidisciplinary program: the diversity of the students. It takes more than a multidisciplinary curriculum and faculty to foster among the fellows an understanding of the convergence and interdependence of health policy disciplines. Bringing together fellows from different sectors with different expertise created the necessary depth and breadth. Patricia Butler described her class at Michigan:

**The PHPP idea of what constituted multidisciplinary training was that each of the disciplines had to be represented in each student.**

> *There were a couple of folks from state government, we had a state legislator, we had someone who worked in the foundation community, a hospital administrator, a person in the insurance industry who also had physician assistant training [and two folks from academia], very interesting people that contributed to the very rich discussions. . . . We weren't all of one mind. As long as you can keep an open mind, you can learn a lot from people like that.*

The concept of multidisciplinary education or training can take on several different meanings, depending on where one sits. Steve Crane explained that the PHPP approach to being multidisciplinary certainly did not mean having people from many different disciplines sitting in the same room or housed in offices next door to one another. Rather, the PHPP idea of what constituted multidisciplinary training was that each of the disciplines had to be represented in each student. This gets back to the reasoning that problems in the health care system are not strictly discipline oriented. Many problems have economic, sociological, psychological, and political components. Furthermore, health care issues span many sectors and involve many different actors. Effectively trained change agents have acquired the knowledge and the skills to understand and apply the many different perspectives required to analyze complex health care system problems. Furthermore, the problems in health care are not institutional in nature, and they are not even mostly state oriented, explained Steve Crane. The problems in health care

are nationally oriented, cutting across all political boundaries. There continues to be a dire need in the health policy community for people who can see the big picture and apply that vision in an effective way, the way that the Pew fellows were trained to do:

> A lot of programs produced people just for the public sector, or just for the academic sector, but rarely just for the private sector. What we wanted to do [at BU] was to have someone who had not only the vocabulary, but the knowledge to cross-walk academics, public service, private sector and not-for-profit. . . . I think [this] need still exists and most of the academic programs are still turning out discipline-focused individuals. Brandeis-Heller is an exception. What we need are people who can understand problems from a multiplicity of viewpoints, who can create solutions that cut across disciplinary and sector perspectives. We are still short on people who can do that.

Stan Wallack discussed the importance of training students to look through the various "lenses" of health policy. He explained how the Brandeis curriculum was multidimensional in terms of political science, economics, and sociology and how a specialization in health was built in using the lenses of the economist, the political scientist, and the sociologist. Stan stated that it is essential for these different paradigms and other perspectives to be incorporated in any program teaching health policy.

Despite the importance of multidisciplinary education and training for policy research, policy making, and change, the integration of different disciplines and experiences into advanced graduate training is still quite rare. Nonetheless, Dan Rubin from Michigan hopes that the prestige of the schools and the success of the programs will ultimately work to disseminate the interdisciplinary training approach at the doctoral and postdoctoral levels. Kathleen Eyre stated that it was this aspect of the curriculum—the integration of the different social sciences into a health policy framework—that distinguished the Pew approach training from the traditional training approaches.

Hal Luft explained that the innovative training approach used by PHPP enabled the fellows, once they entered the field, to continue interacting and communicating with professionals from other disciplines in their own or other sectors. Communication of this nature is fostered during the training years when the academically focused and nonacademically focused fellows merge their expertise to work on projects and solve problems. As a result of this training approach, explains Hal Luft, fellows who go on to become policy analysts in the government can call upon their colleagues in academia for advice in ways that would not have been possible had they not gone through joint training.

Al Williams underscored the value in exposing fellows to projects where they would have to work together with professionals with expertise in various areas. This kind of preparation significantly affects the future success of the fellows. The general consensus was that the health policy field needed broadly trained health policy professionals to effect change. PHPP prepared its fellows for this challenge. In reference to the doctoral program in particular, Dennis Beatrice stated that through this innovative multidisciplinary training approach, "Pew educated a new kind of PhD, one better prepared and more relevant for today's world."

## LEADERSHIP ROLES

It is interesting and noteworthy that IOM had an interest in the Pew Health Policy Program from the start. Marion Ein Lewin remembers that when the Pew Charitable Trusts began looking for an organization to direct the program, IOM had responded but had not won the proposal. The Pew Health Policy Program was brought to IOM from the American Enterprise Institute in 1987; however, it was not officially called the Program Office until 1988. It was on the recommendation of Bill Richardson, who conducted the program evaluations, that IOM was named the official Program Office.

*Pew educated a new kind of PhD, one better prepared and more relevant for today's world.*

### Role of IOM

Marion Ein Lewin describes the role of the IOM office as one that develops the joint activities of all the programs, plans annual meetings and meetings for new fellows, develops the directory and semiannual newsletters, monitors the budgets, and makes sure that all the programs are performing according to the requirements of the program. Perhaps most importantly, IOM is responsible for the network and the "family" of Pew fellows over and above their connection to the individual programs and institutions. The success of this aspect of the IOM Program Office's responsibility can perhaps be best described by a quote from Jonathan Howland, a BU/Brandeis Pew alumnus who also had the unique experience of directing the Pew program at BU for a time.

*The Pew fellows' identity was so transcendent and we all felt like Pew fellows, and that had a higher profile than what school we were at.*

## Creating a Vision for a National Training Program

The definition of "success" varies across graduate programs. Traditionally, successful doctoral or postdoctoral programs would seed the academic field with their graduates, and successful midcareer programs would seed the management field. PHPP however, aimed to seed the whole field of health policy, encompassing the academic world, the health care management world, the various levels of government, the corporate world, and the public and private sectors. How can one program, however, produce successfully trained health policy professionals to meet the needs of so many different areas of the health care field? One way is for each program to establish a strong multidisciplinary core, a sense of urgency, and a national identity that rises above all of the programs and the fellows' individual aspirations and career paths.

## A Transcendent Pew Identity

The leadership of PHPP was able to foster this sense of belonging through an empowering Pew identity, but it was not easy. IOM and the program administration went to great lengths to instill in the Pew fellows a sense that they were all, regardless of their backgrounds and expertise, working toward a common goal, that is, to be more effective change agents in the health policy arena. Marion Ein Lewin reflected on the painstaking but enormously rewarding process. She stated that in the beginning none of the students thought of themselves as "Pew fellows"; rather, they looked at themselves as individuals all getting degrees or going through training programs at individual sites across the country and that Pew was only a financier. During the first year or two, the fellows thought that the source of program funding was the only common bond between their programs. As Marion Ein Lewin stated:

> At that time there were a lot of fellows who were community activists and who wanted to be change agents but in a way that said, we have our values, we have our agenda, we know what we want to accomplish, and we don't care what the rest of the world says, we don't have to communicate with the rest of the world. I remember that I felt that we [the program directors] really had our job cut out for us. If you're going to be a change agent I think the first lesson is that you have to be able to dialogue with the people who are in power even if you disagree with them. If you're just going to wall yourself up as the strong opposition, you're not going to understand where these people are coming from and you're never going to be an effective change agent.

In an effort to counteract this early hostility, the program administration incorporated controversial presentations into the Houston national meeting in 1989, and tried to teach the fellows how to communicate effectively with people who have varying perspectives. Marion Ein Lewin describes what happened:

> *Some of the fellows didn't like some of the panelists because they didn't care for their views. . . . Leon Wyszewianski from the Michigan program got up and said that the purpose of being a Pew fellow is that you gain an understanding about how to be effective change agents in the world of health policy and the purpose of the Pew Health Policy Fellowship Program is for people to become good communicators and to work in the real world, not in some ideological world.*

Marion Ein Lewin explained that this was a real turning point for the program because it was the first time that there was a discussion about what it meant to be a Pew fellow, that it was something above and beyond just financing an education. The fellows began to learn that the program had a purpose and that it wanted to create a cadre of similarly trained people who could work effectively in health policy at all levels and in all sectors.

Many others claimed that the program office helped the individual academic programs to achieve their goals. The goals of program leadership extend beyond integration and the fostering of community. They included motivating fellows to complete their challenging and difficult programs. Joan DaVanzo discussed how the dedicated leadership of the program sites and IOM set the PHPPs apart from other doctoral programs:

> *Doctoral programs are usually very hard to finish, and there are a whole bunch of ABDs around. At RAND/UCLA the motivation to finish was very strong. The Pew programs created a real strong motivation to finish, and they did that in a variety of ways. Some of it being networking with alumni and seeing these people in these neat jobs and writing these great papers and you wanted to finish and join them. . . . A lot of the motivation is created by the program.*

Likewise, Linda Simoni-Wastila discussed how the leadership motivated her to finish her doctoral program at Brandeis:

> *The support of people like Marion Lewin motivated me to want to finish and contribute to the field. . . . My experience with Pew continues to motivate me. When I get the Pew newsletter and I see where everyone is and what they are doing, I think wow, that's great. It makes me want to go out there and publish more and contribute more and do more. In that way Pew has touched me professionally. It has made me more enthusiastic about what I do, not that I wasn't before, but it has given me that extra boost.*

> The fellows began to learn that the program had a purpose and that it wanted to create a cadre of similarly trained people who could work effectively in health policy at all levels and in all sectors.

Following along the same idea articulated by both DaVanzo and Simoni-Wastila, Jonathan Howland discussed how the program leadership distinguished PHPP from other traditional doctoral programs:

> In other doctoral programs there is more of an adversarial relationship between the doctoral candidate and the faculty. You may have your mentor, but as a whole, the department's view is that you have to prove that you are worthy of our bestowing this doctorate from our department. There is this kind of onus on the individuals to prove themselves. In the Pew program, the faculty had a real stake in getting people through, and high attrition rates were not a good thing. . . . Faculty were stakeholders in the success of the program. . . . Every failure is a failure of the program.

Howland explained that there are two sides to this leadership approach, one positive and one an area for concern. On the positive side, the fellows had access to a "very user-friendly faculty" who believed that there was value in appropriately training fellows and allowing them expeditious entry into the field. On the less positive side, this approach allowed some fellows to be irresponsible in terms of course selection, the amount of work that they did and what learning they did. Nonetheless, overall, the fellows were mature enough to take on the challenge of a nontraditional, accelerated program, and the supportive environment succeeded in producing effective health policy professionals focused on real-world issues.

**Overall, the fellows were mature enough to take on the challenge of a nontraditional, accelerated program, and the supportive environment succeeded in producing effective health policy professionals focused on real-world issues.**

## Role of the Trusts

The Pew Charitable Trusts were also commended for their strong commitment to leading and administering the Pew Health Policy Program. According to Marion Ein Lewin, the Trusts' faith in the program never wavered. She explains that the directors at the Trusts had an uphill battle because foundations do not inherently like to fund programs for the long term. From the beginning, the willingness on the part of the Trusts was crucial to the success of the program. Steve Crane reiterated the uniqueness of Pew's commitment:

> The Trusts have been very supportive. They are our colleagues in all of this. They hung with us when things were rough. They celebrated our victories. The Pew Trusts deserve a lot of commendation for doing this and sticking with it. There are as many lessons to be learned on their side about how you deal with fellowship programs. If this model is to be replicated, what the foundations are going to need to know about is not only how it works at our end but how it works at their end.

## THE "PRICE" OF INSTITUTIONALIZATION—FINANCING ISSUES

The Pew Charitable Trusts' decision to discontinue financial support for the health policy programs with the final grant in 1991 was based on the premise that over the 15 years of funding, three very distinct and highly successful models had been developed, and these models should become institutionalized and adopted by other institutions (Pew Charitable Trusts, Rimel and Asbury, 1995). The Trusts' claim that the last grant was, in part, a transitional effort to enable the sites to develop "how to" materials and to explore alternative approaches to financing their programs in the future. The Trusts, however, recognize that with potential reductions in health services and policy research funding these models may be difficult to sustain in the future.

### University of Michigan

In 1993, the Michigan Pew Program Advisory Committee assessed the feasibility of continuing the Michigan program if and when the Pew funding was discontinued. They determined that the university would probably not be able to retain the many faculty members supported by Pew money. They were also concerned that only those students who could afford to self-fund their education would apply to and enroll in the program. They hypothesized that such a situation might lead to a more homogeneous cohort of students, a loss of diversity in backgrounds and perspectives, a more regional student body, and a loss of national focus. The advisory committee feared that the university would be faced with the decision to retain a program of greatly reduced quality and scope or to end the program completely. This was of grave concern because the Michigan program is still the only nonresidential (on job/on campus) doctoral program in the United States. Ending the program would clearly leave a devastating void (Site Visit, 1993).

The Pew doctoral program at the University of Michigan selects midcareer professionals who are active in policy formulation and upgrades their knowledge and skills, thus enabling them to participate more effectively in the policy process. Approximately two-thirds of these individuals receive salaries that make the costs of tuition, fees, travel, and books for the program unaffordable without assistance. Patricia Butler commented on the problems of sustaining a midcareer nonresidential program like the Michigan program without funding and the changes that reduced funding would likely bring:

> The Trusts recognize that with potential reductions in health services and policy research funding these models may be difficult to sustain in the future.

*Most of us were midcareer and many of us live in places where there isn't even a graduate level health policy program offered . . . that's why I am so grateful to the Pew Charitable Trusts for supporting this kind of program. I am disappointed and concerned about what happens when the money goes away, as it has basically begun to do. I think it's a unique and extraordinary opportunity and one that I think should be available to others in the future. I am particularly concerned that as Michigan tries to make its program self-supporting, as they need to do without an outside source of revenue, then they're going to get mostly people who have deep-pocket employers who can send them and that will tend to be more people in the private sector, more health services administrators as opposed to health policy folks from public agencies . . . more residents of Michigan who don't have to pay the out-of-state tuition. I think it's fine that Michigan gets to take advantage of this thing, but it was such a unique national resource that I am sorry to see the dollars go away.*

Pew funds have also enabled the University of Michigan to support visiting faculty. The program coordinators have found that students benefit greatly from lectures by specialists on important topics not necessarily on the research agenda of the University of Michigan faculty. The experience has also been enriched by faculty brought in from other institutions to develop courses or to fill in for local faculty who are unavailable to teach a necessary course (Michigan Proposal Narrative, August 1994). This flexibility in program offerings is very important in maintaining the quality of the Pew experience; however, it is in jeopardy as funding ceases.

On a more positive note, the faculty and program directors at the University of Michigan are committed to sustaining the nonresidential doctoral program on their campus. Their primary concern, as highlighted previously, is maintaining the rich diversity that makes their program so valuable to the health policy field. Bill Weissert commented:

*There is no question that the [Michigan] program will continue. We have expanded it and bought off on it and found we can sustain it. The big problem is that we will not have funding and therefore we'll have a limited ability to reach people who need to be here with fellowships. We just don't have the money. To the extent that you're trying to reach people in the policy process, [it] is pretty important because it's a field where people are not particularly well paid. Thus, without the proper funding, we reduce our likelihood of influencing the policy process. But we will continue to get people who are either able to afford the program because they are MDs or who are supported by their organization or interest group.*

## University of California, San Francisco

The 1990 Hamilton evaluation states, "In all cases, the acid test of legitimization at the grantee institution itself is whether the activities survive after the PCT [Pew Charitable Trusts] umbilical is cut." Indeed, all the Pew program sites have passed the test. At UCSF, the support for infrastructure and related training and research resources earlier in the history of the program were instrumental in acquiring permanent university funding for the Institute for Health and Aging. Hal Luft reflected on the structures now in place at UCSF as a result of the Pew program and the indirect benefits that PHPP has brought to UCSF.

> *I suspect at UCSF that we would not have had a postdoctoral program had there not been the Pew funds to get it started. We would not have had the AHCPR [Agency for Health Care Policy and Research] training grant because that built on our experiences with Pew. And, I suspect that there would not have been as nearly as strong an application from Berkeley and UCSF for the Robert Wood Johnson Health Policy Scholars. I suspect the same thing would have been true at Michigan. All these things can be linked back to the Pew program.*

The Health Policy Management Program at UCSF that was funded during the first cycle by Pew was continued on a permanent basis with funds supplied by the UCSF hospitals and clinics to support one to two fellows a year (Richardson, 1990). Other efforts to institutionalize the Pew program have continued. At an advisory board meeting in 1993, Phil Lee and Carroll Estes reported that the seminars that were developed for the Pew program have been institutionalized at the Institute for Health Policy Studies.

A major objective of the UCSF Pew postdoctoral program has been to develop the capacity to provide full financial support for core faculty and staff. However, this has been extremely difficult. Prolonged economic recession in California continues, as does an even more prolonged crisis in funding the state of California budget. Due to substantial cuts in state funding, the University of California as a whole, including UCSF, is undertaking major reductions in its workforce and salaries. In this climate of spending reductions, the university is loathe to take on additional responsibilities for new administrative or faculty expenses. Given the structural economic and government funding problems, there is little prospect in the foreseeable future for a substantial reversal in UCSF policy.

At the same time, none of the other fellowship funding agencies fully pays for the real expenses incurred for core fellowship program faculty and staff. Most of these agencies appear to assume that they are involved with a normal university disciplinary department, with faculty paid for through the university's annual budget, rather than two research institutes that depend almost exclusively on external sources of funding. The institutes do not have the financial resources to engage in cross-subsidization of the fellowship program activities for any significant period of time, since virtually all reserve comes from research contracts and grants, and discretionary funds are very limited.

Thus, UCSF finds itself in the paradoxical position of training an increasing number of exceptionally qualified fellows while receiving a declining amount of support for core faculty and staff. Although the institutes will look to other foundations for financial support for training-related costs, it is not clear whether these foundations will be willing to pay for nonstipend fellowship costs. Without a solution to this problem, UCSF might be unable to avoid a substantial reduction in the size of what may be the most important postdoctoral and midcareer fellowship training program in health policy and health services research in the United States (UCSF Annual Report 1992–1993).

UCSF continues to take great strides in making PHPP self-sufficient. UCSF faculty have implemented major steps toward the institutionalization of training. A series of new formal courses was developed and the curriculum has been enriched. Several courses have reached the stage of having structured syllabi with regular annual and biannual scheduling, and they attract a wide range of students and fellows from UCSF, the University of California at Berkeley, and other campuses. During the third cycle of Pew funding (1992 to 1995), a major part of the UCSF program's mission was to expand the support bases by attracting new sources of funding and mid career fellows who were able to bring stipend support as well as pay the program for the cost of training.

> **UCSF finds itself in the paradoxical position of training an increasing number of exceptionally qualified fellows while receiving a declining amount of support for core faculty and staff.**

### Brandeis University/Boston University

The Pew doctoral program at Brandeis has enabled the Institute for Health Policy to broaden the health policy specialization in the Heller School curriculum. As of 1993, at least four courses developed through Pew funding were institutionalized at Brandeis (Advisory Board meeting, February 18, 1993). Because of the excellence of the Heller School's PhD program and the national reputation of the Pew doctoral program, many more students who are interested in careers in health policy research are becoming attracted to the program (Raskin et al., 1992). However, since the Pew program funded only six students per year, many of these applicants have accepted the Heller School's offer to matriculate in the doctoral program and specialize in health policy.

Because of this expanded interest in health policy, the institute has developed the Institute for Health Policy Fellows Program to help support some of these strong doctoral candidates. Selected students are required to follow the health policy core curriculum and participate in the weekly Seminar in Health Policy Research. In addition to the academic requirements, Institute fellows are required to work 1 day a week at the institute in exchange for a $7,500 annual stipend (Raskin et al., 1992).

In 1994, the Institute for Health Policy adopted the strategy of seeking health services research (as opposed to health policy research) training grants from the federal government to complete the transition to alternative funding. The Heller School was awarded training grants from the Agency for Health Care Policy and Research (AHCPR), and in 1995 the Heller School enrolled its first fellows in this program. The health services research training program's curriculum is very similar to that of the health policy research training program's curriculum, and the Heller School faculty believe that their success with the Pew programs greatly assisted them in receiving the AHCPR grants.

> Joe Newhouse, who was on the faculty at RAND, built upon the RAND Pew experience in his new PhD program at Harvard University.

The Pew program for corporate midcareer people that was housed at BU has been maintained; however, with the retirement of its director in 1996, its future is questionable. This was the only program of the joint BU-Brandeis program that was maintained at the BU campus, but this is less a result of discontinued funding and more a conscious decision by the university.

## RAND/UCLA

According to Al Williams, the experience of the RAND/ UCLA Pew program represents the real test of whether or not the Pew programs can be maintained after funding ends. The RAND/UCLA programs were defunded after the second funding cycle for the reasons discussed earlier. Although the schools were unable to maintain the midcareer program without support for the fellows, the Pew doctoral program in health policy studies became part of the regular doctoral program at the RAND Graduate School. RAND continues to train health policy fellows by using a multidisciplinary approach and with new funding streams. Furthermore, the success of the RAND/UCLA program has spawned new

*The University of California at Berkeley may have been influenced somewhat by the Pew programs. Two former Pew fellows are teaching at UC-Berkeley and have carried over some of their graduate training experiences.*

health policy graduate training programs. Joe Newhouse, who was on the faculty at RAND, built upon the RAND Pew experience in his new PhD program at Harvard University. The University of Minnesota has also developed a stronger policy focus over time, and it may have been influenced by the Pew programs as well. Leighton Ku stated that the Johns Hopkins University's health policy program, a well-established program, has grown tremendously since the beginning of the Pew programs. Although he stated that he had no evidence that the Pew programs specifically influenced that growth, Ku speculated that some of the newer programs have likely been modeled on the Pew experiences. He also discussed the fact that the University of California at Berkeley may have been influenced somewhat by the Pew programs. Two former Pew fellows, James Robinson and Helen Schauffler, are teaching at UC-Berkeley and have carried over some of their graduate training experiences.

Al Williams stated, "Imitation is a form of endorsement," and Dan Rubin agrees. Rubin asserts that, as a result of the theory of innovation diffusion, the prestige of the schools involved with the Pew programs and their subsequent successes with the innovative, nontraditional approaches to health policy training may have encouraged other universities to emulate their programs.

# Part III.

*Determining the Legacy*

**T**he Pew Health Policy Program (PHPP) network is now 306 fellows strong, with representation in 35 states, the District of Columbia, Puerto Rico, and five foreign countries (Pew Fellows News, Winter 1996). Fellows and alumni are actively engaged in many dimensions of the historical changes taking place in the U.S. health care enterprise. If key roles at national meetings and significant representation in the peer-reviewed literature and major studies are reliable indicators, then Pew fellows, old and new, appear to be deeply involved in some of the leading analysis, demonstrations, and policy and political work that will help determine the landscape of tomorrow's health care system (Pew Fellows News, Winter 1996).

> Fellows and alumni are actively engaged in many dimensions of the historical changes taking place in the U.S. health care enterprise.

## Career Trajectories[5]

Richardson's 1990 evaluation of the PHPPs established that the majority of alumni were involved in health-oriented professions (Richardson, 1990). Most of the alumni entered the PHPPs with considerable experience in health care and health policy; therefore, their overwhelming representation in health-oriented fields is not surprising. Nevertheless, it is interesting to explore the specific subfields of health that alumni chose to work in following completion of their fellowships.

Richardson (1990) states that when the PHPP was being developed in the early 1980s, there were general perceptions of the nature of the positions that program graduates would seek. Some Advisory Committee members thought that many doctoral program graduates would seek faculty positions, whereas other committee members expected graduates to look for positions in the legislative setting, as policy analysts, or as general policy experts. Richardson

---

[5] *The data used in this section come from the directories of Pew fellows and alumni, the Richardson and Hamilton Evaluations, and other archival material. Fellows were not asked about career trajectories. All information is exptrapolated from the mentioned sources.*

(1990) reported on the distribution of program alumni by the nature of their positions, classified as policy analysts, general policy, faculty, and administrative. He found that the majority of alumni were in general policy positions. The general policy category used in his analysis was broad in scope, incorporating everything from hospital association vice president for governmental affairs to a senior policy analyst in the Health Care Financing Administration (HCFA) to a program officer at a foundation.

Richardson (1990) interviewed the alumni to determine what extent their professional positions included the health policy domain. He found their overall policy orientation to be very high. Richardson (1990) also asked to what degree PHPP influenced subsequent professional activity. He found that doctoral students from the Boston University(BU)/Brandeis University program and the University of California at Los Angeles (UCLA)/RAND program considered PHPP's influence to be greater than postdoctoral and midcareer alumni did, which stands to reason because the individuals in the latter two groups were already engaged in careers at the time of their graduate training.[6]

Of the 301 PHPP participants in 1996, 54 are postdoctoral alumni from the University of California at San Francisco (UCSF) program and 152 are doctoral alumni from all four program sites: the University of Michigan (46 participants), Brandeis (44 participants), BU (22 participants), RAND (18 participants), UCLA (15 participants), and UCSF (7 participants). Twenty-seven are policy career development fellowship alumni from RAND, 18 are midcareer fellowship alumni from UCSF, and 6 are management fellowship alumni from UCSF. The remaining 44 fellows are considered current fellows, meaning that they entered the programs between 1994 and 1996. Of the current fellows, 7 are doctoral fellows at Brandeis, 13 are postdoctoral fellows at UCSF, and 24 are doctoral fellows at the University of Michigan. As of 1996, 59 percent of all Pew participants are women.

[6] *Unlike Richardson (1990), all program alumni were not interviewed for this report. The information gathered came mostly from demographic databases and interviews with a few alumni. Our tables and charts are crude representations of career trends.*

## Professional Distribution

Figure 1 presents the professional distribution of PHPP alumni by program site as of 1996. Table 2 provides a breakdown of the career categories used to demonstrate the professional distribution of PHPP alumni. For four PHPP sites, the largest number of fellows graduate into academic positions. UCSF alumni have the largest representation in academia, with 46 percent of their alumni holding university-based positions. Thirty-seven percent of all BU/Brandeis alumni and 33 percent of all RAND/UCLA alumni enter academia upon completion of their programs. Although academic positions represent the largest percentage of all positions held by Michigan alumni (28 percent), positions in health care management represent a close second (26 percent of all Michigan alumni). Consultant positions account for the second largest group of BU/Brandeis fellows (13 percent of all current alumni), with the health care management sector and the private research sector representing the third largest groups (10 percent of all alumni each). Seventeen percent of UCSF alumni are in health care management, and another 17 percent are in government positions, representing the second and third largest groups of alumni, respectively. The second largest percentage of RAND/UCLA alumni (20 percent) are in private research positions, 16 percent are in health care management, and 12 percent are in government.

Pew alumni hold highly influential positions in strategic and highly visible areas of academia, consulting firms, health care management positions, all levels of government, private research organizations, professional associations, and various

**Figure 1.**

*Professional Distribution of PHPP Alumni by Site, 1996*

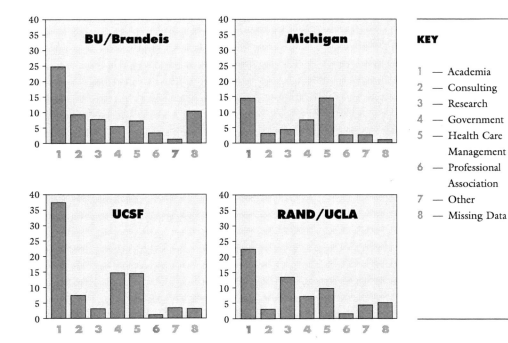

KEY

1 — Academia
2 — Consulting
3 — Research
4 — Government
5 — Health Care Management
6 — Professional Association
7 — Other
8 — Missing Data

other fields. Table 2 presents the actual number of alumni currently in each sector. As of 1996, 37 percent of all Pew alumni are employed in academic positions as faculty, researchers, and academic directors. Many of these positions are in health policy departments and institutes, although a specific teaching or research focus was not determined. The second largest sector as a whole to employ Pew alumni was health care management (17 percent). Fellows employed in this sector primarily manage hospitals, direct private health organizations, and manage clinical departments. Fourteen percent of all Pew alumni are employed in government positions. At the federal level, alumni hold positions in the Office of the Assistant Secretary for Health of the U.S. Department of Health and Human Services, the Agency for Health Care Policy and Research, and the National Institutes on Aging and Drug Abuse, to name a few. Alumni also hold positions in the U.S. General Accounting Office, the U.S. Public Health Service, and in the Medicare and Medicaid programs in the Health Care Financing Administration.

Ten percent of all Pew alumni are employed in the non-university-based private research sector as of 1996. Another 8 percent of alumni work as health policy consultants, some in private firms, others with public organizations, and several in private practice. Three percent of Pew alumni are employed by various professional associations including the National Women's Health Network, the Oregon Nurses Association, and prestigious foundations. Four percent of Pew alumni are working as health care providers and health lawyers, and a few are in non-health-related sectors. Current employment data are missing for 7 percent of Pew alumni.

It should be noted that although the tables and figures differentiate between professional positions, the categories are not always mutually exclusive. For example, there are cases in which university-based faculty are also involved in health policy making at the government level. Furthermore, the "other" category should not be considered less health policy related, because many alumni in law and other sectors could be directly involved in health policy analysis and development. At least two Pew alumni practice law in non-health policy-related firms but focus exclusively on health-related or health policy-related issues. Leighton Ku made some insightful comments regarding this issue that should be taken into account when reading the information in the tables and graphs. Ku is working at the Urban Institute and is involved in health policy and health services-related research. He explained that comparing his position to that

> Pew alumni hold highly influential positions in strategic and highly visible areas of academia, consulting firms, health care management positions, all levels of government, private research organizations, professional associations, and various other fields.

## Table 2.
### Breakdown of Career Categories, 1996

**Government (35)**
*Federal Offices*
Directors
Project Leaders
Health Policy Analysts
Examples:
U.S. General Accounting Office
U.S. Public Health Service
U.S. Congress
Health Care Financing Administration
Environmental Protection Agency
Agency for Health Care Policy and Research
National Academy of Sciences
National Institute on Aging
National Institute on Alcohol Abuse and Alcoholism

*International*
Director of Health
National Expert
Examples:
Aga Khan Health Services, France
European Commission, Luxembourg

*State: Departments of Health*
Health Commissioners/Directors
General Counsel
House Chairman
Examples:
Rate Setting Commission
Offices of Statewide Health Planning & Development
Departments of Health
State Medicaid Programs
Local and County Health Departments
Joint Committee on Health Care

**Academia (98)**
Faculty: Assistant, Associate, Full
Deans
Department Chairs
Research Associates (university-based)

**Consulting Services (22)**
Consultants
Examples:
Private Independent Contractor
On Lok Senior Health Services

The Lewin Group
The MEDSTAT Group
Interactive Technologies in Health Care
California Advocates for Nursing Home Reform

**Research (Non-university based (28)**
Research Associates/Scientists
Examples:
National Institute of Health Care Management
RAND
Latino Health Institute
Sarah Shuptrine and Associates
The Urban Institute
Multicultural AIDS Coalition
New England Research Institute

**Other (10)**
Occupational Health, *Industrial Hygienist*
Business (non-health)
Physicians & other providers (non-academic)
Lawyers

**Professional Associations (8)**
Directors/Chairs
Examples:
The Milton S. Eisenhower Foundation
National Women's Health Network
The Cleveland Foundation
Washington Health Association
Oregon Nurses Association
Carpenter's Health and Safety Fund
National PACE Association
Blue Cross Blue Shield of Michigan Foundation

**Health Care Management (45)**
Assistant Hospital Administrators
Hospital Administrators/Directors
Chief Executive Officers
Clinical Directors
Hospital Presidents/Vice Presidents

*NOTES: Examples of categorical titles are derived from the directories of Pew fellows and alumni (see Appendix D for examples of exact titles). Alumni from classes entering 1983–1993 are included. Insufficient data were available for 18 alumni. Number in parentheses are numbers of alumni.*

of someone working in government might lead to the conclusion that he has less influence over policy; however, this would be incorrect. Among Pew fellows, Ku had a unique perspective on how to have an influence while working outside government:

> [W]hen you're in government . . . you're always sort of fitting in and just trying to keep up with a broader administrative agenda for the administration and/or for Congress. You can shape things, but you're shaping things within that context. If you're on the outside doing policy research, then you can try to shape the agenda somewhat. Whereas when you're working in government, the way the government is set up, it's very hierarchical. Basically speaking, most government people work in relative anonymity and information goes up the administrative hierarchy and then occasionally goes across into other policy circles, whereas if you're on the outside at a place like the Urban Institute you can deal on lots of levels with policy makers in government, in the executive branch, in Congress, at state levels, and with some other associations.

## Movement Between Professional Fields

Table 3 depicts the movement of all fellows between professional fields before and after their participation in PHPP. This matrix allows the reader to determine the percentage of fellows who were in a particular field before the Pew program and then the percentage who changed fields after completing the program. The shaded diagonal represents the percentage of fellows who are employed in the same field in which they were employed before starting PHPP. The career categories used in this matrix are the same as those listed in Table 2. It is noteworthy that 70 percent of all fellows who entered the Pew programs from academic positions remained in academia after completing the program. On the other hand, only 20 percent of all fellows who were employed in the private research sector before entering the program remained in that field. Sixty percent of these fellows entered either government or academia upon completion of the program (30 percent each). Thirty percent of all fellows who were in government positions prior to entering the Pew program remained in that sector. However, as with all categories, this does not imply that they remained in the same position. Appendix D provides some examples of career trajectories and title changes. It should be noted that the titles presented in Appendix D and those used to determine categorization are the fellows' titles immediately before they entered the program (retrieved from the directory published during the year that the fellow entered the program)

# Table 3.

## Professional Distribution of PH/PP Alumni at the Start and End of Program, in percent

| | Distribution at Start of Program | Academia | Consulting | Research | Government | Health Care Management | Professional Associations | Other | Missing Data |
|---|---|---|---|---|---|---|---|---|---|
| Academia | 28 | 70 | 5 | 9 | 5 | 7 | 1 | 0 | 3 |
| Consulting | 5 | 34 | 25 | 25 | 0 | 0 | 8 | 8 | 0 |
| Research | 4 | 30 | 0 | 20 | 30 | 20 | 0 | 0 | 0 |
| Government | 21 | 22 | 7 | 18 | 30 | 11 | 2 | 2 | 8 |
| Health Care Management | 20 | 15 | 15 | 9 | 11 | 38 | 2 | 2 | 8 |
| Professional Associatons | 2 | 17 | 0 | 0 | 17 | 0 | 50 | 0 | 17 |
| Other | 12 | 34 | 6 | 3 | 9 | 19 | 3 | 22 | 3 |
| Missing Data | 9 | 35 | 4 | 0 | 8 | 19 | 4 | 0 | 30 |
| Distribution at End of Program | | 37 | 8 | 10 | 14 | 17 | 3 | 4 | 7 |

NOTES: The shaded diagonal depicts the percentage of fellows who stayed in the same field following their participation in PHPP. The "other" category is defined in the text. All data come from the directories of Pew fellows and alumni.

and then the most recent title listed in the 1996 directory. All positions held between these two points in time are not included in this simple analysis. Nonetheless, it is interesting to see the broad changes in the titles of the fellows before and after participating in the Pew program.

Table 3 does not present title changes by program site; however, a brief discussion of some of the most interesting career trajectories specific to the various programs may be of interest. One of the biggest changes can be found among the Michigan Pew fellows. Before entering the program only 8 percent of all Michigan fellows were employed in academic positions. After completing the program, however, 28 percent of all alumni entered academia. The other large change found among Michigan fellows is in the opposite direction, with 32 percent starting out in government but only 16 percent employed in that sector as of 1996. Several other large changes in career occurred among the BU/Brandeis alumni. Before entering the program, only 21 percent of all fellows were in academia, but after completing the program this number jumped to 37 percent. BU/Brandeis fellows also experienced a 10 percent increase in alumni working in the private research field (0 to 10 percent). Interestingly, before entering the program, 28 percent of all BU/Brandeis fellows were employed in the government sector. After completing the program, however, only 7 percent remained in that sector. A second shift experienced by the BU/Brandeis fellows is in the field of health care management. Twenty-five percent of all fellows were employed in health care management positions before entering BU/Brandeis, but only 10 percent are currently employed in that field.

Fellows in the UCSF and RAND/UCLA programs experienced the fewest career shifts between the time of entry and completion of the Pew program. For the UCSF program this makes the most sense because its largest program was a postdoctoral fellowship, and it can be assumed that most fellows come in from academia and graduate back into academia at higher levels. This is in fact the case, with 41 percent of UCSF fellows starting off in academia and 46 percent of alumni currently employed in academic positions. For the RAND/UCLA fellows there was no change in the percentage of fellows who began the program in academic positions and the percentage of those currently in academia: 33 percent at both the start and finish. There was a large jump, however, in the number of RAND/UCLA fellows who are currently in the private research field (20 percent) as opposed to the percentage of fellows originally employed in that sector (9 percent). Again, it should be noted that these percentages are not based on matched groups. The 33 percent of RAND/UCLA fellows who were employed in academia prior to beginning PHPP may be a set of people completely different from the 33 percent currently employed in academic positions. For a sample of match career trajectories, see Appendix D.

## IMPORTANCE OF DOCTORAL PROGRAM COMPLETION
### Doctoral Completion Rates

Table 4 depicts the doctoral degree completion rate for all programs as of 1996. BU/Brandeis and Brandeis alone (after 1991) offered a doctoral program every year that they received Pew funding. The last year that Brandeis granted Pew fellowships was 1995. BU's average completion rate as of 1996 was 59 percent; for Brandeis it was 70 percent (81

**Table 4.**

*Proportion of Pew Doctoral Fellows Who Completed Degree, by Program Site, 1996, in percent*

| Entry Year | Boston University | Bradeis University | University of Michigan | RAND Graduate School | UCLA | UCSF |
|---|---|---|---|---|---|---|
| 1983 | 66.6 (2/3) | 100 (3/3) | | 66.6 (2/3) | 100 (3/3) | 100 (2/2) |
| 1984 | 100 (3/3) | 66 (2/3) | 55.5 (5/9) | 100 (2/2) | 100 (1/1) | |
| 1985 | 66.6 (2/3) | 100 (3/3) | | 100 (3/3) | 50 (1/2) | 50 (2/4) |
| 1986 | 66.6 (2/3) | 75 (3/4) | 55.5 (5/9) | 50 (1/2) | 75 (3/4) | |
| 1987 | 66.6 (2/3) | 66.6 (2/3) | | 100 (3/3) | 100 (2/2) | |
| 1988 | 50 (2/4) | 66.6 (2/3) | 67 (8/12) | 100 (1/1) | 100 (2/2) | 100 (1/1) |
| 1989 | 0 (0/2) | 100 (3/3) | | 100 (4/4) | 0 (0/1) | |
| 1990 | 0 (0/1) | 50 (1/2) | 25 (2/8) | | | |
| 1991 | | 100 (6/6) | | | | |
| 1992 | | 25 (2/8) | 38 (3/8) | | | |
| AVG. | 59 (13/22) | 71 (27/38) | 50 (23/46) | 89 (16/18) | 80 (12/15) | 71 (5/7) |

SOURCE: Data are from the 1996 Directory of Fellows and Alumni.
NOTE: Fellows entering between 1993 and 1995 are not included.

percent if the entering class of 1992 is excluded). The University of Michigan offers doctoral programs every other year that it receives Pew funding, with the 1997 year being the last. Their average completion rate as of 1996 was 50 percent. UCLA and RAND offered doctoral programs up to the completion of the second funding cycle. Their completion rates as of 1996 were 80 percent and 89 percent respectively. UCSF phased out its doctoral program early on; however, it offered doctoral training to seven fellows, and its completion rate was 71 percent. The doctoral completion rate for the entire PHPP as of 1996 was 66 percent (97 of 148 fellows in the classes of 1983 to 1992). This overall completion rate compares quite favorably to national completion rates. According to Bowen and Rudenstein (1992), about 50 percent of all students entering PhD programs eventually obtain doctorates, many after pursuing their degrees for anywhere from 6 to 12 years. The completion rates for fellows in PHPP as a whole and the individual PHPPs have therefore exceeded the national average.

Raskin and colleagues (1992) state that although most of the Pew students at BU/Brandeis completed their course work and qualifying examinations within the first year and a half, few fellows actually completed their dissertations within the projected 2-year period. Of 60 doctoral fellows admitted from 1983 to 1992, only 4 actually completed the doctorate within the 2-year time frame. As of 1996, the average time for completion of the program at Brandeis, including the dissertation, was 3.8 years. For BU the average time to achieve the doctoral degree was 3.7 years, for RAND the average was 4.7 years, and for UCLA the average was 5.2 years. Perhaps the most impressive time to completion was for Michigan fellows, who work full-time while in school full-time, which was an average of 5.2 years.

## Effect of Program Noncompletion

The completion rates for fellows in PHPP as a whole and the individual PHPPs exceeded the national average.

The faculty who were interviewed were confident that the fellows who did not finish their doctoral degrees were still better prepared to face the challenges of today's health policy world because of their experience with PHPP. All of the fellows who had not completed their doctorates were engaged in important work. Nonetheless, all of the interviewed fellows who had not yet completed their degrees said that they fully intended to finish (and several did between the time of the interview and the completion of this report). Interestingly, many of the fellows who had not finished were in positions that they intended to stay in, even after they received their PhD or DrPH. This implies that for many fellows the completion of the doctorate was motivated by personal needs and not because it would change their status or rank.

Dan Rubin believes that he is better at what he does today because of his Pew doctoral training at Michigan. Even though he has not yet completed his degree, he is in an influential, professional position where he uses his interdisciplinary policy analysis skills every day. His job is to connect pieces of government roles that relate to health care quality and information use. Rubin's professional activities require him to use his judgment about what needs to be related to what and how this can be done in an efficient and politically acceptable way, rather than about how to assemble a research plan for a study; yet, he has every intention of completing his dissertation and thus his DrPH. Why?

> [T]he intellectual closure of doing extended work. One of my personal reasons to do the program was for me to see what it really took for me to do extended work. The bread and butter of government work is not extended, analytic ventures. Sometimes there is extended writing and certainly extended thinking about a topic. But, the kind of effort involved in writing a dissertation is very important for me to learn, and for me to learn about myself.

In thinking about the value of a program like this for people who choose not to complete the dissertation, Rubin stated that if what was learned was a new interdisciplinary perspective, it would be of very high value. For someone like himself who had master's training in policy analysis that was interdisciplinary in nature, stopping the doctoral program after classes would still enrich his knowledge base, but in a very expensive and inefficient way for the Pew Charitable Trusts.

## Other Comments About Doctoral Program Completion

Keeping in line with Dan Rubin's comment about the Trusts, other faculty and fellows spoke about the importance of finishing their degree not only for themselves but also because that was the "contract" that they had made with the Pew Charitable Trusts. Jonathan Howland stated that the foundation was paying the tuition for the fellows and granting them a stipend *in exchange for something*. Thus, not completing the degree was in essence not taking that "deal" seriously. He laments the fact that some fellows do not see the issue from

Fellows spoke about the importance of finishing their degree not only for themselves but also because that was the "contract" that they had made with the Pew Charitable Trusts.

the perspective of a program that invested in them to do something rather than from a purely personal point of view.

Pamela Paul-Shaheen started her doctoral program in 1984 and completed her degree June of 1995. She explained that there were two reasons why she kept at it:

> *First of all, because if I start something, unless there are things in life that I cannot change, I will finish. Also, because people made a commitment to funding my education. Had I not finished I would have reneged on a commitment I made.*

Patricia Butler explained that at Michigan, the goal of the program was to train the fellows to be policy analysts rather than health services researchers. Therefore, she acknowledges the fact that in her subsequent professional activities she will probably never again conduct research quite at the level of the dissertation. However, she believes that it is extremely important for policy analysts to be able to understand the process of collecting original data, how to work with secondary databases, and how to use the data:

> *Because of my age and because of my existing experience, I don't happen to think the degree is that important. But I do plan to get it because I've come this far and because I feel that it is an indication of successfully completing something. The dissertation is a wholly different experience making me understand just how laborious the research experience is. . . . Prior to this I had no true appreciation of what it was like to start from an idea and think about data sources and take it all the way. Understanding of the research process is very valuable to me. (Patricia Butler graduated in May 1996).*

Steve Crane underscored Butler's point about PHPP goals not being to have the fellows go on and get a tenured track position per se but, rather, to be capable of effecting great change. When asked whether this meant that in fact the PhD degree was an inappropriate degree for this type of programs, Crane said:

> *Ah, that's the big question. We ran into a lot of problems because it was a traditional PhD as opposed to a DrPH, as opposed to a super master's degree. What was important about the level of education that we were talking about were a couple of things: (1) emphasis on research methods and being not only a consumer of research, which you become with a master's degree, but a producer of research, which is signified by a PhD. People needed to have that knowledge whether or not they needed the degree for their careers. . . . From a marketing point of view, the PhD was really important. I think Michigan folks will feel a little badly about the DrPH because it's considered to be a professional degree, which in the end is probably a more appropriate degree for this program. So on balance I think the PhD has real*

*value, signifying both the level at which you're working and your capability for independent research.*

Nonetheless, Crane commented that whether the fellows finished the degree or not, the Pew program accepted them as an "equal part of the club." He explained that the programs do not discriminate on the basis of whether someone completed the degree, although completion is certainly celebrated. He attributes this acceptance to the fact that Pew's "focus was more on what you're going to do, not on who you're going to be."

Marion Ein Lewin reiterated Steve Crane's final comment about Pew's philosophy on fellows who have not completed their degree. She stated that those fellows that went through the whole 2 years or so of course work and then did not get the degree are still considered Pew fellows in discussions and are included in the Directory. She believes for the most part that there really is no distinction between the completers and nocompleters, even though the purpose of the program is clearly for people to get their degrees:

> *My feeling is that programs like these have a halo effect. Even if you didn't finish, you participated at least for a time in a very exciting learning activity, you met the people, you got a lot of value even if you didn't get the degree. If you look through the list [of fellows] in an analytic way, there are a lot of people who haven't gotten their degrees who are playing very important roles. We accept them in the "family."*

Some fellows and faculty, however, believe that the fellows who do not complete the dissertation miss out on the real or whole value of the program. According to Linda Simoni-Wastila, the course work was the easy part and merely forms the foundation for the dissertation process. She stated that it's not the courses or the comprehensive exams that pull all the knowledge together; rather, it's the dissertation. Stan Wallack agrees that it's the dissertation that really forces the fellows to take a problem and analyze it completely.

Still, there are others, like Dennis Beatrice, who did not finish the program but who feel that they gained a better understanding of how to use analysis and graduate education training in nonacademic settings. Dennis Beatrice stated that "there is great utility in Pew training," regardless of whether a fellow completed the program.

**It is extremely important for policy analysts to be able to understand the process of collecting original data, how to work with secondary databases, and how to use the data.**

## UNCOVERING THE PHPP LEGACY

At the Pew Health Policy Program Advisory Board Meeting in January 1992, participants raised the topics of program institutionalization and legacy. Grantees were informed that they should all be exploring and negotiating for heightened institutional support for the future. Participants at the meeting discussed the fact that even if the current programs were not able to attract sufficient external funds to continue their full operation, they should be able to show that the program has enabled the development of an advanced health policy curriculum and that it has influenced the outlook and teaching of program faculty. The program should be able to show that it has provided students with a much needed source of funding that enabled them to concentrate their dissertations on health policy rather than health services research (for which funding is available by more classically oriented federal funding agencies). The programs should be able to show that their fellows have had substantial interaction with policy makers through the meetings for new fellows in Washington, D.C., and other efforts at the funded sites. The programs should be able to show that the annual meetings have facilitated an important network and critical mass for interacting and discussing key issues. Another indicator that the program had an impact would be to show that the program influenced universities to value health policy research and to develop a high-level mentoring network. Program enhancement activities that build on the activities of professional associations such as the Association for Health Services Research (AHSR) foster the legitimacy of policy research by providing a forum for presentations and journal publications.

Therefore, what can be said about the success of the programs? Many of the challenges stated above were indeed met by the program sites, as indicated throughout this report. Many of the programs far exceeded the initial goals by instituting the curriculum and the training philosophy and by applying for and getting new funds, such as Agency for Health Care Policy and Research (AHCPR) training grants, to maintain their programs. What can be said, however, about the actual impact that the Pew program has had on the field, on the educational landscape, and on the fellows? Interestingly, all faculty and alumni interviewed were initially skeptical about making statements about the Pew legacy. Most were unsure about whether Pew's legacy could be defined or measured. Many felt that it was too early to determine what the program's legacy is and that this review should be conducted again in 10 years. However, after stating their hesitancy at making causal assumptions, all interviewees offered suggestions about how one could measure the value added by a program like PHPP, and many gave examples of how PHPP has affected the health policy field and education and even provided ideas about what they thought best represented the Pew legacy.

Hal Luft, Stan Wallack, Stuart Altman, and Al Williams commented that measuring success for programs like these is difficult. One way they suggested that success, and thus the value added to the field, could be measured would be to look at where the alumni are, look at what they are doing, and determine if they are doing the things that the program wanted them to be doing. Hal Luft stated that most alumni are doing things related to health policy in various kinds of settings. He believes that many of these people would not be doing this type of work if they had not gone through the Pew program. According to Dr. Luft, that is the "best implicit measure of success."

Leon Wyszewianski stated that looking at alumni representation in the literature is one way to measure contributions to the field; however, Steve Crane is concerned that this would miss other aspects of the influence of the fellows. He stated that it's not the degree or the peer-reviewed publication that measures success; rather, it's the softer measure of what's being contributed to the field and the extent that the alumni are in demand in the system. Leon Wyszewianski does not disagree with this and recommended that another way to measure value added to the field would be to see if alumni changed direction from non-health-related policy work to health policy-related work and to determine if what they do currently differs from what they did before their Pew experience (see Table 3 and earlier discussion).

**Many of these people would not be doing this type of work if they had not gone through the Pew program. That is the best implicit measure of success.**

## Informants' Reflections on the Meaning of Legacy

To understand the meaning of "legacy" the interviewees were asked to frame their experiences in terms of the legacy. Steve Crane said:

> *The Pew legacy is really trite but true, and you've heard it before, the people who were trained. Even though we took in more mature students, some of whom are now in their 50s, they're still a huge crop of people coming along who are going to make a huge difference. I'm not sure that we've seen yet the contributions to health policy that the Pew students are going to make. It takes awhile. But as these folks come up and go through leadership positions, I think we'll see more and more. That emphasizes the importance of trying to keep this group together as well as having them interact with some of the other program fellowship people who are around (e.g., the Johnson program and the Kellogg pro-*

*gram). All these people are unique, they are leaders and they are going to make a contribution. The group effort is only going to enhance their already evolving skills.*

Almost every person interviewed stated that it was indeed the fellows themselves that best represented Pew's legacy to the health policy field and to health policy education. Leighton Ku articulated a commonly held view of the legacy as "nothing brassy and shiny"; rather, it's "the people." Many agreed.

### Legacy as Bridging Theory and Practice

In an effort to tease out exactly how the alumni translate into value added for the field, it was necessary to think about what was happening in the field prior to the Pew programs. Bill Weissert commented on the fact that the true legacy was in the trainees' accomplishments and in the higher level to which they are bringing the health policy debate:

> *There is an awful lot about the policy process that is still happen-stance and convenience regarding who is around. You can only improve the chances that rationality will play a part in policy by having a lot of people around who are trained rationally. So, the more people you put out there, the better chance you have to for-mally or informally influence the policy process. We train a lot of people who are interlopers or daily workers in the policy process; therefore, we increase the chances that what comes out the other end will be better informed than it would have been if people had been shooting from the hip. Yet, its awful hard to quantify.*

Furthermore, Bill Weissert believes that the Pew program made a lot more people aware of the power of the literature to answer a lot of questions in a systematic way rather than guess-ing as they were doing before. Hal Luft believes that the Pew program has influenced health policy in several subtle ways:

> *It is hard to identify specific policies that have changed one way or the other as a result of the Pew program, per se. I'm not clever enough to picture an alternative universe in which there wasn't a Pew program and what would have been different. But I do have the sense that some of the fellows have been doing very excit-ing things that are having impacts on the way the health care system and health policy is being done and how health care sys-tems are changing with health services research, etc., that prob-ably would not have happened had those people not gone through the Pew program.*

### Legacy in Terms of Scale and Scope

Several people interviewed mentioned the "scale effects" of the Pew program's legacy. John Griffith stated that the community is so big and diverse that it is difficult to speculate about the value added by training a small cohort of people. He stated, "the community is many times bigger than the output stream." Nevertheless, says Griffith, in the 15 years since the program started, there has been a noticeable increase in the willingness to use empirical data as a basis for conclusion. He also indicated that even though the cohort may be much smaller than the community to which it is attempting to infiltrate, it must be remembered that health policy is a context in which a critical few in strategic locations can make a big difference.

Stuart Altman appreciates the difficulty in quantifying the actual impact that the Pew program has had on the health policy field; however, he does believe that the program was successful:

> *I think [the Pew programs] demonstrated that these programs are important, that they can produce value added. I know the most difficult aspects of evaluating a program, Pew or any other program, is determining what is the "value added." What is the value added to the individual and what is the value added to the system. Now, it's a little presumptuous of us to think or attribute to any one program, even one that has trained a couple of hundred people, what impact it has had on a one-trillion-dollar industry that affects every American, that employs one out of seven people; let's face it, we are dealing with a gigantic industry. We have to evaluate its impact on the margin. [However] Pew clearly did demonstrate the importance of interdisciplinary research.*

Joan DaVanzo acknowledges that the policies that the Pew fellows are ultimately aiming to change or influence in some way are far-reaching and that the health care field is indeed very large. However, the circle of actual policy makers and policy researchers is much smaller, and it is this sector of the health care field the Pew alumni can affect:

> *Pew brought a broader range of individuals to the field, so [the legacy] is a thing about people. The Pew model, and I don't know [how] much of the curriculum at the schools was the same, but it seemed to me that . . . we all had a fairly similar analytic strategy, if you will, across the set of programs. . . . I don't know the influence of having this bulk of people that have that same view of the world dropped onto the health policy arena. I would think that it shapes the construct, enriches it, and gives it more depth. On one hand it's a grandiose statement to make; on the other hand it's really not. If you think about the economics of the health policy field, it's really a small field, and if you get that many people, what about 200 or so, with the same combination of skills, yet with varied backgrounds and expertise, the scene is hit from many different levels.*

**Even though the Pew cohort may be much smaller than the community to which it is attempting to infiltrate, it must be remembered that health policy is a context in which a critical few in strategic locations can make a big difference.**

### Legacy as Information Processing and Dissemination

If the term *legacy* can be defined as "accomplishments," then Kate Korman believes that the most important contribution of PHPP may be its success at seeding the health policy field with fresh, talented change agents able to communicate effectively with all players in the health care system:

> *The most important contributions may be the richness of the health policy community today, which boasts 250 additional minds responsible for health policy decision making in a wide variety of venues: local, state, and national government, private foundations and institutions, and universities and research institutes. The ripple effect of this knowledge and expertise is found in the lives and future endeavors of those whom past fellows influence. Whether it be a change in policy at the local level or the influence of a teacher for a student to pursue a change in career in health policy, the ramifications are far reaching.*

Marion Ein Lewin agrees that PHPP has enriched the field of health policy research in a remarkable and significant way, both in the quality and in the level of people that it was able to attract:

> *This program came along at a time when health policy research was becoming increasingly recognized as an important discipline and health care programs and budgets were becoming a significant aspect of public, federal, state, community, and private-sector budgets. Until the Pew Health Policy Program came along there were not many people who were good at both policy and who had the analytic skills to really understand what these dynamics were all about; how to develop a changed agenda. My feeling is that this program really enriched the field. To the degree that it was multidisciplinary and to the degree that there were individual programs, that was also a very significant and valuable accomplishment.*

Marion Ein Lewin explained that all the fellows in all the programs were trained in statistics and analytic skills and were given a knowledge base in policy research, but as discussed earlier, all brought different expertise to bear on an issue. What resulted, says Lewin, were complementary programs that had the magnitude and depth to enrich the field and inform the debate. Furthermore, says Lewin, when you look through the literature at how the fellows are represented and when you look at what areas and activities the fellows have participated in, you see a reflection of the world of health policy and health care reform in the last dozen years.

### Legacy as Professionalization of Health Policy

Many others agreed that the Pew program was instrumental in raising the awareness of health policy as an important area

**What resulted were complementary programs that had the magnitude and depth to enrich the field and inform the debate.**

for advanced graduate training. Al Williams commented on how he views Pew's impact on the field:

> *I think as a whole the Pew fellows have gone toward policy in a more focused way than people in the past. [Pew] emphasized policy. The emphasis was different across the set of programs, but the policy side was more focused than I think is common. When Paul Ginsburg was running PPRC [the Physician Payment Review Commission], he hired several of our graduates and specifically noted that he preferred our graduates because while he needed people with strong analytic skills, he also needed people who had a background in the health care system and health policy. We created that mix of skills that set our fellows apart.*

Kate Korman explained that fellows have faculty positions in universities throughout the country and are in the process of passing on to new health policy analysts the gems of their training. Pew-trained faculty are replicating PHPP at new sites, thus the true definition of "seeding the field." Carroll Estes agrees:

> *I think the Pew program has very successfully seeded the field with competent well-trained scholars at government levels, nonprofit and foundation levels, and university levels. The flowering and capability of those fellows and their contribution are beginning to be recognized at fairly significant levels. . . . The most important contribution of the fellows is a passionate commitment to health policy and health services research that is objective and has an impact and the ability to carry out that work either directly themselves or to stimulate organizations and institutions to do it where they are.*

Leighton Ku has also observed changes in the health policy program scene and attributes that partly to the accomplishments of PHPP. He states that there are many more health policy programs than there were prior to the initiation of PHPP. He believes that the Pew program helped to take academic health policy out of the traditional areas with which it has been predominately associated: hospital administration and economics. Ed Hamilton also discussed Pew's legacy for the health policy field in his 1995 evaluation:

> *[T]he Pew Charitable Trusts-funded effort was one of the early and influential stimulants to what became, over time, a sizable expansion of rigorous health policy training during the past dozen years. This has, in turn, elevated the technical debate about health policy options and implementation to a markedly more sophisticated level. . . . [T]he PCT was ahead of most other major private funders in perceiving the importance of cross-disciplinary training in this area, and its 245 trainees, while not a substantial fraction of all individuals employed by public and nonprofit entities in positions like the ones they occupy, seem like-*

The Pew program helped to take academic health policy out of the traditional areas with which it has been predominately associated: hospital administration and economics.

*ly to make up a non trivial element of the vanguard of such people who have emerged as the health policy debate has gathered strength.*

### Legacy as Offering New Conceptual Models

Kathleen Eyre explained how she believed the legacy for the midcareer programs differed slightly from that for the other programs, in that it introduced a paradigm, or a new way of thinking, for existing professionals:

*We all came out of professional positions . . . came in with our own professional set of skills and analytic tools and what we were introduced to for the first time was a rigorous policy analysis paradigm and way of thinking, the kinds of questions to ask, the different disciplines that influence policy, and we, in our brief year, were exposed to all kinds of different academic settings and disciplines.*

**This is a high-quality way to approach policy, and it does not mean that policy is not carried out in a political context.**

Terry Hammons expanded on this, discussing how at RAND the principle accomplishment was to have pulled a number of experienced people into an environment where they were able to become valuable contributors to health care policy in both the private sector and the public sector. What made this accomplishment so valuable for the field, explains Hammons, is that the fellows were trained to do this in a way that grounded policy making in research. He believes that this is a high-quality way to approach policy, and it does not mean that policy is not carried out in a political context.

### Legacy as the Future Impact

According to Pamela Paul-Shaheen, the legacy diffuses "through the individuals who were involved"; however, she provided a reminder that the most important contributions to policy may not yet be noticeable. Paul-Shaheen stated that the "proof" will be even more noticeable in the next 20 years as the fellows mature into the elite policy positions. The fellows need time to move through the system. Nonetheless, she believes that some of Pew's effect can already be seen:

*In the aggregate, in terms of the totality of the program, the jury is still out. But clearly the program has put a number of people into key policy positions. You can see the success of the program as you look across a spectrum of alumni and the roles that they are playing across the nation, regardless of whether they completed the program totally or not, many have moved into reasonably influential positions.*

## The Legacy in Summary

Steve Crane summed up what he thought represented all the legacies that are attributable to the Pew program: (1) the quick PhD was pioneered by the Pew programs, and as many problems as successes were found; (2) the focus on change; (3) the multidisciplinary and multisectoral approach; (4) the importance of discussion; and (5) the ability to take the mature learner into the system and have him or her succeed.

In a recent article written for the anniversary of the Institute of Medicine (1996), Stuart Altman described PHPP as a program that "tackles what some believe is the great divide between health economists and other disciplines, bringing the synergy of an interdisciplinary approach to problem-solving." He believes that the Pew program offers a truly unique opportunity for advanced interdisciplinary training in each of the four sites. Integrating fellows from various disciplines, including economics, political science, sociology, law, medicine, and other health-related professions, "fosters a cross-fertilization of different theoretical perspectives, as well as different methodological approaches in solving concrete policy problems." Altman provides an example:

> [T]he deeper appreciation of the dynamics of competing political interests and how these interests are played out in the policy process offers a useful complement to an understanding of the economic implications of a specific financing strategy proposed for Medicare. In the same way that the RWJ [Robert Wood Johnson Foundation] program provides an environment of understanding between hands-on managers and clinicians and those familiar with the policy process, so too the Pew fellowships offer a creative linkage between the old vanguard of health policy analysts and those with a more interdisciplinary approach.

Altman acknowledges the tension between depth and breadth in a program such as PHPP, incorporating an interdisciplinary approach. He recognizes that one might argue that doctoral-level training should be grounded in one particular discipline. However, Altman states that as a result of the Pew training approach, the fellows are "better trained to bridge the gap between policy research and policy making." The value of interdisciplinary training has been underscored by the fellows themselves throughout this report.

In his 1990 Report to the Pew Charitable Trusts, Bill Richardson discusses the degree to which the various PHPPs complement each other. He states that although each institution provided a unique setting and structure, each served a common set of interests and goals. Hal Luft agrees:

As a result of the Pew training approach, the fellows are better trained to bridge the gap between policy research and policy making.

*Among the main things [that Pew accomplished] is that we've developed an integrated program across three or four sites that involve a wide range of people from fresh graduate students to fairly senior career people. We have placed those people into various settings ranging from the university to major health policy kinds of settings. The fellows are doing a great job. We have also established three programs that are likely to survive past Pew.*

Clearly, a major goal of PHPP was to create a critical mass of highly trained health policy professionals. It is commonly agreed that this goal has been achieved. Carroll Estes attests to the success of the Pew programs:

*I think the Pew program has very successfully seeded the field with competent well-trained scholars at government levels, non-profit and foundation levels, and university levels. The flowering and capability of those fellows and their contributions are beginning to be recognized at fairly significant levels.*

**Clearly, a major goal of PHPP was to create a critical mass of highly trained health policy professionals. It is commonly agreed that this goal has been achieved.**

Another major goal of PHPP was to establish innovative training models that would one day stand on their own. In some cases this goal has been achieved in its entirety; in other cases it has been achieved only partially. However, a recurring theme found in all the interviews and evaluations is that the Pew program did make a difference. The Pew program has changed each institution in some way. Many aspects of the Pew program have been institutionalized, and the Pew program's ideas are standing and will continue to stand.

Linda Simoni-Wastila used a research analogy of start-up funds to describe what she believes is part of Pew's legacy in health policy:

*What Pew had also done was to make sure that programs like the Brandeis program and UCLA and UCSF have the programs even without funding. They all have a real strong interest in continuing programs like this through other funding sources, like AHCPR. They all continue to build this health policy arena, broadly speaking. Pew really enabled a few programs to develop educational programs in health policy and gave people fantastic skills. And now they are ongoing. It was like seed money. It's really important. . . . Health policy keeps on growing. Pew fostered that, and that's the legacy.*

Simoni-Wastila also pointed out that although it's true that Pew succeeded in seeding the field with health policy professionals, they are not all the same type of professional. Clarifying this distinction magnifies Pew's potential impact in the health policy arena. She cited that although the Pew program has put many fellows in high-profile positions where they are able to make real contributions to the field, it has also placed with equal emphasis many background people who do the actual research. These people build the foundation of knowledge. Pew's legacy is thus multifaceted.

One of the remarkable things that came out of the interviews was the consistency with which the faculty and fellows discussed the various issues. There was a clear consensus among those interviewed that PHPP was not only a success but is also a valuable asset to the health policy community and research.

Although there are many who worry that the programs were defunded too early, the 15-year commitment on the part of the Pew Charitable Trusts has enabled the development of the infrastructure, the institutional memory, and the invaluable training of potential mentors. As Marion Ein Lewin stated, "right now the right things are in place."

## ANSWERING FUTURE NEEDS AND OFFERING ADVICE

Because of the intensification of health care reform issues, health policy research is playing an increasingly vital role in generating the knowledge necessary to assist health policy makers in making informed policy decisions. There will be a continuing need to expand the supply of trained researchers schooled in health policy. Several of the schools have targeted experienced health professionals to achieve this goal. Many are also redefining the doctoral degree to make it more applicable to the current health care world. Dennis Beatrice stated that the job of training this new breed of PhDs, multidisciplinary health policy professionals, is not yet done:

> *PhDs need to change because the environment needs more academic types in government. Government people can no longer shoot from the hip. The stakes are too high. We need to bring those two worlds together. We need to continue to educate, train, and out put a "different" kind of student.*

In the case of postdoctoral training, both Hal Luft and Carroll Estes agree that the job is not done. They stated that there is still an environmental need for advanced training in health policy. Hal Luft reflects on the evolution of the program at UCSF and the changing environment:

> *When our program started there were very few integrated postdoctoral fellowship programs. I think now there are more of them, some funded by AHCPR, the RWJ Clinical Scholars, the new Johnson Policy Scholars, etc. So there are definitely more opportunities and programs for postdoctoral fellows. On the other hand I think the need for training and the demand for well-trained people has been increasing even more rapidly. I still*

The 15-year commitment on the part of the Pew Charitable Trusts has enabled the development of the infrastructure, the institutional memory, and the invaluable training of potential mentors.

We have gone from a fragmented delivery system to a system integrated horizontally and vertically. Policy makers need to better understand how their actions affect these changes, and the organization community needs to learn more about how its members affect policy and how policy affects them.

*don't see a lot of programs that are really focused on integrating people from multiple disciplines. For instance, the Johnson Policy Scholars are for economists, political scientists, and sociologists; the AHCPR program, while broader, tends to have very few people at any one site and is often more predoctorally focused. And, there is not much integration across sites, so that they don't get enough blending. Bottom line: there is still a real need. I don't think the job is done.*

In terms of the important issues plaguing the heath policy world before 1983 and the pertinent issues of today, Carroll Estes doesn't think much has changed:

*We were very concerned about access, cost, and quality when we started, and we are still concerned about access, cost, and quality.*

Stan Wallack thinks the need does continue to exist; however, many of the hot issues have changed to some degree. He explained that in the 1980s the issues at hand were the rapid growth of the private sector and the beginning of the emergence of managed care. This environment is no longer in its early stage. Today, the hot topics are the future of organizations and organizational change, who will survive and who will not. How will vulnerable populations fare in the new era of cost-conscious care? Wallack stated that we've gone from a fragmented delivery system to a system integrated horizontally and vertically. Policy makers need to better understand how their actions affect these changes, and the organization community needs to learn more about how its members affect policy and how policy affects them. Stan Wallack stated that the "link between policy and organization is really key" in today's world and starting a program like PHPP today would need to reflect these changes. He stated that the way that PHPP was structured was appropriate for the time:

*Most traditional PhD programs are teaching methods and theory. . . . Health is a problem area. Health policy programs are different in the sense that they focus on the problems trying to find solutions. It's a different niche. Pew did do something different in developing people who were in that niche in the 1980s focusing on problems and their solutions. It was really appropriate for the time.*

Stuart Altman agreed that there is still a need in the health policy arena for individuals who have a broad sense of what the issues are and who do not come from narrowly based disciplines. There is still a need for professionals with analytical training that allows them to think clearly and to do research. He reiterates what this document has stressed, that the problems in health care are still multidisciplinary with many dimensions and require individuals who can function effectively in this environment. Outside of the Pew programs, relatively few places in the country provide the type of training that is needed.

Steve Crane underscored Stuart Altman's and Hal Luft's point, emphasizing the importance of continuing to bring in students from different areas of the health care field. He stated that the problems of today are not oriented toward institutions, the nation, or the states; rather, they cut across all conventional boundaries and we need to continue to train people to take that view and to learn how to promote change and dialogue within the sectors.

In terms of giving advice to leaders of future programs, the Pew community had much to offer. First, having the start-up money is imperative. Funds are essential to bringing the best students out of the work force and back into school where they can be "retooled" and better prepared to deal with health care policy-related issues. Second, Carroll Estes stated that it is also essential that the leadership of the university support the program and provide the time for faculty to develop and maintain the caliber of teaching and mentoring:

> *I think you need an excellent faculty and a strong research program because the training has got to be hands-on with experience and supervision. I would also say how important a writing seminar would be and explicit allocation of resources to assure that there is training in writing, proposal development, and publication. It's just essential.*

Hal Luft stated that any future program would have to think through the nature of the faculty, for the reasons mentioned above by Carroll Estes. It is important to understand the incentives to faculty and how they would benefit in the development of such a program. Hal Luft explained that the UCSF model is very faculty intensive, but that little funding is provided for faculty. Therefore, the programs have to be creative and figure out how else they can make it work. Each program will find its own solution:

**It is essential to bring the best students out of the work force and back into school where they can be "retooled" and better prepared to deal with health care policy-related issues.**

> *Our program is a little bit like an individually designed house that was built into the side of a mountain. You really need to understand the local geology. . . . When you do it's wonderful, but you can't take those blueprints and use them somewhere else.*

Leon Wyszewianski and Bill Weissert agreed that having up-front commitment not only from faculty but also from the institution is quintessential. They explained that a substantial investment needs to be made at the outset and that continued investment needs to be made throughout the program.

In summary, the general consensus is that there is still a need for advanced health policy training and that the PHPP approach works well. The programs have succeeded in raising the level of acceptance for academically based health policy programs and in demonstrating their importance and value to the field.

# Part IV.

## Summarizing the Legacy: Some Conclusions and Thoughts for the Future

*The best investment around is the professional school.*
—Peter Drucker

*Bottom line: there is still a real need. I do not think the job is done.*
—Hal Luft

*The greatest thing about the Pew program is that it got people excited. . . . Wow, we can change the world!*
—Linda Simoni-Wastila

This fourth and final section of the report attempts to draw the many loose threads together. Based on archival work, the external evaluations, the 25 interviews and narrative accounts, the roundtable discussions and focus groups, and the authors' observations, the Pew Health Policy Program (PHPP) evolved from a unique, ambiguous idea to a highly successful, highly sought after, and well-respected academic program. The demographics are mesmerizing: hundreds of graduates have been placed into a wide variety of health policy jobs and they are now university professors, researchers, consultants, federal and state policy makers, and health care managers.

Some questions remain. From a strategic standpoint, what are the elements of successful programs? How are the collective accomplishments summarized? What lessons have been learned about niche educational programs in health policy? Where do we go from here?

Part four of this report addresses these questions in four sections. The first section develops (with the aid of an analytic framework) strategic guidelines to help foundations and

> The Pew Health Policy Program evolved from a unique, ambiguous idea to a highly successful, highly sought after, and well-respected academic program.

academic institutions to implement niche educational programs. The second section highlights the lessons for other academic institutions learned from the Pew experience. The third section summarizes (in a nonscientific way) impressions of the collective accomplishments and program impacts. To accomplish these three final tasks, the focus is shifted away from the voice of the participants to a more conceptual plane that makes sense of the Pew legacy as a "lived experience."

As Hal Luft, Stuart Altman, Marion Ein Lewin, and others have said, we have learned how to do this, and this work needs to continue. Therefore, it is appropriate for this section to consider the future not only in terms of knowledge creation and vision but also the degree of future participation in policy making and policy training. It is unlikely that market forces will mobilize the loosely coupled community of Pew scholars into an active network. There is a need for a few leaders in the group to create a strong organization. The fourth, and final section concludes by offering the Pew fellows thoughts about a path for the future.

## A STRATEGIC FRAMEWORK FOR ANALYZING THE PHPP EXPERIENCE: BASIC AND INTEGRATIVE ELEMENTS

This section analyzes the PHPP from a strategic standpoint by employing a analytic framework developed by Heskett.[1] According to Heskett (1986) there are four basic elements for success in implementing any service. They are targeting markets, well-defined service concepts, focused operating strategies, and well-designed service delivery systems. Heskett also argues that the four basic elements mentioned above are mediated by three integrative elements: positioning, leveraging, and integrating the operating strategy with the service delivery system. In fact, each of the PHPP sites spent the last dozen or so years honing health policy programs around these basic and integrative elements.

Each of the sites assembled its programs around the four basic elements for strategic success (Heskett, 1986). Sites targeted internal (faculty) and external (fellows) "market" segments and focused on understanding their needs. Each site also carefully crafted a distinct educational service concept in terms of the results that they could produce for fellows and faculty. A third basic element during implementation was developing a focused operations strategy, and the fourth element was designing a system (pedagogy and methodology) for providing educational services.

---

[1] *This section is based on the framework developed by James Heskett (1986) in his book* Managing in the Service Economy.

Each program eventually developed a distinct market niche in health policy by positioning itself to serve faculty, students, and the health policy world. Irrespective of how programs position their educational concept, they must leverage their activities so that the education is valued by the fellows. This was especially important for the midcareer and on-job/on-campus students. Finally, all of the programs in varying degrees, had to integrate and coordinate their operating strategies with their other educational programs (delivery systems) to insure a high quality education at reasonable costs, an engaged faculty, and internal consistency (Heskett, 1986). These ideas are portrayed in Figure 2.

## Figure 2.
*Developing Niche Educational Programs: Basic and Integrative Elements*

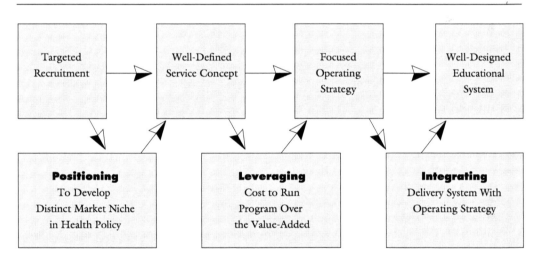

*Adapted from Heskett, 1986.*

## DEVELOPING STRATEGIC PROGRAM VISIONS: BASIC ELEMENTS
### Recruiting Faculty and Fellows:
### Examples of Internal and External Targeting

To launch an educational program, there is a need to do internal faculty recruitment and external fellow recruitment. There is a synergy between the two types of recruitment. To have a successful program, a strong and committed core faculty had to be enlisted and deployed. To attract a strong faculty, excellent students are needed.

Involving faculty members in new activities is difficult, requiring resources and resourcefulness. Two examples illustrate the idea. At the University of Michigan program, they found that running an off-site weekend program required obtaining an "up-front" commitment of faculty willing to teach adult learners on Saturdays and Sundays for 5 months of the year. Traditional ways of hiring faculty did not work, because a new breed of faculty member was needed. According to Richardson (1990), "the faculty selected to teach this group of adult learners" had to be carefully screened and oriented because many Pew fellows were experts in their work domains. Over time Michigan learned how to develop and deploy an outstanding faculty.

At the University of California at San Francisco (UCSF), for example, the problem of engaging the faculty required "selling them" on the benefits of working with postdoctoral fellows. When the program began attracting exceptional Pew fellows, a committed faculty quickly surfaced. RAND/University of California at Los Angeles (UCLA) was able to build on the strengths of the faculty at each school to create a singularly rich training program.

> The faculty selected to teach this group of adult learners had to be carefully screened and oriented because many Pew fellows were experts in their work domains. PHPP averaged students with 12 to 14 years of work experience before they came to the Pew program.

Targeting excellent fellows to keep the faculty interested and involved was not unique to UCSF but occurred at every site. There is strong evidence that all of the program sites managed to attract high-quality fellows from a strong applicant pool. Throughout the program, the outside evaluators found the quality of the fellows to be "very strong"; moreover, there were noticeable improvements in the quality of fellows from 1982 to 1985, 1985 to 1989, and 1989 to 1994. PHPP averaged students with 12 to 14 years of work experience before they came to the Pew program. The postdoctoral fellows were PhDs, and clinicians. The predoctoral fellows often had Master's degrees or professional graduate degrees from excellent schools.

In doctoral and postdoctoral programs, the attrition rates are surprisingly high (Bowen and Rudenstine, 1992). PHPP hypothesized that attrition may be related to the ability to recruit high-quality students. Therefore, the Pew program focused on "quality students" along two dimensions: (1) finding the best and brightest candidates and (2) finding people motivated to complete these challenging programs.

Recruitment of high-quality, highly motivated fellows was not the only recruitment characteristic. Each program also had to discover ways to single out groups of applicants (i.e., student segments) with common characteristics whose educational needs could best be met by a particular program in terms of the results they could deliver. So, in recruiting fellows, each program had to learn how to screen for fellows motivated and capable of completing the degree and who fit well with the educational services that the program could deliver.

Discovering ways to single out segments of applicants was not a trivial problem for a niche program in health policy. The Michigan program, for example, was a nonresidential doctoral program in health policy for working people. This meant locating prospective fellows who wanted to pursue a full-time doctoral program without giving up their full-time professional lives.

To increase the chances of locating highly qualified fellows, schools need to select from a large applicant pool. Recruiting from a national (as opposed to a local) market yields a larger pool. Michigan learned that its program had great appeal to high-profile, midcareer professionals from government and health care management, which offered a large, national segment to draw from. Recruiting Michigan fellows from this pool, however, was tricky because Michigan fellows had to be good at both work and school. To complete a doctoral degree, Michigan had to identify fellows who could master the craft of being a good student. By and large, great leaders are not great students; moreover, older students do not do well on standardized tests. To insure that fellows who were selected would complete the program, Michigan used college grades, past work accomplishments, and Graduate Record Examination (GRE) scores as criteria for final selection.

Each of the programs found different ways to group applicants into segments with common characteristics. At first, Boston University (BU)/Brandeis sought people who had had some governmental or health care management experience and who wanted advanced training in health policy. At BU, the Center for Industry and Health Care aimed at increasing the involvement of the business community in health policy by establishing corporate coalitions, so they targeted students who were planning careers in business and public service. Over time, Brandeis singled out people who were interested in issues of social justice for vulnerable populations–violence, people with AIDS, chronic disease populations, veterans, and so on. The UCSF program targeted a high-quality national pool, consisting of a mix of applicants who wanted advanced training in research: MDs with specialties in primary care and preventive medicine and PhDs (in social science and other areas) from academia.

*To increase the chances of locating highly qualified fellows, schools need to select from a large applicant pool. Recruiting from a national (as opposed to a local) market yields a larger pool.*

## An Evolving Educational Service Concept

To recruit bright and motivated fellows who are willing to leave their jobs and careers to go back to school and to attract a dedicated faculty willing to allocate their time and attention, an educational service concept must be defined. This educational concept must be defined not as offering a degree or a high quality educational experience but in terms of opportunities and potential advantages for the fellows and the faculty. At the outset of a program, it is rare to have clarity in an educational concept; concepts evolve.

*The program had a commitment to excellence and ability to take corrective action when the external program evaluations uncovered weaknesses.*

In 1981, the staff at the Pew Charitable Trusts believed that there was a lack of depth and breadth in health policy research, analysis, and management, and they believed that multidisciplinary educational concepts might address this problem. Each of the sites offered variations on the traditional educational concept: providing a high-quality educational experience for students. One key result area, implicitly promised by the Pew Program was in an area in which graduate education fails to achieve, academic survival and success.

Over time, the programs sharpened their definitions of these concepts. In part, this occurred as a result of the programs, commitment to excellence and ability to take corrective action when the external program evaluations uncovered weaknesses. Defining the concept became an evolving process, in which programs learned the results that can be achieved and they adapted the current concept in that direction.

UCSF initially offered three types of 2-year fellowships: predoctoral, postdoctoral, and management. The predoctoral and management programs, although highly successful, were discontinued so that resources could be concentrated on developing a strong postdoctoral program. The educational concept was a multidisciplinary postdoctoral health policy program in which fellows worked with faculty on research projects. The faculty would commit to an active involvement with fellows as mentors and colleagues. Faculty would participate in annual fellow reviews and mentorship meetings.

The BU/Brandeis program initially contained two elements: a Pew scholars program and a Pew fellows program. The Scholars Program was an on-campus, post-master's, multidisciplinary accelerated doctoral program which aimed at reducing the time, cost, and incompletion rates to produce educated individuals effective in the health policy system. The Pew fellows program aimed at mid-level and upper-level managers and trained them in health care management and cost-containment strategies.

Michigan offered a unique, nonresidential 3-year doctoral program in health policy. The central educational concept was that fellows could get their doctorates while keeping their jobs. The OJ/OC doctoral program provided 20 4-day sessions and two 4-week sessions. Upon completion of the program, fellows received a doctor of public health degree.

In 1982, a joint venture between RAND/UCLA offered a 3-year interdisciplinary program in which fellows could obtain a PhD in policy analysis at RAND or a PhD in several different areas, such as public health and epidemiology at UCLA. The program also had a 10-session lecture discussion series to introduce medical students to policy issues and a 1-year nondegree policy career development program.[2]

**Each of the programs developed a strong core curriculum that taught students to appreciate and synthesize the clinical, sociological, political, economic, and behavioral implications of the policy process.**

## A Focused Operating Strategy

Heskett (1986) argues that that to deliver on the promises implicit in the educational concept (while achieving the internal operating goals) a focused operating strategy is needed. This especially makes sense for an educational program since faculty and other resources are so scarce. So, to develop into a high quality educational services program, the PHPP leadership had to concentrate its attention in a few strategic areas, which included:

1.  developing a strong curriculum with a well-integrated learning sequence,
2.  the deployment of faculty,
3.  the creation of a small "service-oriented" organization, and
4.  the control of costs.

### Developing a Strong Curriculum That Ensures Academic Success and Survival

The multidisciplinary nature of the curriculum was mentioned throughout the interviews and evaluations as one of the greatest strengths of PHPP. In each of the programs, the social sciences, economics and clinical "disciplines" began to be seen as "tools" to help policy makers solve problems. Each of the programs developed a strong core curriculum that taught students to appreciate and synthesize the clinical, sociological, political, economic, and behavioral implications of the policy process. (The actual curriculas are in Appendix B.)

For example, one of the major strengths of the Brandeis program was its broad multidisciplinary approach. The doctoral program required course work in the basic social sci-

[2] *By 1991, it was decided that three educational concepts should be maintained: postdoctoral education in a policy-rich environment, an accelerated doctoral program, and a doctoral program for people with full time jobs.*

ences, statistics, research methods, and policy analysis and advanced course work in health policy (Issues in Health Policy; Health Care Organization and Politics; Social, Ethical, and Legal Issues; and Health Economics). At least one course in special populations was also required.

However, to ensure academic survival and success in postdoctoral work, midcareer programs, and the accelerated doctoral program, new mechanisms were needed. The dissertation seminars at BU/Brandeis and Michigan became a pedagogical mechanism not only to help students structure and manage the dissertation process early on but also to provide the psychological support to build and connect the fellows into a committed group of mature scholars. An innovative mechanism was needed to get students to start thinking about a dissertation on the first day of the program. The dissertation seminar also became an opportunity to integrate the multidisciplinary curriculum.

The promise of survival and success in a postdoctoral program also required a strong core curriculum. In addition to developing a strong health policy curriculum, UCSF developed a weekly health policy seminar, writing seminar, and journal club to sharpen the fellows' communication skills. These seminars became mechanisms for bringing fellows closer to researchers and policy makers, while providing psychological support and assisting in their "socialization" in health policy.

To help ensure academic survival, RAND/UCLA employed an innovative strategy that included an early dissertation focus with an research apprenticeship model. Not only did this innovation get students to experience real research and to develop professional relationships with faculty; these projects often turned into dissertations.

> The dissertation seminars at BU/Brandeis and Michigan became a pedagogical mechanism not only to help students structure and manage the dissertation process early on but also to provide the psychological support to build and connect the fellows into a committed group of mature scholars.

### Faculty Deployment

To meet the fellows' expectations for an exceptional education, there was a need to provide adequate contact with faculty. At UCSF the operating strategy focused on a highly structured learning sequence and a model of mentoring. The mentoring at UCSF worked well. The model required each student to work with two faculty members in an apprenticeship model. Pew, through its habit of systematic program evaluations "prodded," the programs to develop more structure.

All of the Pew programs compensated the faculty for their contribution to the program in one of two ways:

(1) remuneration for time spent or (2) the opportunity to be a mentor for and collaborate with some excellent fellows. Although money alone does not motivate faculty, asking faculty to teach additional courses in health policy without pay "can be difficult."

At UCSF, the model was very faculty intensive, with one or two faculty mentors assigned to a fellow. Hal Luft said that getting fellows involved with faculty research did work. Faculty liked working with Pew fellows, who were seen as good colleagues. Although faculty were not compensated with salary, the faculty were motivated by intrinsic rewards, such as the value of working with a good research assistant.

### Changing Behavior Patterns via Service-Oriented Culture

The organization of most graduate schools offering predoctoral and postdoctoral education is a hierarchical, loosely coupled set of rituals and routine activities that more or less accomplish the task of enrollment management. The premise of most graduate programs is that given enough time, students will find their way around. They will link up with faculty, select the right courses, and connect with interesting and important research. The process is haphazard, and not student centered.

For the PHPP to work, people had to go out of their way to help students connect with faculty and offer greater flexibility when problems arose. Not every program succeeded in creating a service oriented culture; in fact, fellows complained about the need for more attention. But every program did create a small, effective staff usually involving one faculty member as program director, one or two key faculty, and one or two support staff to serve faculty and fellow needs. Program champions also emerged at each site.

**Faculty liked working with Pew fellows, who were seen as good colleagues.**

### Cost-Effectiveness

Although every program had to control costs, because of its unique service concept and national targets, Michigan had to focus on controlling costs. Since Michigan chose to target fellows from a national (not local) pool, the program managers had to control (1) travel costs, (2) communication costs, and (3) the massive investment in regular and adjunct faculty, all within the regular tuition structure. Therefore, the Michigan program not only managed costs but also became cost effective.

## Developing an Educational Program into a Well-Designed Delivery System

To offer an educational program, facilities must be designed to work well with the operating strategy. Programs must consider the important characteristics of the educational program as a service process. In fact, the development of an educational service delivery system was an important feature of each program's evolution. Explicit consideration had to be given to the role of key people, physical layout, and changing procedures.

### Role of Key People

To deliver on the strategy of a service-oriented culture, each of the programs needed an incredibly dedicated program staff to serve faculty, students and program leadership. At RAND/UCLA, Kate Korman was cited as "an indispensable linchpin with respect to tying together diverse interests and activities." Throughout the interviews, Marion Ein Lewin, Steve Crane, Ted Benjamin, and David Perlman were all mentioned as being extraordinarily supportive.

### Physical Layout

**Every program created a small, effective staff usually involving one faculty member as program director, one or two key faculty, and one or two support staff to serve faculty and fellow needs. Program champions also emerged at each site.**

Placement of people in offices (or the lack of office space) affects people in a number of ways. Physical layouts are an indicator of social distance and membership (Schein, 1985). The allocation of space (crowding students into rooms, size of the office, and quality of the furniture) symbolizes the rank of the people and affects their feelings of inclusion. Finally, organizational research has shown that the probability of weekly interactions drops to zero when people are more than 40 meters apart. Being on different floors (or buildings) is like being in different cities.

Each of the programs was challenged by the physical locations of the fellows, especially in relation to faculty. Some programs, such as Brandeis, were never able to offer their fellows office space, which undermined communication. To compensate, Brandeis provided weekly dissertation seminars and biweekly colloquia which were opportunities for concerted group action. In a bid to promote communication among off-site participants, Michigan used electronic communication.

UCSF found that to the extent that fellows were located off-site, interaction with faculty and other fellows was hindered. The situation improved when office space became available. They found that when they brought the fellows into office space with the faculty, mentoring relationships improved.

### Changing Rules and Procedures

At Michigan, they discovered that the OJ/OC weekend mode resulted in the accumulation of many incompletes because of the working students' inability to complete term papers. Over time, these incompletes became obstacles to completing the dissertations. The remedy was the creation of new procedures aimed at discouraging major papers due at the end of a course. The procedures encouraged the faculty to assign deliverables over the terms rather than a major paper at the end of the term. As a result of those procedures, the rate of incompletes dropped. Incompletes were only given if a serious personal problem (such as a death in the family) had occurred. The procedures helped to reduce the risk of low completion rates.

To decrease feelings of elitism and to increase integration among Pew and non-Pew students, BU/Brandeis changed the rules to allow any student into the dissertation seminars. To help fellows complete the program in 2 years, Brandeis changed its procedures to allow Pew fellows to take their qualifying examinations in the first year.

At UCSF, formal procedures were developed to improve faculty-fellow interactions and mentoring. Incoming fellows received a detailed orientation to the faculty. Fellows had scheduled meetings with their primary research advisers. Finally, guidelines listing goals and expectations of the faculty mentors and fellows were developed.

### DEVELOPING STRATEGIC PROGRAM VISIONS: INTEGRATIVE ELEMENTS

#### Positioning Each Program

Positioning in education means identifying academic needs that no one is serving. Before each site could position itself it needed a deeper understanding of: (1) what other health services research doctoral programs were offering, (2) the needs of potential employers in the policy world and (3) how to serve the educational needs of the students. Although there was a clear need for many more people broadly trained in health policy, each program had to focus its attention on what it could do differently from other graduate programs in health services. Most programs focused on teaching policy analysis and advanced research skills from a single perspec-

> Although there was a clear need for many more people broadly trained in health policy, each program had to focus its attention on what it could do differently from other graduate programs in health services.

Traditional doctoral education takes a long time to complete, and relatively few survive. Doctoral education is plagued by low completion rates, often 50 to 60 percent in the social sciences and those who complete all but the dissertation have an 80 percent chance of obtaining the PhD. The doctoral completion rate for PHPP as of 1996 was 66 percent.

tive–public policy, public health, political science, health administration, or health economics. Few programs positioned themselves where health policy and advanced theoretical and research training intersect. They also had to find ways to customize the training and education to enhance the value-added per fellow.

If the PHPPs were to differentiate and distinguish themselves, they also had to understand the new world of health policy. New policy units had emerged in the 1980s, such as the Physician Payment Review Commission (PPRC). These new policy centers needed well-educated people with strong analytic skills and a deep understanding of the health care context. The new world needed a mix of analytical and methodological skills with a context-specific policy knowledge base. The context-specific (as opposed to context-free) education set the Pew graduates apart from graduates of other programs.

The Michigan program positioned itself to appeal to high quality people who never could have obtained a PhD because traditional programs require leaving a job for at least 2 or 3 years.

To understand how PHPP carved health policy niches, one must consider what graduate education is all about. Traditional doctoral education takes a long time to complete, and relatively few survive. In general, doctoral education is plagued by low completion rates, often 50 to 60 percent in the social sciences and those who complete all but the dissertation have an 80 percent chance of obtaining the PhD. The median time between entry to graduate school and being awarded the PhD is 6.7 years (Bowen and Rudenstine, 1992).

Why does this occur? There is no theory about student survival rates, but several plausible hypotheses are offered. First, doctoral education has very high opportunity costs for the average student. In addition to doctoral expenses, students lose the money they would have earned had they not been a student. Many students work at part-time (and some at full-time) jobs throughout their education. Many keep their job responsibilities while they are students. Others take odd jobs, work as consultants, and so forth.

A second hypothesis is that other aspects of a student's life begins to take over after 2 or 3 years. For example, once the course work is completed, many full-time doctoral (having completed all but the dissertation) students take on full-time jobs. They assume that since they have managed to complete the examinations and dozens of courses, they can write their dissertations around the edges of their lives. Many find that time passes as relentlessly as a Boeing 747; 5 years have gone by and they have written a few pages since they left the program. Given the high costs of the education when the student is "All But Dissertation," the value of finishing the degree often depends on the current reputation of the school in the national competitive arena.

A third hypothesis about why it is hard to finish has to do with the very nature of academia and beliefs about the amount of time people need to master the knowledge and to think about opportunities to make contributions. Traditional predoctoral education allows students to limit their commitment to the sequential completion of required tasks. First, take courses and other requirements, next take general examinations, then one can think about the dissertation proposal. The learning sequence plays out as rigid rules.

Throughout the course work, the responsible faculty member distracts students (in a positive way) by suggesting another course, more reading, rival theories, other perspectives, and so on. The underlying assumption is that learning what we know and what we don't know requires lengthy time periods.

Finally, the core doctoral faculty take a passive rather than an active stance with students. They wait for students to "find" them; access to faculty regarding student's research interests is often sporadic, haphazard, and peripheral to the doctoral "program." Some programs talk about mentoring, but few have developed formal mentoring components, such as UCSF (see Appendix C).

Table 5 reveals some of the ways that PHPP positioned its predoctoral education. The positioning required a focused operating strategy on unlearning old ways of doing things and organizing for innovation. For PHPP to succeed, it had to change the nature of academia and break some of the rules of traditional doctoral education. The individual programs not only had to promise a high probability of academic success and survival, but to do so in an accelerated time period. There would be full tuition scholarships; in addition, the opportunity costs would be offset by allocating stipends to doctoral fellows. In addition to a standardized general curriculum, there would be an early dissertation and research focus and flexibility with respect to requirements so as to allow the development of highly individualized learning plans. A "high-touch" philosophy would be implemented by encouraging the faculty to take a more active stance, and in most, if not all, cases faculty mentors would emerge.

For PHPP to succeed, a national identity had to be created. PHPP created a kind of "membership in a club" relationship between the fellows and the national office. The value of an individual to the policy world would be augmented by one's status as a Pew fellow.

**Table 5.**

*Positioning of the Pew Health Policy Program Versus Traditional Doctoral Programs*

| Traditional Predoctoral Approach | PHPP Approach |
|---|---|
| Lengthy time to completion | Accelerated time to completion |
| Moderate to low survival rates | Higher survival rates |
| High opportunity costs | Moderate opportunity costs |
| Some outside income required | Fellowship includes stipends |
| Sequential attention to tasks | Early dissertation/research focus |
| Rigidity to rules | Flexibility |
| Passive faculty stance | More active faculty stance |
| Informal access to faculty | Formal mentoring requirements |
| Dependence on school reputation | Development of national identity |

## Leveraging Program Costs Over the Value of the Program to the Fellows

If niche programs are to be institutionalized, the educational service concept must be positioned in a way that a margin (student tuition minus relevant unit variable costs) covers faculty and staff costs and future program costs. For this to happen, niche programs must leverage program value over cost. That means that educational service concepts and operating strategies must be developed in ways that strongly appeal to faculty and fellows in the program, while keeping costs to provide the program reasonable (Heskett, 1986). Each of the programs leveraged the program in one of four ways: (1) building on a core competency, (2) adding value via network effects, (3) combining standard curriculum with customized elements, and (4) deep involvement of fellows.

### Building on Core Competencies

Each of the programs identified its core competencies and built the program on the distinguishing competencies. These competencies were not always obvious to the programs at first. Some programs tried to develop new strengths, but over time they came back to those things that they did best.

UCSF built its program on the strength of its medical school, nursing school, and Institute for Health Policy Studies. The faculty from those places believed that research was a team effort and they also believed in the learning by doing model. All of these strengths came together in the UCSF Pew program, which was designed as a postdoctoral program for advanced research studies that would team up MDs with PhDs in social science. Although there were no preexisting health policy courses in which fellows could enroll, with Pew support they were able to leverage the faculty to develop some excellent courses.

At RAND/UCLA, leverage came from building on the workshop model, which it had used in the graduate school. When the Pew program began, it modified workshops or seminars on broad policy domains with a set of modules. Policy exercises were required which made the fellows think analytically about a contemporary health policy problem via a policy memo or class presentation. The RAND program, whose predoctoral programs had a high completion rate, created an on-the-job component in which fellows spent half their time working with faculty on real research projects. In many cases these projects resulted in a completed dissertation.

Michigan also built its program from a core competency. It had developed an innovation nearly 30 years ago—a midcareer, weekend program in which everyone took the same courses. PHPP built on years of experimenting and improving the OJ/OC educational concept.

Leverage at Brandeis came from two places. First, the faculty at the Heller School at Brandeis was world renowned for its pioneering studies in social policy. The doctoral program incorporated this research and knowledge to create a multidisciplinary curriculum different from those of other doctoral programs. Since the Brandeis Pew program targeted and attracted students interested in vulnerable populations, social justice, and social change, a strong curriculum in social policy had already been developed. Now a very strong curriculum in health policy was needed.

> For PHPP to succeed, a national identity had to be created. PHPP created a kind of "membership in a club" relationship between the fellows and the national office.

The second source of leveraging came from the Health Policy Institute, which had been established in 1978 and became one of the largest academically based health policy research groups in the United States. The institute became an excellent laboratory for fellows who were interested in sharpening their health policy research skills.

## Adding Value via Network Effects

PHPP was positioned to become a national program, in which being a Pew fellow would not only mean something to Washington, D.C. policy makers but also to state health policy experts. Over a period of several years, the Pew program developed an outstanding nationwide network of highly trained people. Although PhPP's original mission was to develop policy makers, fellows ended up in a wide variety of health policy positions. As a result, Pew fellows have become extremely mobile. The network is the amalgamation of four or five different program experiences representing dozens of different disciplines and hundreds of personal experiences. As Steve Crane said, "These people understand and know each other, and they can get things done."

According to a 1994 survey of fellows, the greatest value of the program to the fellows was the opportunity to "meet and network with talented scholars and prominent faculty and influential policy makers." For many people, these connections have lasted and have resulted in research collaborations and friendships.

### Combining a Standard Curriculum with Customized Elements

In designing a niche program each school must ask: How can we adapt our curriculum and requirements to meet the needs of a mix of individuals with diverse backgrounds? Requiring students to take the required curriculum and participate in dissertation and writing seminars and so on increased program effectiveness and common knowledge bases while creating the sense of a shared experience among fellows. On the other hand, there is a need to customize a niche program to allow fellows to explore new areas of interest.

Although the sites ranged from a lock-step structure at Michigan to near complete academic freedom at BU, each of the programs took steps in which a highly individualized learning program could be offered. The programs learned that too much leniency and flexibility hampered the students' ability to finish the program. As programs moved toward increasing the structure, the challenge became balancing structure with flexibility.

At Michigan, for example, competency examinations were used to gauge the student's level of preparation in statistics, economics, politics, and organizational behavior. These requirements achieved three results. First, they forced students to study these subjects before starting the doctoral program. Second, since students were studying for these examinations, they were entering the Michigan program with similar levels of preparation. This increased the job satisfaction of the faculty who in the early years of the program had found it very difficult to teach students with diverse levels of knowledge. Third, the competency exams communicated to the students that they were entering a rigorous program that required them to do some serious work.

The BU program offered the greatest freedom. Although BU did not tell the students what courses they

**Pew fellows have become extremely mobile. The network is the amalgamation of four or five different program experiences representing dozens of different disciplines and hundreds of personal experiences.**

must take, students were advised to take a social science core. To facilitate faster-track fellows, BU allowed them to do course work and the dissertation at the same time. Although the freedom did not work for everyone, several students completed the program in 24 months or less.

UCSF developed a structured curriculum in which all fellows took the same core seminars. UCSF customized the curriculum on the basis of the type of career trajectory that the fellow desired. Each fellow's needs were assessed through extensive discussions with mentors. Fellows who wanted academic careers were encouraged to publish; fellows who wanted to be become policy makers were encouraged to do research that resulted in reports rather the publications. UCSF learned that allowing people flexibility to search for their own mentors rather than assigning mentors increased the likelihood of survival and success.

**The greatest value of the program to the fellows was the opportunity to meet and network with talented scholars and prominent faculty and influential policy makers.**

### Deep Involvement of the Fellows

Program costs decrease if fellows can become more involved in the program. Learning is also enhanced when students are deeply involved in their own education. Throughout the program Pew fellows were asked to give lectures, run seminars, and help with planning and organization. Each year many of the sessions at the annual Pew meeting were organized by fellows and chaired by fellows, and many of the presenters were fellows.

### Integrating the Operating Strategy and the Educational Program

For a niche health policy program to be successful, the operating strategy must be integrated with the delivery system. Integration occurred in three ways: learning how to match faculty and fellows, creative uses of technology, and use of integration mechanisms developed by the Institute of Medicine (IOM), as the central program office.

### Matching Fellows with Faculty

All of the programs found that matching faculty with students was very challenging. At first the programs tried selling faculty to students or vice versa; for example, at RAND/UCLA the students had to market their expertise to the faculty. Although this approach was not ideal, it helped students to assess their strengths and weaknesses.

At UCSF some of the fellows had trouble deciding which of the faculty to work with. The program leadership learned that organizing a 2- or 3-day faculty presentation was not a good way to expose faculty and their research. Over time UCSF learned how to manage the matching process. Recently, it developed a faculty handbook that contains the type of research that all of the health faculty are involved with.

### Application of Computer Technology

The sites ranged from a lock-step structure at Michigan to near complete academic freedom at BU, yet each of the programs took steps in which a highly individualized leaning program could be offered.

The use of technology to electronically link fellows was limited. However, one of the innovators of this approach was the Michigan program. Michigan had to learn how to allow fellows to acquire a doctoral education without interrupting their jobs and careers. To offer fellows a high-quality PhD program in health policy without having to leave their jobs, the program had to find innovative ways to foster and improve communication.

The Michigan program developed on-line computer networks that electronically connected fellows with Michigan health policy faculty. Extensive computer linkages and conferencing between faculty and students had a great impact on the quality and productivity of the off-site program. The use of computer conferencing helped to integrate the Michigan Pew students with their cohorts and the faculty.

### Integration Through IOM

Perhaps the most significant way that integration was achieved was through the work of Marion Ein Lewin at IOM. IOM planned annual meetings, developed an annual directory, published a newsletter, and monitored the mission, goals and progress of the various sites. Through the national office, PHPP developed into an integrated program across four sites with a national identity. Moreover, through the efforts of IOM, Washington, D.C. as a laboratory became more accessible to the fellows.

## IMPLICATIONS FOR DEVELOPING HEALTH POLICY PROGRAMS AS A NEW EDUCATIONAL NICHE

The previous section analyzed the elements of programmatic success from a strategic standpoint. This section summarizes the implications of the Pew Legacy as a new educational niche programs in health policy. Three questions are addressed: To create a niche educational program, what kind of planning process is needed? During implementation what were the obstacles and how did they influence performance? What lessons were learned from the four Pew programs over the last decade? Answering these questions may provide some useful insights for schools attempting to develop niche educational programs in health policy and other areas.

Many schools of public health, schools of public and social policy, medical schools, business schools, schools of health administration, and schools of social work have begun to offer various programs in health services research. Educational programs cannot pretend to offer an excellent program in a field like health care because it is too large. Therefore, answering these questions can help schools to consider concentrating their resources by developing a niche educational program. These questions are addressed by identifying the activities needed to develop a niche educational program.

To help answer these questions, the experience of the creation of PHPP as a developmental process is examined. To help organize the thinking, the Program Planning Model (PPM) developed by Delbecq and Van de Ven (1971) is adopted as an analytical framework. PPM identifies five overlapping phases, each with a distinct set of activities that must be managed. They are as follows:

**Program costs decrease if fellows can become more involved in the program. Throughout the program Pew fellows were asked to give lectures, run seminars, and help with planning and organization.**

### Phase 1: Planning Prerequisites

*To initiate a new program, PPM suggests beginning a planning effort by defining a policy committee and a planning staff.*

### Phase 2: Problem Exploration

*The planning staff begins to collect data on the nature and complexity of problems in the area that the new educational program is attempting to address. The problems are cast from the perspective of the key stakeholders.*

### Phase 3: Knowledge Exploration

*Experts analyze the data on problems and alternatives are generated in a report that is reviewed by the planning committee and circulated among phase 1 and 2 participants.*

### Phase 4: Program Design

*The problems and expert opinions are summarized and workshops and problem-solving meetings are begun with all relevant stakeholders. A demonstration of the program is funded for a trial period.*

### Phase 5: Program Evaluation, Implementation, and Operation

*After a new program is under way, it is periodically evaluated so that corrective action can be taken.*

Although PPM was developed for human service organizations, it can help to guide the design and development of niche graduate educational programs in the future. The remainder of this section explores factors associated with implementation success based on the collective experience of PHPP participants.

### Interpreting the Pew Experience

There is very little evidence that there was much systematic planning and goal setting before the start of the Pew program. In 1982 the Pew Charitable Trusts launched the health policy program and made its first awards in 1983. PHPP did not begin with a clear set of well-defined goals. The mission of PHPP was as follows:

> *To stimulate the development of multidisciplinary health policy educational programs that will equip a cadre of leaders with the required skills to deal effectively with the nation's complex current and future health policy issues.*

**The original solicitation was unique and impressive because it was based on the recommendations of a small group of advisers to the Pew Charitable Trusts who believed that important policy issues were developing in health care. The foundation, however, made no attempt to define precisely what these health policy issues would be.**

During one of the interviews, Stuart Altman commented that the original solicitation was "unique and impressive" because it was based on the recommendations of a small group of advisers to the Pew Charitable Trusts who believed that important policy issues were developing in health care. The foundation, however, made no attempt to define precisely what these health policy issues would be. Since each of the program sites was allowed to set its own goals, each program truly "owned" these goals and was committed to their achievement.

Through a solicitation process, the foundation targeted 15 institutions and four nonacademic health centers to receive the request for proposal. The foundation selected four university-based centers and 1 nonacademic center as training sites and granted them the autonomy to (1) define these health policy issues and (2) design a training program to address those issues. The foundation allowed the program sites an opportunity to define the major health care problems and to discover a program methodology by experimenting.

According to PPM, success in program development often depends on the amount of professional consultation or technical assistance during planning and implementation phases. During the planning stages, little technical assistance was offered. However, during implementation (under Marion Ein Lewin's leadership) the foundation offered IOM as a "process consultant."

As process consultant, IOM did not focus on improving the content of the educational activities; rather it focused on the cohesiveness, communication, and group dynamics of the fellows and training directors. IOM also engaged each of the program directors at each of the program sites in task-oriented team-building activities during retreats and off-site meetings, held in Washington, D.C., at IOM or a mutually convenient location. The program directors would spend a day working intensively; reflecting on PHPP, its problems, and solutions to those problems; and planning joint activities.

During implementation, several problems arose: faculty recruitment, faculty complacency and motivation, lack of space, insufficient financial resources, and a general resistance to change. All of the PHPP sites encountered some of these problems. The experience with the Pew program suggests that allowing each program site to define tasks by experimenting with various service concepts and operating strategies worked.

For example, recruitment of faculty and matching students and faculty was one of the most frequently mentioned difficulties. Over time, with the help of the outside evaluations, each program learned how to enlist an excellent faculty. In the beginning the programs aimed for a minimal set of procedures. Structural and procedural ambiguity allowed each program to adapt to student needs. All of the programs discovered that development of new procedures made the programs more effective.

During the early years of implementation, the emphasis of the foundation was on program accomplishments and not on program efficiency (or measures such as total program costs per fellow). At the director's meetings and in the annual reports of the program sites, the focus was on the educational innovations, fellows' accomplishments, number of publications, number of PhDs granted, and so on. Although efficiency is an important criterion for a mature program, the Pew Charitable Trusts displayed great wisdom in its tolerance for ambiguity and its realization that a premature focus on the total cost per fellow in a niche educational program would be a misleading indicator of program success. Had the program directors' meetings or the annual reports focused on efficiency, attention would have been refocused on ways to save money rather than on learning how to run an effective program.

Finally, the experiences of PHPP do not suggest an inevitable move from financial dependence to independence. Neither BU nor the RAND midcareer programs continued

As process consultant, the Institute of Medicine did not focus on improving the content of the educational activities; rather it focused on the cohesiveness, communication, and group dynamics of the fellows and training directors.

after Pew funds were withdrawn. Interestingly, the doctoral program at RAND has continued.

There is not enough information on what happened after Pew support was withdrawn, perhaps because the funding did not last long enough for some of these programs to take root. Although many of the formal mechanisms that helped to coordinate the PHPP structure (orientation meeting in Washington, D.C., annual meetings, directors' meetings, directories of fellows and alumni, and routine newsletters) will end, the surviving sites claim that some type of institutionalization has taken place. Time will tell.

## SUMMARIZING THE LESSONS LEARNED: MAXIMS FOR OTHER SCHOOLS

This final section suggests some implications for designing health policy programs in the future. Technically the findings are based on the experiences of the four PHPP sites. Although the findings are preliminary impressions and speculations, the experience can shed light on how a foundation's strategic choices can affect the success of new educational programs.

### Bold and Ambiguous Goals Encourage Active Experimentation

Although efficiency is an important criterion for a mature program, the Pew Charitable Trusts displayed great wisdom in its tolerance for ambiguity and its realization that a premature focus on the total cost per fellow in a niche educational program would be a misleading indicator of program success.

One of the fascinating lessons learned arises around the bold and ambiguous goals set by the Pew Charitable Trusts. First, they wanted to stimulate development of multidisciplinary programs in health policy to train a cadre of leaders. Second, they wanted an accelerated timetable, the tradition of a 6 or 7-year doctoral program was insufficient. Third, they wanted these programs to institutionalize and become self-sufficient, although they would be financially dependent on the Trusts. The goals required everyone—fellows, faculty, and program leaders—to stretch for these goals. Requiring everyone to stretch led to higher levels of performance.

The creation of new multidisciplinary health policy doctoral programs aimed at producing health policy leaders is an ambiguous goal. The Pew program had no historical precedent, so it was guided by ongoing adaptive choices. Ambiguity allowed active experimentation and adjustments when strategic intent and program activities veered away from the core competency of a school. Program site goals were negotiated by the interaction of IOM, the evaluators, the Trusts, and the sites.

## By Encouraging the Programs to Focus on a Single Niche and Educational Service Concept, the Program Flourished

Each of the programs offered a variety of advanced training service concepts in health policy to management fellows, pre-doctoral fellows, and postdoctoral fellows. Although serving a broader set of needs was successful, the Pew Charitable Trusts decided to have each program focus all of its energy on a single concept: nonresidential predoctoral fellows, residential predoctoral fellows, and postdoctoral fellows.

The world of health policy is changing because the needs are changing. If PHPP had attempted to satisfy all the diverse needs through one large program, it probably would have failed. Now one can appreciate the wisdom of having multiple program sites with very different program concepts. Although none of the program sites could claim a program that could do it all—produce great academic researchers, teachers, great policy makers, and great practitioners—collectively the Pew program sites were able to serve the needs of the health policy world. The programs learned that focusing on fellows with an operating strategy and a service delivery system specifically designed to meet their needs worked better when a single educational niche was the target.

The creation of new multidisciplinary health policy doctoral programs aimed at producing health policy leaders is an ambiguous goal. The Pew program had no historical precedent, so it was guided by ongoing adaptive choices.

## Importance of Money in Securing the Basics: Space, Stipends, and Faculty Compensation

Without the generosity of the Pew Charitable Trusts, there would be no Pew health policy legacy to speak of. It is difficult to maintain graduate programs in health policy in the absence of strong funding for research and training. New programs are not capable of overcoming the faculty routines, commitments, and lifestyles; institutional memories; and traditional ways of doing educational things.

The conclusion is that money matters. Targeting of excellent students requires the ability to offer them a valuable education (beyond their basic expectation), easy access to the best faculty, and protection from line responsibility. Budgets provide office space, attract high-quality people, concentrate attention resources, encourage innovation, and promote coordination and networking. Building a new program requires large initial investments and reinvestments in academic programs.

Although money matters, focusing prematurely on the dollars spent per student is misleading because it will lead to less success.

### Program Expectations Guide Students

Bowen and Rudenstine (1992) once observed that, "doctoral programs do not run themselves. . . .much depends on the care with which they are designed and the expectations that are established concerned the character and quality of the work to be done by those admitted" (p. 250).

In traditional graduate programs, expectations are formed haphazardly out of a mixture of official statements, course requirements and waivers, examinations taken or avoided, peer and faculty pressures, myths and half-truths, and so on. The Pew programs learned that leniency and flexibility are not the same thing. Performance improved when expectations were clarified and when specific expectations were set.

Some of the mechanisms that helped to set expectations in the Pew predoctoral programs were competency examinations and dissertation seminars. The dissertation seminars emphatically stated that that the goal, although not hard and fast, was to help students get started on a dissertation topic in the first semester of the program so that they could defend their dissertation in two or three years. Fellows explained the importance of demystifying the dissertation process. The PHPP approach made a commitment to managing everyone's expectations.

### External Program Evaluations Are Real When Financial Dependence Exists

PHPP wanted to stimulate the development of multidisciplinary health policy education programs to produce leaders capable of taking leadership roles in policy development in government and industry. To help understand the degree of success achieved, three formal program evaluations were contracted out. These evaluations helped to focus attention on some of the problems that fellows were having with the way that the programs were being implemented.

These evaluations helped to shape and change the evolution of the programs. They focused managerial attention on (1) how the practices of each of the programs compared, (2) what innovations and outcomes were achieved, (3) how well the programs were serving "Pew fellows as students," and (4) how were the funds being spent. The result was that a balanced scorecard was achieved. There was a focus on four areas: (1) learning and innovation, (2) faculty and fellow satisfaction, (3) business operations, and (4) financial performance. For example, the program that had the weak-

The world of health policy is changing because the needs are changing. If PHPP had attempted to satisfy all the diverse needs through one large program, it probably would have failed.

est fellows according to the 1985 external evaluation had the strongest fellows by 1989. In general, program weaknesses cited in the first evaluations were corrected by the second evaluation.

Because a commitment structure was established by the foundation through financial dependence, the pressure from these external evaluations led to significant efforts to improve the program. In other words, the programs took these evaluations seriously for fear of being shut-down.[3] The evaluations advanced the learning from experience. The reports led to continual moves to improve the curricula and to make them more multidisciplinary, more distinct, more rigorous, and better integrated. The evaluations helped to teach the program sites what seemed to be "good" about the program. Thus, they provided the program sites with a type of feedback, unavailable when programs monitor their own behavior.

Over time the programs focused their efforts on the needs and perceptions of the fellows and building on the internal core competence of each school. Perhaps the best example of this evolution occurred at the Michigan program. . . ."One of the most striking features today is the degree to which the faculty and the program leadership have learned from earlier experiences, adjusted various aspects of the program, and refined the model to eliminate a variety of dysfunctional characteristics that were noted in the first evaluation" (Richardson, 1990, p 7).

As an aid to developing new programs, schools need systematic ways of analyzing ongoing programs. Without realizing it the external evaluations helped to pressure the programs toward self-improvement, a responsiveness to students, and continuous improvement.

> Targeting of excellent students requires the ability to offer them a valuable education (beyond their basic expectation), easy access to the best faculty, and protection from line responsibility.

## Managing the Tension Between Recruiting Experienced Leaders versus Young, Eager Learners

People with prior experience in complex organizations have developed political and social skills. Often they possess very different kinds of intelligence than the typical doctoral student, who has high verbal and mathematical-logical skills but who lacks extensive real-world experience. Older students with distinguished careers probably have learned a self-awareness and have developed an ability to manage conflict and negotiate with others. PHPP learned that there was a place in the doctoral world for the mature learner. The mix of experienced students with inexperienced students results in a rich, dynamic, and diverse learning environment.

[3] *Funding was discontinued largely for geographic reasons, not performance.*

## It Takes Three Years, Not Two

In the absence of a strong structure, the main questions that pre- and postdoctoral students must answer are: "Where do I focus my attention?" and "Where do my research interests lie?" There are infinite ways to address these questions, given the experiences, capabilities, and interests of the individual and given the particular school and educational context. The traditional way to organize doctoral education is to have students learn many research techniques, and to allow them to be distracted by many ideas. In this way, the students' research attention is dominated by coursework in a sequenced curriculum. The result is that the completion rates are poor, and it may take between 5 and 7 years to complete the PhD degree.

The promise of a 2-year program to complete the dissertation attracted many students. Although four Pew fellows finished in 23 or 24 months, the notion of a 2-year accelerated doctoral program was problematic. At BU/Brandeis the average time to completion of the dissertation was 3 to 4 years (Raskin, et al., 1992). The program offered 2 years of protection from job responsibilities; however, after the 2 years the funding ceased and many students, forced to go back to work, were distracted and prevented from achieving "accelerated" completion. An accelerated doctoral program in health policy required 3 years of full-time work with funding.

PHPP uncovered ways in which the predoctoral program could be completed with accelerated timetables. If Pew fellows were to compete their dissertations in less than 2 years, they have to think about a proposal before they take their qualifying examinations in January of their second year. Fellows had to assemble a dissertation committee, and conduct a literature review prior to taking the qualifying exam. This fast track meant that students had to make decisions about how they spent their time. The costs were more serious than the benefits, because a 2-year program meant that Pew fellows had to miss many of the special seminars and colloquia and other learning opportunities.

## To Create a National Identity, Joint National Meetings Made Sense

Each Pew fellow had very different professional backgrounds and experiences. Since the programs wanted the participants to create an identity that transcended the boundaries of their program sites, there was a need to meet and talk about

> There was a place in the doctoral world for the mature learner. The mix of experienced students with inexperienced students results in a rich, dynamic, and diverse learning environment.

shared experiences (Weick, 1995).  IOM, under Marion Ein Lewin's leadership, brought people together for retreats providing them with common experiences.  These centrally organized events become the glue of the "Pew Culture."

For example, during the first year of the program every fellow went to Washington, D.C.  The fellows were exposed to the world outside of their particular program.  They discovered that there were hot issues and policy wonks, gurus, and experts attached to those issues.  Each year an annual meeting was hosted by one of the programs.  These meetings brought the fellows together to talk about health policy and participate in "moments of conversation" with leading-edge thinkers and practitioners.  These sessions became major learning opportunities.

Without these joint national meetings, there would have been no shared stories, no common experiences, no postmortems on their programs, no sharing of frameworks, and no hope for a network that might outlive program funding.  Finally, there would have been no warm sentiment attached to the response, "Oh yeah? I was a Pew health policy fellow, too!"

> The promise of a 2-year program to complete the dissertation attracted many students; however, the notion of a 2-year accelerated doctoral program was problematic.

### Analyzing Softer Influences: The Power of a Program to Generate Enthusiasm and Empowerment

To have a more complete understanding of the Pew legacy, one must consider some of the influences that are harder to measure, but understand the enthusiasm of the program leaders and the students at each of the Pew sites.  Karl Weick (1995) has argued that "enthusiasm can produce wisdom because action creates experience and meaning."  Program enthusiasm partially explains some program success.  Enthusiasm was always generated at the program directors' meetings organized by Marion Ein Lewin.  The enthusiasm of Marion Lewin and her staff at IOM have clearly given the fellows a "special identity and national recognition."

Another subtle influence on program success (based on interviews with Pew fellows) is the extent to which the interviewed fellows seem to express a sense of empowerment and self-confidence.  It was clear that their education gave them an ability to make things happen.  All interviewees felt that they had acquired the knowledge and skills to analyze, make, and implement decisions affecting the policy system.  The 1994 survey revealed that for many fellows, the Pew program "launched them into better and more influential professional positions." In the words of one fellow, the program helped people to break "through the glass ceiling for non-PhDs." In the words of another fellow, the program "empowers individuals in their workplace."

## Success Requires Building on Core Competencies

The success of each program was a result of adopting a core competence perspective that required building on the strengths of each school. For the competency approach to work, the program leadership had to perform three basic tasks: (1) identify the existing distinct competencies, (2) improve and develop the competencies, and (3) deploy the competency in novel ways.

The creation of new educational niches in health policy research requires the development and deployment of at least three competencies: (1) expertise in multidisciplinary policy research, (2) flexible program development, and (3) "faculty focused on students" as a service concept. Turning a new pre- or postdoctoral curriculum into an effective educational program demands an ability to understand the area of study and the educational issues, anticipate student needs, and direct resources to meeting those needs.

The first competency is having a strong knowledge base in health services research and real-world expertise in the health policy sciences. The key indicators of knowledge and experiences are faculty publications, faculty involvement in major policy issues and initiatives, and a strong faculty record in basic and applied funded research.

The second competency for niche creation is "flexible program development." When compared with the lengthy time periods for completion of traditional pre- and postdoctoral programs, niche programs require shorter time periods, higher completion rates, and an ability to accommodate diverse student interests against diverse faculty research interests.

By and large, professional educational programs are built around degree concepts rather than the core competencies of the school. To be successful, the faculty must be focused on the needs of students. Faculty must know what students want, the faculty must accept that student expectations are reasonable, and performance standards must be set. A strong message must go out in the form of a service guarantee everyone (faculty and staff) at the program, without exception, will have a service-oriented attitude (Heskett, 1986).

During the first year of the program every fellow went to Washington, D.C. The fellows were exposed to the world outside of their particular program. They discovered that there were hot issues and policy wonks, gurus, and experts attached to those issues.

**Institutionalization Takes Time and It's Paradoxical**

Funded programs have a life cycle, and death is an inevitable feature. In the case of PHPP, death may not be inevitable. The longer a program survives in a school, the more institutionalized the program becomes—that is, the greater the likelihood that it will survive in the future. Institutionalization means acquiring both stability and status within a school. The degree to which an educational program has achieved institutionalization is defined partly by its age and depends on the degree to which flexibility, autonomy, and coherence have been achieved.

According to Kimberly (1981), "institutionalization is that process whereby new norms, values, and structures become incorporated within the framework of existing patterns of norms, values, and structures" (p. 31). So institutionalization takes time. In the case of the PHPP by the tenth year the programs were just beginning to understand how to make a niche educational strategy in health policy a success. However, innovation and institutionalization often work at cross purposes.

In creating new educational programs, success can be paradoxical (Kimberly, 1981). The problems of getting started and the problems of institutionalization lead to very different attention structures. Being new and different creates short-run opportunities for niche programs because commitment leads to experimentation and tolerance for mistakes (Kimberly, 1981). Eventually, institutionalization leads to formalization and stability, but "diminished innovativeness" (Kimberly, 1981).

> Fellows felt that they had acquired the knowledge and skills to analyze, make, and implement decisions affecting the policy system.

**The Best Lessons Are Often Unanticipated**

As is often the case, program evaluation measures the success or failure based on accomplishing predetermined goals. What's often lost in this type of analysis is an appreciation of the unintended consequences of programs. By observing and analyzing these unanticipated consequences one can also learn some powerful lessons.

At Michigan, for example, the faculty's experience with the off-campus education concept had several positive, although unanticipated consequences for faculty job satisfaction. The faculty found it very rewarding to have these part-time doctoral students coming to the campus to learn and then go back to their full-time jobs to apply that knowledge. Another unexpected consequence was the spill-over effect of the Pew experience to other corners of the school. The financial support from the Pew program made the faculty's policy research and teaching materials available to other health policy students in the school.

## HIGHLIGHTING COLLECTIVE ACCOMPLISHMENTS AND PROGRAM IMPACTS

For many reasons, understanding the collective accomplishments of any new educational program are difficult. Program consequences or impacts are often difficult to link (causally) to specific educational activities, because outcomes are "delayed, confounded, and negotiated" (Weick, 1995). Often people can only understand what they are doing many years after they have done something (Weick, 1995). If one were to fast-forward 10 or even 20 years, what would the Pew legacy be?

One simple, but inadequate, way to assess accomplishment is to count the final outputs produced or services provided. The program produced hundreds of people who have contributed to knowledge creation by publishing hundreds of publications and who will contribute to future health policy visions. Consequences will continue for many years in the future.

Another measure of accomplishment is to track job changes over time. Table 6 lists various health policy fields and Pew fellows' migration paths before and after attending the program. Although the entire program has helped to place many people into a variety of health policy positions, each of the program sites has had different impacts.

The BU/Brandeis and Michigan programs saw significant shifts into academic positions (from 21 percent to 37 percent and from 8 percent to 28 percent, respectively). BU/Brandeis, University of Michigan, and RAND/UCLA had greater shifts into research jobs (from 0 percent to 10 percent, 4 percent to 8 percent, and 9 percent to 20 percent). UCSF had some shifts to consulting (15 percent to 8 percent) and government (12 percent to 17 percent). UCSF and Michigan had small shifts into health care management (from 13 percent to 17 percent and 22 percent to 26 percent, respectively).

When one considers the range of positions occupied by Pew fellows today, one finds that there are few problems in the domain of health policy issues that lie out of some Pew fellows' reach. In one sense the program has fostered an invisible health policy college with a network of potential allies. It is presumed that Pew fellows will continue to improve the formulation and implementation of health policy. Whether this

**Institutionalization means acquiring both stability and status within a school. The degree to which an educational program has achieved institutionalization is defined partly by its age and depends on the degree to which flexibility, autonomy, and coherence have been achieved. However, innovation and institutionalization often work at cross purposes.**

# Table 6.

## Migration Paths of Pew Fellows by Program Site Before and After Attending the Program

| Field | BU/Brandeis | | UCSF | | Michigan | | RAND/UCLA | | Total (all programs) | |
|---|---|---|---|---|---|---|---|---|---|---|
| | Before | After | Before | After | Before | After | Before | After | Before | After |
| Academia | 14/67 (21%) | 25/67 (37%) | 34/83 (41%) | 38/83 (46%) | 4/50 (8%) | 14/50 (28%) | 23/69 (33%) | 23/69 (33%) | 74/269 (28%) | 98/269 (37%) |
| Consulting | 4/67 (6%) | 9/67 (13%) | 1/83 (1%) | 7/83 (8%) | 4/50 (8%) | 3/50 (6%) | 3/69 (4%) | 3/69 (4%) | 12/269 (5%) | 22/269 (8%) |
| Research | 0/67 (0%) | 7/67 (10%) | 2/83 (2%) | 3/83 (4%) | 2/50 (4%) | 4/50 (8%) | 6/69 (9%) | 14/69 (20%) | 10/269 (4%) | 28/269 (10%) |
| Government | 19/67 (28%) | 5/67 (7%) | 10/83 (12%) | 14/83 (17%) | 16/50 (32%) | 8/50 (16%) | 10/69 (14%) | 8/69 (12%) | 55/269 (20%) | 35/269 (14%) |
| Health Care Management | 17/67 (25%) | 7/67 (10%) | 11/83 (13%) | 14/83 (17%) | 11/50 (22%) | 13/50 (26%) | 14/69 (20%) | 11/69 (16%) | 53/269 (20%) | 45/269 (17%) |
| Professional Associations | 1/67 (2%) | 3/67 (4%) | 0/83 (0%) | 1/83 (1%) | 4/50 (8%) | 3/50 (6%) | 1/69 (1%) | 1/69 (1%) | 6/269 (2%) | 8/269 (3%) |
| Other | 7/67 (10%) | 1/67 (2%) | 15/83 (18%) | 3/83 (4%) | 6/50 (12%) | 3/50 (6%) | 4/69 (6%) | 4/69 (6%) | 32/269 (12%) | 10/269 (4%) |
| Data Missing | 5/67 (7%) | 10/67 (15%) | 10/83 (12%) | 3/83 (4%) | 3/50 (6%) | 2/50 (4%) | 8/69 (12%) | 5/69 (7%) | 26/269 (9%) | 18/269 (7%) |

NOTES: The data for classes entering 1983 to 1993 are included. All information retrieved from Pew directories corresponding with year of entry. The "Other" category, described in greater detail elsewhere, includes fields such as: clinical medicine, communications, and business.

potential network is used to help in major health reform or restructuring efforts in the future remains to be seen.

It was found that the program affected the program sites, the fellows, the faculty, IOM, the Pew Charitable Trusts, and the health policy world. Each of these will be discussed in turn.

## Program Sites

If one were to fast-forward 10 or even 20 years, what would the Pew legacy be?

According to leadership at each of the program sites, the schools benefited in a number of ways. Each program site learned how to organize a curriculum and a faculty that satisfied program faculty, students and external evaluators. Each program site also developed a methodology for the multidisciplinary training of predoctoral and postdoctoral students, and they were able to leverage these programs into larger educational domains.

Today UCSF has a health policy specialty that would not have existed without Pew support; it now has seminars and courses that would not have existed otherwise. For example, at UCSF a writing seminar and a health policy seminar that met every week built on the experience of the Pew program to develop an Agency for Health Policy Research training program, and interdisciplinary scholarly work came as a result of Pew. The Institute for Health and Aging would not have existed without the Pew program. The Pew program led to the development of a successful joint University of California at Berkeley/UCSF proposal to the Robert Wood Johnson Foundation for a program in health policy.

Brandeis was also able to extend the Pew experience into a successful new predoctoral program in health services research funded by Agency for Health Policy Research. RAND/UCLA found ways to sustain a commitment to the Pew approach to training and educating doctoral students. Finally, Michigan learned that the OJ/OC concept could work in doctoral education.

## Fellows

Each of the programs contributed to the fellows' professional lives in several ways. Many fellows spoke favorably about the education they received. The education helped many fellows to think about health policy in a rigorous way, expanding their knowledge of policy and their research skills. Fellows also claimed that they learned about the role of science and knowledge in political institutions.

Some fellows felt that they had obtained the credentials to be more legitimate and convincing advocates. The program also introduced fellows to multidisciplinary education. As a result, fellows claimed to have become better "policy colleagues" by developing a greater awareness, appreciation of, and respect for what their colleagues in other disciplines do.

### Faculty

The program also had important impacts on the faculty in every program. UCSF faculty spoke of the Pew experience as "broadening, offering faculty a chance to enrich their workloads and their professional careers." This enrichment occurred in several ways. Faculty claimed that the Pew courses were fun to teach, often exposing the faculty to challenging and stimulating sessions. Faculty, especially in the postdoctoral programs, wrote many papers with Pew fellows. When faculty worked with Pew fellows, they found that they were affected by them. For example, Pew faculty also learned to be better "policy colleagues" by working with fellows from disciplines other than economics—law, medicine, management, political science, and sociology.

Pew fellows will continue to improve the formulation and implementation of health policy. Whether this potential network is used to help in major health reform or restructuring efforts in the future remains to be seen.

### IOM

IOM also benefited from the Pew fellows, who continue to add a fresh voice to the policy work of the program. IOM has hired Pew fellows and commissioned papers and reports from Pew fellows. The rigorous training received by Pew fellows will continue to serve IOM in the years to come as fellows are called upon to help it deal with contemporary issues.

### Pew Charitable Trusts

For all the reasons cited above, it appears that the Pew Charitable Trusts have also benefited from the program. This program was one of the Trusts' first efforts that was national in scope. The program has been considered a tremendous success by the external evaluators and the health policy world. During the last decade, the effort took on all the characteristics of a "signature program" for the Trusts.

### Health Policy World

One can speculate endlessly on the presumed impacts on the policy world. But the most significant impact of the program has been the placement of highly educated people in strategic health policy positions in virtually every segment: academia, research and consulting, government and public health, professional associations, and health care delivery. Each individual has a unique set of special skills, yet each fellow is trained to understand the multidisciplinary nature of health policy. Each one is trained to translate research findings into policy-relevant and managerially relevant language. Each one is given an awareness of how politics, markets, and organizations works in health policy. Each one has an appreciation of the significance of knowledge in making better policy. Each one is committed to life-long learning.

Between 1991 and 1996 Pew fellows and alumni published about 650 scholarly papers and technical reports covering a wide variety of health policy subjects.

| Years | Estimated Number of Publications[a] |
|---|---|
| 1991-1992 | 106 |
| 1992-1993 | 127 |
| 1993-1994 | 159 |
| 1994-1995 | 165 |
| 1995-1996 | 92 |
| **Total** | 649 |

As one considers the contributions to knowledge made by these publications, one is reminded of Peter Drucker's insight into the central role of the individual: "Knowledge does not reside in a book, a databank, a software program; they contain only information. Knowledge is always embodied in a person; carried out by a person; created, augmented, and improved by a person; applied by a person; taught and passed on by a person; used or misused by a person" (Drucker, 1993, p. 210). According to Drucker, knowledge production is enriching, but the advancement of knowledge requires human action, and that requires defining a role for people. Envisioning a role for Pew fellows in the future is the subject of the final section.

[a] These estimates are based on self-reported figures given to the Program Office at IOM. It is likely that the actual number of publications is 20 to 40 percent higher.

## ENVISIONING A FUTURE POLICY ROLE FOR PEW FELLOWS

In the coming years, health policy will continue to be a high-drama, high-stakes, high-social-purpose field. With a growing underclass of vulnerable subpopulations, and with managed care and competition causing strategic re-orientations, alliances, and changes in finance and payment, the world of health policy becomes ever more complicated. Health policy makers will be central characters in this drama.

Today, health services research and health care management have emerged as new disciplines capable of making important contributions to health policy (Ginzberg, 1991). A recent study found that the demand for highly qualified health policy researchers would continue to exceed the supply (Field, et al., 1995). If the health care system needs more health policy scholars, doctoral education and postdoctoral programs focused health policy will remain important social investments. More well-educated people will be needed.

It is hoped that the Pew fellows will become the self-appointed "trustees" of this new health policy world.[5] Amidst the growing complexity, neither government nor the delivery system can afford to shoot from the hip. The health care delivery system of the future will be assigned responsibility for vulnerable populations. These organizations must develop an unprecedented capacity to learn–which includes understanding the issues and framing them as policy questions, discovering new theories, developing and deploying them, and evaluating the outcomes on the populations. To paraphrase a quote made by a hospital chief executive officer in the midst of this sea change:

> *"Today the familiar paths no longer seem to work. This time we will have to* think *our way out of this situation; because we can no longer simply* buy *our way out."*
> —Personal communication with a Boston-area hospital CEO
> [emphasis added is the authors']

The most significant impact of the program has been the placement of highly educated people in strategic health policy positions in virtually every segment: academia, research and consulting, government and public health, professional associations, and health care delivery.

That quote suggests that innovations in health policy will require abandoning old ways. Thought needs to be given to the knowledge base for policy makers, the need for better-educated policy makers, and the need to get off the treadmill to begin generating new ideas.

As one reflects on these lessons, one can see the need for health reform to be greater than ever. However, the future world of health policy does not need a brilliant leader with a vision. Health reform can be characterized as a massive construction project in need of academically oriented, meta-policy architects:[6]

1. Policy architects who are willing to advocate the social values that underlie desirable consumer and producer behaviors (responsibility, social justice, caring, and so on).

2. Academically-oriented architects who are continually sharing their deep understanding of the evolving needs

[5] *Borrowed from former Ambassador to Great Britain, Kingman Brewster, who asked, "Who are the Trustees of the future."*

[6] *The role of meta-architects was first described by Charles Handy (1990).*

of patient populations and the nature and capacity of the delivery system.

3. Practice-oriented policy architects who are producing knowledge and vision for the health policy world.

For several reasons, there is an opportunity for a collective rather than an individual role for Pew fellows. First, the difficulty of concentrating attention on more than a few policy issues at a time is a severe limitation for the health policy world. If, for example, one were to rely on the media to frame the health issues, the end result would be a faddish and transient agenda rather than an intellectual agenda (Simon, 1983). Without a group whose mission is to systematically identify and solve policy problems, attention drifts away from issue A to issue B to issue C.

Second, since most complex health policy issues are dynamically complex, single experts can have damaging effects on health policy. Rather than contribute to the pool of knowledge, experts and gurus often become symbols representing positions taken (pro and con) for any given solution. Knowledge can take generations to assimilate, but experts become "creatures of media machines" (Rieff, 1972). We prefer groups of people working together in teams because groups (when compared with individuals) have more information to share, have greater breadth and depth of experiences, and have the capacity to use multiple lenses. Therefore, by enlarging the pool of ideas, groups have the potential to produce higher quality and more effective policy decisions.

Third, Herbert Simon continually reminds us that each individual only sees the part of the world in which he or she lives and tends to aggrandize the importance of that part (Simon, 1983). Since Pew fellows are located throughout the policy world, no individual can see the whole world. Each fellow sees that part of the world that he or she knows. There is a need to share information.

Fourth, from a health policy standpoint, the delivery of health care depends on expectations about the future and the market's reactions to those expectations, and these are difficult to study. So, to understand the alternatives and their consequences, policy research and development and demonstrations in health care need to continue. For all these reasons there is a need for sustained attention from Pew fellows as a collective group.

Today there is a living, breathing network of more than 300 Pew fellows with a significant opportunity to influence health policy development. To be effective in health policy,

> Innovations in health policy will require abandoning old ways. Thought needs to be given to the knowledge base for policy makers, the need for better-educated policy makers, and the need to get off the treadmill to begin generating new ideas.

there will be a continued need for Pew fellows to bridge three cultures: (1) academia and intellectual research, (2) polity, and (3) health care delivery systems. The intellectual community must continue to focus on language and ideas, the polity must focus on the realpolitik allocation of values, and the delivery system must focus on people and services. The emotional and intellectual energies of those fellows will continue to make a tremendous difference if actions such as the following are taken:[7]

1. Translate and frame academic knowledge into policy-relevant and managerially relevant language.

2. Develop mechanisms to enlist new health policy fellows by: (a) establishing a new professional association or (b) establishing a virtual or invisible college, perhaps at the original program sites.

3. Launch a "virtual Pew program" in which Pew fellows will continue to share their collective knowledge, ideas, and other resources through distance learning technology, electronic networking, formally organized conferences and colloquia, and possibly, new policy publication outlets.

4. Maintain current information about Pew fellows and their locations in academia, federal and state government agencies, corporate organizations and the delivery system via a home page on the World Wide Web, newsletters, and phone directories.

5. Continue to hold annual reunions aimed at developing commitments to an intellectual agenda.

6. Continue to read, synthesize, contribute to, and disseminate the literature.

7. Continue to validate and refresh the policy-making inputs—the data, information, knowledge, and theories.

8. Track fellows global presence in health policy by developing a capacity to disseminate local knowledge through the Pew network and infrastructure.

For these actions to happen, there will be a need for a leadership group to emerge, with leaders willing to find common values and shared expectations and instill a deep respect for those areas where differences exist. These leaders who will not merely project the current system incrementally into the future, but will play with new ideas, discover new zones of study, and look upon change with what Karl Weick calls "disciplined imaginations."

This report has tried to capture some of the feelings and some of the spirit of the Pew Health Policy Program in its attempt to stimulate multidisciplinary education in health policy. By writing about this experience, it is hoped

Today there is a living, breathing network of more than 300 Pew fellows with a significant opportunity to influence health policy development.

[7] *Some of these ideas come from Hamel and Prahalad (1994) and Handy (1990).*

that something has been done to encourage people to think about the future. Health policy remains a vast subject, with an ability to affect human lives in extraordinary ways. The only possible conclusion that can be reached is that health policy has just begun to be studied. We believe that Pew fellows will continue to play a critical role in leading the effort.

# References

Advisory Board Meeting (February 1992). Minutes of the Pew Health Policy Program, Program Directors/Advisory Board Meeting, Washington, D.C.

Advisory Board Meeting (February 1993). Minutes of the Pew Health Policy Program, Program Directors/Advisor Board Meeting, Washington, D.C.

Altman, S.H. (1995). Value of interdisciplinary training in the health policy process. In *For the Public Good*, pp.156-160. Washington, D.C.: National Academy Press.

Bowen, W.G. and Rudenstein, N.L. (1992). *In Pursuit of the Ph.D.* Princeton, N.J.: Princeton University Press.

Delbecq, A. L., and Van de Veen, A.H. (1971). A group process model for identification and program planning. *Journal of Applied Behavioral Science* 7:466-492.

Drucker, P. (1993). *Post-Capitalist Society.* New York: Harper Business.

Feibelman, P. J. (1992). *A Ph.D. Is Not Enough: A Guide to Survival in the Sciences.* Reading, Mass.: Addison-Wesley.

Field, M. J., Tranquada, R. E., and Feasley, J.C., eds. (1995). *Health Services Research: Work Force Issues and Educational Issues.* Washington, D.C.: National Academy Press.

Ginzberg, E. (1991). *Health Service Research: Key to Health Policy.* Washington, D.C.: Foundation for Health Service Research.

Hamel, G., and Prahalad, C.K. (1994). *Competing for the Future.* Boston: Harvard Business School Press.

Hamilton, E. (1995). *Report on the Pew Health Policy Program.* Prepared for the Pew Charitable Trusts. Philadelphia, PA.

Handy, C. (1990). *The Age of Unreason.* Boston: Harvard University Press.

Heskett, J. L. (1986). *Managing in the Service Economy.* Boston: Harvard Business School Press.

Institute of Medicine (July 1993). Pew Health Policy Program, Narrative Report. Pew Charitable Trusts Grant T91-00482-001. Washington, D.C.: Institute of Medicine.

Kimberly, J. (1981). Initiation, innovation, and institutionalization in the creation process. In *The Organizational Life Cycle: Issues in the Creation, Transformation, and Decline of Organizations.* San Francisco: Jossey-Bass.

Lewin, M.E. (1995). Contributions of the Robert Wood Johnson Health Policy Fellowship and Pew Health Policy Programs. In *For the Public Good,* pp.146-155. Washington, D.C.: National Academy Press.

Institute of Medicine. Pew Fellow News (Winter 1996). Washington, D.C.: Institute of Medicine.

Raskin, K., Chilingerian, J., and Wallack, S. (December 1992). *Evolution of the Pew Health Policy Doctoral Program at Brandeis University.* Waltham, Mass: Institute for Health Policy, Florence Heller Graduate School for Advanced Studies in Social Welfare, Brandeis University.

Rieff, P. (1972). *Fellow Teachers.* New York: Dell Publishing Company: New York.

Richardson, W.C. (1990). Report on the Pew Health Policy Program. Prepared for the Pew Charitable Trusts. Philadelphia, PA.

Rimel, R. and Asbury, C. (1995). Personal correspondence to Marion Ein Lewin.

Rockhart, J.F. (March-April 1979). Chief executives define their own data needs. *Harvard Business Review* 52, N2: 81-93.

Schein, E. (1986). *Organizational Culture and Leadership,* San Francisco: Jossey-Bass.

Schroeder, S.A. (1995). The Institute of Medicine's Review of the Health Policy Fellowship Program. In *For the Public Good,* pp.161-166. Washington, D.C.: National Academy Press.

Simon, H. (1983). *Reason in Society.* New Haven, Conn.: Yale University Press.

University of California, San Francisco (1992-1993). Annual Report, Pew Health Policy Program.

University of California, San Francisco (August 1994). Proposal to the Pew Charitable Trusts for Continued Support for the Pew Health Policy Program at the University of California, San Francisco.

University of California, San Francisco (1992-1993). *Lessons Learned.*

University of Michigan (February 1993). Report of Michigan Site Visit. Ann Arbor, Michigan.

University of Michigan (1994). Annual Report, Pew Health Policy Fellowship Program.

University of Michigan (1994). Proposal Narrative.

Van de Ven, A.H. (1981). Early Planning, Implementation, and Performance of New Organizations. In, *The Organizational Life Cycle: Issues in the Creation, Transformation, and Decline of Organizations.* San Francisco: Jossey-Bass.

Wallack, S.S., and Chilingerian, J.A. (August 1994). Proposal to the Pew Charitable Trusts. Waltham, Mass.: Institute for Health Policy, Florence Heller Graduate School for Advanced Studies in Social Welfare, Brandeis University.

Weick, K. (1995). *Sensemaking in Organizations.* Newbury Park: Sage.

# APPENDIX A.

## *Telephone Interviews*

## Telephone Interview with Bill Weissert
Thursday, August 17, 1995, 10 a.m.

**1a.** *Based on your experience and familiarity with the fellows and the programs, what did we really accomplish? What were the most important contributions?*

We trained a lot of people in research findings from health services research, and we trained the last three or four cohorts pretty well in methods. We helped quite a few careers, and as with any program, we gave some degrees to people who probably should not have them. A program like this is particularly vulnerable because you hope that people will either stay or go into the health policy field instead of becoming academics. This is a real risk when you give a doctoral degree without requiring residence. You wind up giving a degree to people who are not really academics, but who are now qualified to teach. That is a downside of our program and something about which we are constantly vigilant.

The most obvious [contribution] is career development. You can clearly see that and more or less count it. Many alumni were promoted or got better jobs in the policy field as a result.

There is much about the policy process that is still happenstance and convenience—who is around. You can only improve the chances that rationality will play a part in policy by having around a lot of people who are trained rationally. So, the more people you put out there, the better chance you have to formally or informally influence the policy process. We train a lot of people who are interlopers or daily workers in the policy process. Therefore, we increase the chances that what comes out the other end will be better informed than it would have been if people had been shooting from the hip. Yet, it is hard to quantify that.

**1b.** *What is the Pew "legacy" in terms of:*

  *a)* *health policy?*

We made a lot more people aware of the power of the literature to answer a lot of the questions in a systematic way rather than guessing, as they were doing before. We helped with the diffusion of the health services research findings. I am always struck when I go to meetings and talk to folks who are making major policy decisions or influencing policy decisions without reading the literature. These foundation types and policy types have almost never read the literature. It's shocking. They are trying to move forward the state of the art without having found out what the state of the art is. They are verbal people, and they learn by hearing; they don't read. So, the bottom line: the more people who know about the literature and what it says and can relate to it, the more likely you are to influence the policy process. It may be an inefficient way, but I have not found anything that works better. Certainly, sending policymakers the articles does not work.

b) *education (doctoral, postdoctoral, or midcareer programs)?*

c) *your institution?*

For our institution it has led to a new degree program which we will keep. It broadened our presence in training health services researchers at the doctoral level. We had been primarily a master's program with a very small doctoral program; this gave us a whole new program, more bodies, and a slightly different cut of people. People came who were more in the policy process. Pew definitely had an influence on this institution's functioning and its contribution to health services research and health policy. It also made both the program and me more flexible in terms of how policy is defined. Policy is being made even within institutions. For example, I initially opposed a dissertation topic by somebody who was interested in how hospitals allocated the funds they were getting that go to education, how the medical school and hospital fight that out. I had said that wasn't really policy. Well, it is a policy question and now it's the leading policy question.

It has made us more flexible as a program in what we do to support women. When you take women who are in the midcareer process and they come into a long-term program like this, they are going to have babies. You have to be able to cope with that. You have to be prepared occasionally for a baby in the classroom. These are all good things. They make us a better university. I am pleased with that aspect of our program.

2. *How and why did your specific program develop? To what extent will your program continue now that Pew funding has ceased?*

We had an innovation here that dates back 25 years, which is this midcareer weekend program where people come in and take 2 years of the same courses. That was a proven idea that worked and cranked a huge number of people out into the health management community. So, with this program we extended that to the health policy community, and I think it's a good idea. And, it gets better every year. That's how it developed. It was basically an incremental change over a proven program that was and is unique in the country. It was innovative at the time and continues to be innovative.

There is no question that this program will continue. We have expanded it and bought off on it and found that we can sustain it. The big problem is that we will not have funding, and therefore, we will have a limited ability to reach people who need to be here with fellowships. We just don't have the money. To the extent that you're trying to reach people in the policy process, funding is pretty important because it's a field where people are not particularly well paid. Thus, without the proper funding we reduce our likelihood of influencing the policy process. But we will continue to get people who are either able to afford the program because they are MDs or because they are supported by their organization or interest group.

3. *What was the need in the health policy community when your program started, and how have those needs changed today? Is the job done?*

The need is the same. You have to train a lot of people because the path to influencing policy is very murky and difficult to predict so its better to have a lot of trained people around. Certainly, the job is *not* done. I continue to be shocked at the poor quality of policy in some areas, although I think it has gotten a lot better in the 20 years since I've been doing this.

4. *What was it about your curriculum that contributed or did not contribute to your program's success?*

The cohort effect—locking people into being part of a group for 2 years of intensive course work. I think that has a terrifically positive effect, is very successful, and socializes a lot of people. They learn from each other like crazy. The faculty learns as well.

Those things that do not contribute: It's difficult to take people who are midcareer and send them off after 2 years and have them finish their dissertation, although we have worked on that and we are about where we want to be on that. That's been a difficult problem to overcome. Getting back into the work site and not being forced to show up with papers every month. It's difficult not to let job demands take precedence.

There is no solution to this dilemma, however the

degree requirements that are imposed upon us by the accrediting organization of the schools of public health do not contribute to the success of the program. To satisfy the public health requirements, we had to find people to teach from other departments. That can lead to courses of variable quality. We amend this by flying people in from Boston and other universities. Every year it's a struggle.

5a.   *What was the most innovative or unique aspect of:*

a)   *your program design?*

Lockstep. Everybody has to take the same courses; they come in on weekends, they're midcareer, but the demands on them are no less than those on students in on-campus (OC) programs and may be even greater.

b)   *methods of implementation*

One method that works (Leon Wyszewianski's idea, but I implement it) is to give the students the usual statistics courses but have the methods course taught by a practitioner rather than a methodologist. That seems to be one of the most important courses we offer. The idea is that they will know what to do with the knowledge they learn. It's the best idea we have in the program. It takes these people from being theory-trained to appliers.

c)   *educational process?*

Answered previously.

6.   *Based on your experience, what lessons were learned about the educational process in terms of:*

a)   *recruitment?*

We tested the likelihood that we were producing a lot of false negatives. In the past we had been turning down people who might have been able to make it, and this year we let them in. What we found was that with a 10 percent drop in Graduate Record Examinations (GRE) scores we could increase our cohort size by 100 percent. I do not see a substantial difference in performance. We have proportionately more people who shouldn't have been in, but not an increase in the percentage. So, we have the same number of people we wish we had not admitted, but we always have some we wish we had not admitted. Some of those drop out and some don't. It confirms my long-held hypothesis that we only worry about false positives and in the process throw out two or three who could have made it, and this year we included those people and most of them were pretty good choices.

b)   *degree requirements?*

We dropped a bunch of prerequisites this year that we thought were pseudo prereqs. We required people to worry and study to pass an exam that everybody passed or everybody flunked. I just threw out everything that wasn't either statistics or economics prerequisites, and it worked. We got rid of some people who just couldn't cut it in terms of the quantitative stuff. And as for the others, we didn't put them through a lot of Mickey Mouse stuff.

c)   *curriculum and content?*

d)   *integration of fellows with other students, the rest of the university, and the program in general?*

It's approaching zero. We have them here all day in class, and they work and party as a cohort. There is almost no interaction with other university students. I have tried to integrate the OC and off-campus programs, but the OC programs are threatened. Someday we'll get more integrated. The greatest positive of integration would be to give a dose of reality to the OC people and perhaps a little more of the role of cognates in research to the off-campus people.

e)   *relationship between faculty and students?*

I don't think there are programs in which the relationship is better than in this program. The faculty and students are collegial. The students are experienced and not shy. There is a very good relationship.

f)   *completion rates (where applicable)?*

This is something we have worked on constantly. Our penultimate cohort is up to 66 percent with a couple more likely to come through. I don't think doctoral programs ever want to be 100 percent. So I think that's just terrific.

**7a.**   *To what extent do you think there were "programmatic" barriers to student completion?*

We didn't really have anybody whose job it was to make sure the students were equipped to do a dissertation. They had advisers, but they weren't even seeing their advisers once a month. So, we made an institutional change and added a course where someone actually taught the students how to write, one step at a time.

**7b.** *To what extent do you think the program was beneficial for those who did not finish the program?*

Everyone who drops out basically praises what they've learned so far and report that they are immediately applying the stuff. We know from classroom assignments that it is very typical for the students to use what we assign that month or the next in their job. An example would be where we sent them off to do a policy analysis and provide policy options for the Secretary, and the Secretary actually chose one of their policy options. That is not untypical.

**7c.** *How can we measure success for those programs where completion rates do not apply (i.e., postdoctoral programs)?*

Look closely at the people who applied and were turned down. Compare their outcomes and influences with those who got in. Where are they with their careers and what kind of impact have they had on the policy process? Do a comparison group study.

**8.** *How does the Pew fellowship approach differ from a traditional fellowship approach? How have the major outcomes differed?*

The major differences are within the cohort. We examine the product that these people are getting and make changes in faculty and courses in order to change their total product. So, it is not a course-by-course assessment, which is true for traditional OC programs. We look at the product and say, "Are these people getting enough of this particular thing? If not, where in all of their courses can we add it?" Since there is no discretion, we can focus on things they really need.

Major outcomes do not differ very much. Pew people tend to be somewhat more policy focused and more involved.

**9.** *If you were asked to give advice to another university attempting to initiate a similar program, what would you say?*

You need to make sure that the best faculty are willing to teach Saturdays and Sundays. Faculty do not realize that they will be teaching at least 5 of the 7 or 7 of the 9 months on weekends, both Saturday and Sunday. This is a big commitment that needs to be established up front.

**Telephone Interview with Carroll Estes**
Wednesday, August 23, 1995, 4 p.m.

1a. *Based on your experience and familiarity with the fellows and the programs, what did we really accomplish? What were the most important contributions?*

I think the Pew program has very successfully seeded the field with competent, well-trained scholars at government levels, nonprofit and foundation levels, and university levels. The flowering and capability of those fellows and their contributions are beginning to be recognized at fairly significant levels. For example, one of our fellows was chair of one of the White House task forces on benefits in the health reform area (Linda Bergthold). The most important contribution of the fellows is a passionate commitment to health policy and health services research that is objective and has an impact and the ability to carry out that work either directly themselves or to stimulate organizations and institutions to do it where they are.

1b. *What is the Pew "legacy" in terms of:*

a) *health policy?*

There is very specific expertise that is available in the field as a result of the Pew program. I don't think it's enough. I think the program falls short by cutting itself to an end prematurely. I think the Pew Health Policy Fellowship Program needed to be extended a minimum of another 10 years. I look more toward the Robert Wood Johnson Clinical Scholars model. The magnitude of the work and the magnitude of change in the field is such that health policy contributions have just begun to be made, and these scholars will be around as they are becoming policy makers. Nevertheless, there is very important substantive work that still has to be done in health policy, and the training of more leaders continues to be needed.

b) *education (doctoral, postdoctoral, or midcareer programs)?*

There certainly are seminars and courses that exist on our campus that would not have existed on this campus without support from Pew. There are other postdoctoral programs that are multiplier effects from the Agency for Health Care Policy and Research (AHCPR), but now we don't know the extent to which AHCPR is going to be a viable institution to continue what would be complementary

programs of training. There is no question that interdisciplinary, scholarly work in health policy has been forwarded as a
result of the Pew commitment and faculty commitment to
education on a multidisciplinary level has probably grown.
In terms of UCSF (University of California, San Francisco)
there is no question that the Institute for Health and Aging,
which is a major research institute that did not exist prior to
the Pew program, probably exists in large part because of the
support from Pew for both research and the training program. It does research in education and is a multimillion-
dollar-a-year institute that is contributing quite a bit in terms
of disability statistics and health and long-term care policy.

c)     *your institution?*

Answered above.

2.     *How and why did your specific program develop? To what extent will
your program continue now that Pew funding has ceased?*

It developed because we had two people who had significant research backgrounds and experience on which a
successful training program could be built. Furthermore we
had faculty who had many specific methodological substantive skills to offer. Our particular program began with predoctoral, management, postdoctoral, and midcareer components. I think we found that the midcareer program was a
very good route for certain people who were quite accomplished and had a lot to bring to the classroom, but who
needed to acquire the health policy and interdisciplinary
skills. These people already had positions of influence into
which they could carry this. We obviously had a charismatic
leader in Phil Lee. He had great vision of where health policy needed to go, and he served as a catalyst to bring together existing resources and capabilities and make this happen.

     To what extent will the program continue now that
funding has ceased? I think that there are serious institutional problems at the University of California which have to do
with funding problems. There has been a 25 percent cut in
educational resources in the last 4 years alone, with no
appreciable resource increase. The academic health centers
questions with regard to health care restructuring and their
competitiveness in the new managed care world have further
raised resources questions for major medical centers and
health science centers. This just means that the resource base
from general-source supports that one had hoped to institutionalize are more difficult than ever to access due to factors

that have nothing to do with the success of the program and that are totally exogenous. There are and will continue to be research seminars. There will continue to be the search for postdoctoral training programs—individual and institutional—to keep the concept alive. However, the lack of institutional support or the lack of faculty support and uncertain or declining federal training grant support will impede the magnitude or the size of such programs. It's not news. It has been said at every meeting we've had that Pew should not be cutting off at this point.

3. *What was the need in the health policy community when your program started, and how have those needs changed today? Is the job done?*

We were very concerned about access, cost, and quality when we started, and we are still concerned with access, cost, and quality. No, the job isn't done. Access is worse than ever. Quality questions are bigger than ever. There are programs that attempt to cap cost but really don't do cost containment on the system level. The work that needs to be done is bigger and more important than ever.

4. *What was it about your curriculum that contributed or did not contribute to your program's success?*

UCSF has a health policy specialty that it did not have prior to the Pew doctoral program in the Department of Social and Behavioral Sciences. A major success of our program has been the curriculum of the writing seminar and every week a seminar on health policy issues with faculty and fellows presenting on a convening ground. The writing seminar is stunning, and our fellows probably have a much stronger publishing record than they would have had without it. We have been very fortunate to have on our faculty the West Coast Editor of *JAMA,* Dr. Drummond Rennie, who has really done an incredible job with stimulating and encouraging publications.

5a. *What was the most innovative or unique aspect of:*

a) *your program design?*

One innovative aspect is the hands-on research with ongoing faculty investigators who have major programs of research and the competency to direct fellows in wide areas of interest, which allowed for special approaches that fellows might have.

I think the writing seminar was very crucial and very exciting in teaching how to critique and to take critique.

b)    *methods of implementation?*

Implementation was through the colleagueship and mentoring and the coauthorships and separate authorships through these large-scale research projects. The fact the two institutes at UCSF together have about $20 million in funded research every year and probably 40 faculty investigators who are well known in their area has really contributed to implementing very significant training opportunities.

c)    *educational process?*

The Pew conferences every year have been important. Networking and socialization to the field, the norms of work, and networking of colleagues have been important parts of the educational process. I have already mentioned the unique element of the writing seminar, which was very challenging or is very challenging to fellows, while also being very productive. Our weekly seminars are valued and the rooms are packed with a lot of other people wanting to join these seminars.

**5b.**   *What were the biggest challenges or barriers to overcome of:*

a)    *your program design?*

Getting doctors to mix with social scientists, to be open to learning, to be able to do what is basically social science-type research. For the social scientists it's similarly the obverse of learning more about how health care institutions actually work from a health professional perspective.

b)    *methods of implementation?*

c)    *educational process?*

The integration of the disciplines really has worked, the method of implementation was constant, and there are continuing opportunities for interchange and various projects and seminars.

**6.**    *Based on your experience, what lessons were learned about the educational process in terms of:*

a)    *recruitment*

We probably send out 200 institutional letters a year. As everything, the word of mouth in the field and the referral from other fellows is a very important source of recruitment. Obviously, the excellence of our faculty and their reputations were the single most important attraction in recruitment. So, I think you need a sterling faculty and a sterling institution for recruitment.

b) *degree requirements?*

We require a doctoral degree or a health professional degree. We only had a predoctoral program for a couple of years. We missed the predoctoral part and were sad that it was cut out. It was not our choice. I think the degree requirements for a postdoc were appropriate, and basically, taking people who already had some health policy experience was far better than having people who had none or who had some health services contact in education. In a short 2-year program people really needed to have another degree or some courses in the area prior to entrance. Otherwise, it is a much bigger learning curve that is harder to deal with. It also holds back others in terms of the complexity of the material.

c) *curriculum and content?*

We made courses required at certain times in the program. We found it was very important to be explicit and to have some details and firm requirements. All students were required to participate in the writing seminar and Pew seminar. But we learned that it was also important to have flexibility for other aspects of the curriculum, allowing people to search out the curriculum opportunities. Nonetheless, we wanted to create a strong methodological component and we wanted to make sure courses in particular areas such as art and science, proposal writing, and other basic course skills were available, and they were essentially required. The proposal writing piece was very important. A course in economics was essentially required, unless people had comparable experience.

d) *integration of fellows with other students, the rest of the university, and the program in general?*

We definitely integrated our fellows with fellows funded from the National Institute on Aging, AHCPR, and other private foundation training programs. This strategy benefited everyone. We opened up our courses to selected other faculty probably more than to other students, although an occasional exceptional student would be permitted (e.g., nurses working on doctorates). But we really tried to keep our courses small and with a select group of fellows, because it needed to have the collectiveness and a community spirit and connection. We also were intent on training and making sure that content was tailored to the interests and skills of our fellows.

> e) *relationship between faculty and students?*

The relationship was and is extremely close. The relationships developed through collaborations on research projects and the weekly seminars and occasional social events. I do think the conferences have been important in networking. Faculty and students worked together on those conferences and jointly attended them.

> f) *completion rates (where applicable)?*

All our predoctoral students did graduate, and we are very proud of them. In term of our postdoctoral students, this does not really apply.

**7a.** *To what extent do you think there were "programmatic" barriers to student completion?*

This relates more to predoctoral programs.

**7b.** *To what extent do you think the program was beneficial for those who did not finish the program?*

All our fellows finished our program.

**8.** *How does the Pew fellowship approach differ from a traditional fellowship approach? How have the major outcomes differed?*

This is much more of an interdisciplinary experience and much less of a lone wolf researcher experience: do it independently on your own and sink or swim on your own. There is much more of a faculty-planned approach and a commitment to annual reviews, mentorship meetings, preceptor meetings, and scheduled reviews of students. There are more groups meeting with faculty members on programs of activity in what they have accomplished and what they want to accomplish and getting mentorship and advice on papers, research proposals, and jobs. I don't think in most other fellowships there exists that kind of tutorage. There is really a community commitment here, a lot of which is possible because of the general support that Pew provided, which allowed for the support of faculty who otherwise would not have support for any teaching and/or mentorship concern. This will be a tremendous loss for the program because there are no replacement funds for that institutionally or in terms of other federal grants. It would have to be a foundation-type program.

The outcomes have differed dramatically from those from the traditional fellowship approach, for example, the productivity of our fellows in terms of research and publications. We would stand them up against any federal postdoc program, and I think they would be probably have twice the rate in terms of explicit measures of productivity. It is that nurturing, collectiveness, orientation, network, and support that the fellows offered each other.

9. *If you were asked to give advice to another university attempting to initiate a similar program, what would you say?*

There has to be some way of getting the leadership of the university to support faculty time to develop and maintain excellence in teaching and mentoring. I think you need excellent faculty and a strong research program because the training has got to be hands-on with experience and supervision. I would also say how important a writing seminar is, and that there needs to be an explicit allocation of resources to ensure that there is training in writing, proposal development, and publication. It's just essential.

## Telephone Interview with Dennis Beatrice
Wednesday, August 16, 1995, 10 a.m.

**1a.** *Based on your experience and familiarity with the fellows and the programs, what did we really accomplish? What were the most important contributions?*

We mastered the art of cross-training. We trained our fellows in analysis and policy. This approach is more important now than ever because the fine lines between health policy analysts and health policy makers are becoming blurred.

**1b.** *What is the Pew "legacy" in terms of:*

**a)** *health policy?*

The Pew program enabled people who wanted to become program analysts to obtain both the analytic and policy training needed.

Pew put policy types in an academic setting. Pew took people from state and federal positions. A new and different cadre of individuals was put through this program.

The Pew program retooled and juiced up several cohorts of people who would ultimately end up in public policy positions.

**b)** *education (doctoral, postdoctoral, or midcareer programs)?*

Pew educated a new kind of PhD, one better prepared and more relevant for today's world.

**c)** *your institution?*

At Brandeis, Pew succeeded in bringing a different kind of student into the university. The Pew program got Brandeis thinking about ways to accommodate different students in different tracks (practitioner training versus research training).

**d)** *other?*

**2.** *How and why did your specific program develop? To what extent will your program continue now that Pew funding has ceased?*

With the help of the Pew program, Brandeis has initiated Health Institute Fellowships. The very best health applicants are recruited. The institute has committed itself to the training and support of these students. This is the way that Brandeis has kept and will continue to keep the Pew spirit alive.

3. *What was the need in the health policy community when your program started, and how have those needs changed today? Is the job done?*

The job is not done. PhDs need to change because the environment needs more academic types in government. Government people can no longer shoot from the hip. The stakes are too high. We need to bring those two worlds together. We need to continue to educate, train, and produce a "different" kind of student.

4. *What were the biggest challenges or barriers to overcome of:*

a) *your program design?*

How do you create an accelerated program that people can finish without watering down the content? There is tension within this issue. The program works well for some. Some work better at an accelerated pace.

5a. *To what extent do you think the program was beneficial for those who did not finish the program?*

I did not finish; however, I got a better fix on how one uses analysis and graduate education in nonacademic settings. There is great utility in the Pew training.

5b. *How can we measure success for those programs where completion rates do not apply (i.e., postdoctoral programs)?*

What happened to the fellows? That is by far the greatest measure of success. Is there a plausible reason to believe that those who did not finish still benefited from their Pew training and achieved a heightened awareness? This may be a soft analysis. But, there is no proxy measure.

6. *If you were asked to give advice to another university attempting to initiate a similar program, what would you say?*

I would be as explicit as possible. I would emphasize the practical/analytical aspects of the program. Institutions need to be prepared to recruit people who are able to adhere to a very strict, high level of work. Pay close attention to the benefits of "cross-training."

## Telephone Interview with Hal Luft
Thursday, August 17, 1995, 11:30 a.m.

**1a.** *Based on your experience and familiarity with the fellows and the programs, what did we really accomplish? What were the most important contributions?*

Among the main things is that we have developed an integrated program across three or four sites that involves a wide range of people from fresh graduate students to fairly senior career people. We have placed those people into various settings ranging from the university to major health policy kinds of settings. The fellows are doing a great job. We have also established three programs that are likely to survive past Pew.

**1b.** *What is the Pew "legacy" in terms of:*

a)     *health policy?*

It is hard to identify specific health policies that have changed one way or the other as a result of the Pew program per se. I am not clever enough to picture an alternative universe in which there was not a Pew program and what would have been different. But I do have the sense that some of the fellows have been doing very exciting things that are having an impact on the way that the health care system is changing and the way that health policy is being formulated. That probably would not have happened had those people not gone through the Pew program.

b)     *education (doctoral, postdoctoral, or midcareer programs)?*

I suspect at UCSF (University of California, San Francisco) that we would have not had a postdoctoral program had there not been the Pew funds to get it started. We would not have had the AHCPR (Agency for Health Care Policy and Research) training grant because that built on our experiences with Pew. And, I suspect that there would not have been as nearly as strong an application from Berkeley and UCSF for the Robert Wood Johnson Health Policy Scholars. I suspect the same thing would have been true for Michigan. All these things can be linked back to the Pew program. It is hard for me to say what would have happened at Brandeis or Michigan without the Pew program, but I can say that at UCSF, without that sort of core training program, our postdoctoral program probably would not have gotten started.

c) *your institution?*

What has developed here is a clear commitment to postdoctoral training. The training program itself has helped bring together faculty and research projects. We now have quite a few faculty at UCSF who were trained in the Pew program who would not be doing what they are doing at UCSF had they not been Pew fellows. So, in a sense it is being institutionalized through the faculty.

d) *other?*

There is a network of people out there who will probably continue to interact. Something needs to be done to encourage that, to retain that in the future. The Pew network of fellows will continue to draw upon each other in a way that would have not been the case had they just been independent postdocs.

2. *How and why did your specific program develop? To what extent will your program continue now that Pew funding has ceased?*

Phil Lee's commitment to training, to doing health policy and health policy research, and to incorporating a wide range of people with different backgrounds and expertise was crucial. Another aspect to it was that prior to the program, UCSF had gotten a grant from the Mellon Foundation to set up a clinical epidemiology program affiliated with the institute. That served as a basis for people thinking about the development of postdoc training programs. Mellon had a very clear vision of institutionalizing the program by training faculty who would then stay at that campus and become the leaders of the future. Although staying at the site was not a goal of Pew early on, the idea of training people and returning them to the field helped to shape the Pew proposal.

Another aspect was that unlike the other programs, the institute is essentially a freestanding research group, not a department—we don't grant degrees. Our faculty saw the opportunity of developing a postdoctoral training program as a very exciting opportunity to do some teaching, to get involved with students in ways that were not normally available. We're not apt to do a lot of teaching in the medical school or nursing schools. Here was a program where we could really do something.

The third piece was that many of the faculty involved in the institute come out of a multidisciplinary background and believe that good integrative health policy research and policy analysis is something that is valued and is good to do, and this gave us an opportunity, in a sense, to reproduce. There is a certain, almost biological urge, but it made a lot of sense. It allowed us to build a program that fulfilled a need in the field, one that we weren't seeing being filled.

There remains a certain amount of uncertainty surrounding the maintenance of such a program because we don't have any major grants. We are waiting to hear about AHCPR. There are active discussions going on among some leadership people within the university to try to develop a new postdoc program, and so we are working on that and thinking about various ways of financing it. Can I say that we have something in place? No. Are we working on it? Yes, with a strong commitment to make something happen.

3. *What was the need in the health policy community when your program started, and how have those needs changed today? Is the job done?*

When our program started there were very few integrated postdoc fellowship programs. I think now there are more of them, some funded by AHCPR, Robert Wood Johnson Clinical Scholars, the new Johnson Policy Scholars, etc. So there are definitely more opportunities and programs for postdoc fellows. On the other hand I think the need for training and the demand for well-trained people have been increasing even more rapidly. I still don't see a lot of programs that are really focused on integrating people from multiple disciplines. For instance, the Johnson clinical scholars are for clinicians, the Johnson Policy Scholars are for Political Scientists and Sociologists, and the AHCPR, while broader, tends to have very few people at any one site and is often more predoc focused rather than postdoc focused. Furthermore, there is not much integration across sites and not enough blending.

Bottom line: there is still a real need. I don't think the job is done.

4. *What was it about your curriculum that contributed or did not contribute to your program's success?*

There are two major things: (1) mentoring. The model that we chose worked well, and that's a model where the fellows basically get involved with one or two faculty members, work on some projects, and get that hands-on experience. It's more of an apprenticeship model than a classroom model. (2) I think over time, admittedly with some prodding from the Pew Charitable Trusts, we developed a more structured set of seminars and courses. I think the health policy seminar had always been successful, but by making it more formal, by structuring sequences within it, I think it has become much better. I think the writing seminar that Drummond Rennie led worked extraordinarily well. It helped the fellows produce publishable papers and learn how to do high-quality work in a supportive but critical environment. My art and science class filled a niche that other people seemed not to get training in.

The curriculum might still have benefited from tighter structure; it is far from rigid. We are tightening up some of the mentoring relationships, doing more reviews, and making sure people are moving along the way they ought to be moving along in terms of productivity. We continue to improve it year by year.

**5a.** *What was the most innovative or unique aspect of:*

**a)** *your program design?*

The apprenticeship model. It is a postdoc program, but its a structured postdoc program with people working on projects with faculty members.

**b)** *methods of implementation?*

In a sense this is also a response to the kind of situation that we're in where almost all of our faculty are on soft money with research projects. Asking them to teach lots of courses without paying for it can be difficult. Getting fellows involved with them in research projects does work. It's a win-win situation. We have learned how to build a model that works in that kind of environment.

**5b.** *What were the biggest challenges or barriers to overcome of:*

**a)** *your program design?*

**b)** *methods of implementation?*

**c)** *educational process?*

In general, one of the biggest challenges early on was space. When we were located in our old site, on the main campus, there wasn't even enough room for faculty. So there was no place for the postdocs. They were hanging out in weird and bizarre places. They were often off site in office space provided, but this hindered interaction. When we moved 5 years ago we provided real office space for all the fellows as part of the unit. They were integrated with the faculty, with the unit. It works a lot better.

Matching fellows with faculty has always been a bit of a challenge. Because of the nature of the educational model you need to get a good match. We struggled back and forth in terms of how does one develop that match. Sometimes it becomes a problem because the fellows feel like they are in a candy store: there are all these great things to choose from. They sort of freeze. We are now restructuring that a little bit. This year we'll provide a handbook describing each of the faculty and what he or she is doing. We have always had faculty presentations, but it goes by too quickly and is often too intense. Three days of hearing 30 to 40 faculty members speak. . .it all blurs together. We are now having present only those faculty seriously interested in having fellows participate.

While I think we have attracted and recruited very good fellows. With one or two exceptions where the fellow had decided to move on to another position early on, I don't think we ever washed anybody out. Sometimes one might question that. It's not like you have a graduate program with exams that people just don't pass. There isn't a clear criterion for dropping somebody after a period of time. It's fuzzy. I'm not sure I would recommend major changes, but I think in the future there might be somewhat more careful review so that people have a more clear sense that the second year is not guaranteed.

6. *Based on your experience, what lessons were learned about the educational process in terms of:*

   a) *recruitment?*

Identifying a good match is one of the key things that needs to be done. It's not just saying that this person has the right degree of horsepower and interest, but how is he or she going to fit into the program? Are there a couple of good potential matches with faculty members and their ongoing projects? Working that through is very important.

At the postdoc level we find ourselves sometimes attracting people who are also looking at starting faculty positions at the same time. The timing of that is not always ideal. They may or may not be getting an offer from somebody, and how are we going to ask them to make a decision by "Friday" when they may or may not have a firm tenure-track offer from a great university in 3 weeks. Are you going to hold them to that or not? What that process then does sometimes is extend the admissions process for those candidates (often the best candidates are the ones in this position), and then if they finally say no, then you may end up going fairly far down your list because other people have already excepted other positions. How to play that through? We need to be working on this.

    b)    *degree requirements?*

We don't have a degree. In terms of what is expected of the fellows we have been fairly flexible. We have some people who are on trajectories toward faculty positions, so they really need to be publishing and we are encouraging them to do that. There are others who are much more policy oriented, and for these fellows publication is secondary. We encourage research for them as well, but we have them working on other kinds of projects, doing other kinds of reports. This flexibility has worked well. It is not a problem; rather it is a matter of learning how to have everybody understand that to some extent we are willing to tailor the program, but that does not mean that we are willing to be pushovers.

    c)    *curriculum and content?*

The core seminars are basically the same for everybody, although sometimes we have some flexibility. For example, we encourage fellows to take a research design course, but some fellows who have come in with good research skills ask to take other courses, and we are flexible with that.

    d)    *integration of fellows with other students, the rest of the university, and the program in general?*

This has worked out very well in terms of our postdocs at the Institute. Part of that has been a conscious strategy of using Pew funds to supplement other fellowship funds so we'll have people who were fully funded by Pew and others who basically got $1,000 all mixed together in the same classes. We did not establish a pecking order. We set a standard for fellowship applicants and say this is the standard all our applicants have to meet, and then once they are in that acceptable pool, who we ill give what kind of dollars to out of what pot partly depends on the constraints of the pots. For example, the AHCPR program really is more interested in people who are going to be academics rather than people going into policy careers. So, we have shifted the AHCPR dollars toward them and the Pew dollars go for the people who are more policy oriented. There are some Pew dollars going to the research people and some AHCPR dollars going to the policy people to bring them up to the same stipend level. Everybody is on equal footing. That integration has worked very well. I frankly cannot remember who of our fellows have been primarily Pew and who have not. We are fully integrated.

In terms of interaction with the rest of the university, that is becoming better. In the last couple of years we have expanded the program in some way. Each year for the last 3 or 4 years we have had at least one clinical fellow spending all of his or her research time with us. They go to our seminars, they get involved with a faculty member research project, and they are basically integrated into the fellowship program, but they are paid for by somebody else entirely. These are people who would have otherwise been doing bench research on pulmonary function, for example. They are now doing work on risk adjustment models and health care costs of AIDS, etc., exactly the kinds of things the Pew fellows do. In this way we are integrating our fellows with other people in the classic fellowship programs on this campus.

e) *relationship between faculty and students?*

The relationship works very well. There have been some situations where the match has not been perfect. In general, people like having fellows. In many instances the faculty see the fellows more as colleagues than as students. We have also had situations where faculty have research assistants who then start functioning as fellows. In other words, what we do is pay them for 70 percent of their time, and the other 30 percent of their time they do fellowship activities. Often we will include them in the Pew program as Pew fellows. This is another way in which we have institutionalized things. My guess is that many of the fellows don't even know whether the person sitting next to them is funded out of fellowship money or project money. We have done that by having a set of criteria where we say this person is eligible for a fellowship. Now, how do we fund him or her?

f) *completion rates (where applicable)?*

Basically everyone has completed the program with the exception of one or two who left early on for wonderful opportunities elsewhere. We have had a few fellows who have taken more than 2 years, and usually it was because they got additional fellowship support for the third year and it made sense for them to stay the third year either for a spousal connection or another reason. I would not call that a lack of completion.

**7a.** *To what extent do you think there were "programmatic" barriers to student completion?*

It's more PhD related.

**7b.** *How can we measure success for those programs where completion rates do not apply (i.e., postdoctoral programs)?*

I think that this is probably the hardest thing. One way to look at it would be to look through our alumni lists and look at where they are. Do you get a warm, fuzzy feeling? Are they doing the kinds of things that you would like them to be doing? If you look at it from the perspective of the Robert Wood Johnson scholars which basically prepares fellows to be the future chairs of medicine, you probably wouldn't think someone who just went into private practice to be a huge success. On the other hand, I know one person who is in private practice but who continues to be interested in health policy issues and who writes articles on health policy issues for the *New England Journal of Medicine*. That's still a success. In terms of our postdocs and where they've gone, almost all of them are doing things related to health policy in various kinds of settings; some of them are academic and some of them are not. I don't think there are very many just sort of doing routine kinds of activities. You would not look at these people and say, "Well, they probably would have been doing this anyway." That's probably the best implicit measure of success.

If you really wanted to put a lot of energy and effort into it, what you could do is ask the fellows what they think their career would have been had they not done the postdoc fellowship and what does it now look like? Of course, you get a certain amount of bias in that. Ideally, what you would have had would be the career trajectories that they would have written prior to applying. I can tell you that I went through a postdoc training program, and had I not done that, I would have had a very different career trajectory.

**8.** *How does the Pew fellowship approach differ from a traditional fellowship approach? How have the major outcomes differed?*

The Pew program has the policy focus and the integration of different experiences, different disciplines and different programs. You have the network, which is very important, making it bigger than any one program.

Outcomes? Hard to say. Most of the Johnson clinical scholars, the other major program, have done very good stuff, but they are all MDs. Now, some of our fellows are

MDs, but most of them are not, so it is hard to separate. Its hard to know how much of that is Pew and how much is MD versus PhD. But I think the Pew program has really been more policy oriented and not wholly academically focused. I think that's a real plus. It also means that some of the academic fellows get to know and rely on the nonacademically focused ones, and vice versa. So, then, people who go and become policy analysts in the government can then call on their colleagues for advice in ways that would not have been done had they not gone through that joint training program.

9. *If you were asked to give advice to another university attempting to initiate a similar program, what would you say?*

You really need to think through the nature of the faculty, what their incentives are, how they would benefit in the development of a program like this, and how you can bring them along in terms of doing it and structure it very carefully to fit that setting. Our model is very faculty intensive with little in the way of dollars. So, you have to have a whole series of other things that make it work. It's not like we are a PhD program where faculty are going to get teaching credits for doing the teaching as a fairly structured kind of thing where you can say here is the syllabus, go do it. Our program is a little bit like an individually designed house that you need to build onto the wall of a mountain. You really need to understand the local geology. When you do its wonderful. But you can't simply take those blueprints and use them somewhere else.

**Telephone Interview with Doctoral Alumnus
John McDonough**
Tuesday, September 5, 1995, 10 a.m.

**1a.** *Based on your experience and familiarity with the Pew program, what did the fellowship really accomplish? What are the most important contributions?*

Personally, the Pew program gave me a lot of skills that I did not have before. It exposed me to folks in the health research community who have been very important and helpful and who I would not have otherwise had the opportunity to meet. It exposed me to an outstanding network of people.

In the aggregate, I think it has done roughly the same for an awful lot of other people from many different walks of life.

**1b.** *What is the Pew "legacy" in terms of:*

    **a)** *health policy?*

    **b)** *education?*

    **c)** *your future?*

Not really knowing a large number of other Pew fellows, I think it would be the combined legacy of what people have been able to do with their degrees, and I assume that it's substantial, but I don't know that for sure.

**2.** *What was the most innovative or unique aspect of your program design and implementation?*

Figuring out a way to allow people to pursue an advanced degree without having to interrupt their job career.

**3.** *What was it about the curriculum that contributed or did not contribute to the program's success?*

The very small student-to-faculty ratio (8:1), the intensive investment by the Michigan faculty, and the multidisciplinary nature of the curriculum.

**4.** *How was the Pew approach different from the traditional teaching approach?*

The intensive weekend was unlike anything. The extensive computer linkages among and between students and faculty was terrifically sophisticated.

**5a.** *How has your professional life changed as a result of the Pew program? What value has Pew training added to your life?*

I can't say, as is the problem with all these types of programs: How much of it is because of the program and how much would have happened anyway? I don't think you can really know that. When I started the program I was in a minor leadership position in the Massachusetts House of Representatives; since I joined the program I served a period of time as the House Chairman for the Committee on Insurance, where I dealt extensively with health-related manners, and more recently I've become the House Chairman of the Joint Committee on Health Care, where I have very extensive involvement in all health policy. The best contribution of the program to what I do is the giving of more critical policy analysis skills that I didn't have before.

**5b.** *Has your career trajectory changed as a result of your time spent in the Pew program? If yes, how?*

I don't know how much is a result of Pew. I think quite honestly I might be here anyway. I feel primarily that what I'm doing now, I will be and am better at because of the program. I can't really say that the program is what put me here. It has, however, made me infinitely better equipped to handle the responsibility.

**6.** *If you did not complete the program, do you plan to? If yes, why? If no, why?*

I will definitely complete the program. There is no question. I am right on target with my dissertation, and I should be done next spring. I got a Health Care Financing Administration dissertation grant to help me finish.

## Telephone Interview with Postdoctoral Alumna Lisa Bero
Wednesday, August 24, 1995, 2 p.m.

**1a.** *Based on your experience and familiarity with the Pew program, what did the fellowship really accomplish? What are the most important contributions?*

It helped me complete a career transition that I had planned from basic science to policy research, and I'm sure that without the fellowship I would not have been able to do that. It also helped me develop a lot of contacts in the health policy world and to learn how to develop policy-relevant research questions.

In general, Pew has succeeded in sending out some highly trained people to a whole variety of positions around the United States to do policy-relevant research. I know one of the goals of the Pew program was to seed the field, and I think it has accomplished that.

**1b.** *What is the Pew "legacy" in terms of:*

*a)    health policy?*

It established a network of highly trained individuals who will stay in touch forever. That will be really important, as it helps people in different agencies and in different states as they approach similar problems with different perspectives.

*b)    education?*

The Pew program has trained fellows in health policy, where there has not been a lot of programs available. From a more personal perspective, the postdoctoral training has really been a lot more valuable because there are just more programs for undergraduate training. That is not to say that we have enough of either. But for the postdoctoral training it filled a very large gap. There just wasn't anything out there, and what that was able to do was to educate people who had fairly advanced training in some specific discipline and then help them target their current training for health policy.

*c)    your future?*

The program positioned me for doing a lot of international work. I had my first contact with the World Health Organization while I was a Pew fellow. That rocketed me into doing international health policy work, which was great. I got a real jump start on that through the fellowship.

It enabled me to make a career transition, as discussed previously.

2. *What was the most innovative or unique aspect of your program design and implementation?*

The most unique aspect was that it was very tailored to the individual fellow. Every fellow came into the program with different experiences. We had some core courses, but most were tailored to the individual, and the faculty spent a lot of time talking to each fellow to find out specifically what their needs were at the beginning, It was a needs assessment. We were asked: Where do you want to go? What do you need to do that? And then efforts were made to give the fellows what they needed to get to where they wanted to be. This individual attention was by far the strongest point.

You really had to be a certain type of individual. If you needed a lot of direction the implementation didn't work too well. You had to be very self-motivated. It wasn't just like you had to go to class and sit in on lectures and get your grade and come out. You had to decide with your mentor what classes you were going to and what you were going to get out of them. A lot of people audited classes, which gives you the opportunity to sort of blow off the class. You had to be self-motivated in the actual implementation.

3. *What was it about the curriculum that contributed or did not contribute to the program's success?*

The writing seminar. It was interesting. I was in the cohort where the writing seminar changed directors right in the middle of my fellowship. It was two very different types of writing seminars. They were both great. It helped us learn how to write for a variety of audiences, not just the academic journal audience, and it also helped us learn to be good and fair critics of our colleagues and to offer advice in a constructive way. The writing seminar was great.

The health policy seminar series was great, especially for somebody like me who didn't know a lot about what was happening in health policy. A lot of different speakers, people from government, foundations, and private industry came through, and discussed a whole area that I had never experienced. It was great to listen to these people for an hour and then chat with them informally afterward.

The third thing was the optional part of our curriculum; not everybody had to take this. I took it as part of my tailored curriculum, and that was a research design epidemiology workshop which really helped me as an academic into that sort of thing.

4. *How was the Pew approach different from the traditional teaching approach?*

The individual curriculum made it different. It was much more interdisciplinary, and that made a huge difference. It was interesting to me because I came from basic science, and I thought that I was coming from such a narrow background that no one would understand me and that I would not understand anybody else. I thought all these sociologists would be much better off than me, but as it turns out we were all in the same boat. I didn't realize that every discipline was so narrow in terms of PhD training. The sociologists and the economists were thinking the same thing. And so we had to learn to understand each other and to really gain an appreciation for all these other disciplines, and I think it was really a win-win situation. We all shared that relief that we were now outside those strict departmental lines. That approach was very different from all the traditional training we had.

5a. *How has your professional life changed as a result of the Pew program?*

It allowed me to make a career transition. It also allowed me to explore nonacademic job options, which I never did go for, but before I started the Pew program, I would never even have interviewed for nonacademic jobs. I was very interested in being an academic, and after my fellowship I interviewed and actually was offered jobs in nonacademic settings. Still, I wound up staying in academia, and I am very happy here, but on the other hand, I am also in a multidisciplinary setting and I am kind of an odd academic. I do a lot of work on government committees and international committees. Had it not been for the Pew program I would have been a much more typical academic.

*What value has Pew training added to your life?*

It basically allowed me to do exactly what I wanted to do. I'll never forget when I started the Pew fellowship, the person in charge of the admissions at that time called me up and told me I got the fellowship, and I was working in this lab and I was just so happy. For over a year I had been pondering how I was going to get where I wanted to go. I had this general idea of what I wanted to do, but I had no idea how I was going to get there. I had obsessed on this fellowship to get me there, which it did!

5b. *Has your career trajectory changed as a result of your time spent in the Pew program? If yes, how?*

As discussed previously, it allowed me to make a career transition from basic sciences to health policy and to consider nonacademic jobs, which I still would not rule out. For example, when I do a sabbatical I'll almost definitely do it in a nonacademic setting. Also, I do a lot of technical assistance and policy work that is kind of off the traditional academic track, which hurts me a little because you don't get a lot of brownie points as an academic for doing that. On the other hand, it makes me feel like what I'm doing is relevant and somebody can use it tomorrow rather than 10 years from now.

6. *If you did not complete the program, do you plan to? If yes, why? If no, why?*

Not applicable.

## Telephone Interview with Leon Wyszewianski
Wednesday, August 16, 1995, 2 p.m.

**1a.** *Based on your experience and familiarity with the fellows and the programs, what did we really accomplish? What were the most important contributions?*

We heightened the visibility of health policy. We forced people in academia to address the questions "what is health policy," "what tools do we need to deal with health policy" and "how can we learn to do a better job at formulating and analyzing health policy?"

**1b.** *What is the Pew "legacy" in terms of:*

**a)** *health policy?*

It is hard to say. It is beyond my knowledge. I can only speak about the Michigan fellows. There definitely was a contribution to the health policy field, and those fellows who wanted to go into health policy were able to go into health policy. Training and/or a degree from Michigan enabled fellows to become health policy people when they were not health policy people before. And then there were those who were already in health policy who I would like to believe are now doing a better job as a result of their training.

I often see UCLA (University of California, Los Angeles) or Brandeis alumni in the literature. The RAND people are particularly strong in that area. That's another example of contributions to the field. But I'm not in a place to judge whether or not they would have done differently had they not been part of the Pew program.

**b)** *education (doctoral, postdoctoral, or midcareer programs)?*

Comments about education come up later.

**c)** *your institution?*

In terms of Michigan, there has been a major contribution in that we now have a program in health policy that we most assuredly would not have if there had not been Pew funding. There are other derivative benefits in having the program here, such as attracting faculty, creating a nucleus of interest around health policy at Michigan, etc.

**2.** *How and why did your specific program develop? To what extent will your program continue now that Pew funding has ceased?*

It was an interesting case at Michigan. We had been thinking about setting up a program in the OJ/OC (On-Job/On-Campus) weekend mode in the area of health policy at the doctoral level. We had been exploring and thinking about such a program; however, we saw ourselves unable to launch such an effort for lack of financial resources. It was therefore a real godsend when the Pew Charitable Trusts decided to help us set up a program exactly along those lines.

The germ of the idea was already there, but the impetus was certainly the result of the Pew Charitable Trusts. I doubt we would have ever started the program without that.

There is a real commitment and aggressive effort at Michigan to continue the program.

3.  *What was the need in the health policy community when your program started, and how have those needs changed today? Is the job done?*

There was this very large group of people out in the health policy field already, in responsible positions, who felt inadequately prepared to deal with a lot of their tasks. They wanted to do a better job at what they were already doing and were looking toward our PhD program as a place to learn that. And, it was inappropriate. PhD programs are programs to train researchers and faculty, and therefore have a very strong emphasis (as it should) on methodology, research skills, and other scholarly kinds of work, but these people were not looking for scholarly training. More later.

4.  *What was it about your curriculum that contributed or did not contribute to your program's success?*

At the very beginning there was this view that the curriculum would be a division between more purely didactic courses and what were called policy seminars. At the seminars the emphasis would be on discussion and on interaction. It turned out relatively early in the game that the fellows really did not want all this free-form seminar discussion; rather, they wanted discussion in the context of much harder-hitting didactic material. They did not want to just walk in and have some policy questions thrown at them. So, we pared back on those policy seminars.

Another change that I was heavily involved with was beefing up substantially the methodological aspects of the curriculum. We started out with having the students pass a graduate-level statistics exam, and in addition to that, they got one course in methods, and that was it. What they came out with was knowledge that they did not know how to apply to their day-to-day work. So, we instituted entrance exams to show competency up to a certain level in statistics, microeconomics, government, and organizational behavior. This started everyone at the same level. The faculty had been complaining that the students were all at different places. The entrance exams forced the students to bring themselves up to graduate-level knowledge before coming into the program. And then we gave them a statistics course (science, methods, how do you know what you know?, threats to validity, etc.). We then followed that up with two more courses: applied statistics and applied methodology. These courses were coordinated so that the students were doing things in the methods course that was related to the other course. That was the major change. It was a welcomed change. We are not trying to make them into methodologists, we are not even trying to make them into researchers, but we certainly wanted to put them in a position where they could do good-quality analysis and certainly write a good-quality dissertation that had proper methodological components.

We also set up specific dissertation seminars where the students were led into finding a topic and how to go about defining a topic. It provided structure. We initially thought that we would bring in all these very bright successful people who would have no problem writing a dissertation because they would just thirst for learning. Well, even with their thirst for learning they needed structure due to the heavy demands of their full-time careers. They were too busy. These were people who were working 50 to 60 hours a week and trying to go to school full-time. We should have realized the need for structure. We have a lot of experience with this type of student. We somehow forgot that at the beginning of the Pew program, but we soon remembered and then set up the program much as we had done for our master's-level program. This worked much better. We concentrated on the dissertation early on rather than just assuming that somehow the students will know how to find a topic, how to find a committee, and how to move along the path. We learned our lesson.

In the beginning there was a very lenient attitude toward the students and their course work, so we found many students hobbled down with huge numbers of incompletes. This hampered the students' ability to get done because not only were they writing a dissertation but they had stale papers to get done from courses long gone. We soon changed the policy to make it very difficult for the students and faculty to get or give incompletes. What we did was to discourage very strongly the faculty from having a major paper due at the end of the course. You just can't do that with this population. Instead, we encouraged the faculty to have the term paper develop in pieces over the course of the term. The students had deliverables that by the end of the course would add up to the product the faculty were looking for. This worked far better than waiting for it to somehow magically appear in the last flurry of the term. The rate of incompletes dropped dramatically. The students learned that incompletes were given only under the most extreme circumstances (e.g., a death in the family), not because they had a big project at work. They had to make the program top priority and a major presence in their lives.

5a.  *What was the most innovative or unique aspect of:*

a)  *your program design?*

. We offered a doctoral program on a nonresidential basis, where students come here once a month for 4 days, 12 times a year. We are still the only game in town. As far as I know we have no competition.

5b.  *What were the biggest challenges or barriers to overcome of:*

a)  *your program design?*

How do you offer a doctoral program to people who are working full-time and who are geographically dispersed throughout the United States?

6.  *Based on your experience, what lessons were learned about the educational process in terms of:*

a)  *recruitment?*

This is an academic program. This is not another job. When all is said and done, we offer pretty standard, straight-forward doctoral-level courses. The students had to have the academic know-how to make it through those courses no matter what their other qualities were or their other accomplishments may have been. We may have lost sight of that in the beginning. We tried to take in people who were very accomplished in the field but who were not necessarily great achievers in the academic realm. It was a disaster. They just couldn't cope with all this. If you're going to work full-time and go to school, you have to be very good at the school business. You have to already have mastered the craft of being a student. Some of the early cohorts had never mastered that craft. We learned to pay a lot more attention to grades, past academic accomplishment, as well as Graduate Record Examinations (GREs). It turns out that if you take people who have GREs in the 80th and 90th percentiles they do much better. Also, we looked for people who have shown that they can handle work and school at the same time. That is a good predictor of success. This was another lesson learned: no matter how applied this is, and even though we were not looking to create scholars, ultimately they cannot take full advantage of what we have to offer if they are not good students. Many of these students' first inclination is to find someone to whom they can delegate the work, but you can't delegate this. This is one of those essential activities that cannot be delegated.

b)    *degree requirements?*

Competency exams were a good screening device. The first day the students arrived they were sat down for 8 hours of exams. That sent a message: we're very serious, this is a serious program, it is *not* like coming to a conference once a month. It made them have to get back into studying even before they got into school. It was a sort of self-selection process; after the exams some people thought twice about whether or not they were going to do this. This also made the faculty happy because it brought all the students in at the same level. A large set of complaints from the faculty disappeared once the competency exams were instituted.

c)    *curriculum and content?*

This was discussed earlier.

d)    *integration of fellows with other students, the rest of the university and the program in general?*

It is a concern. The students are sort of isolated, and they tend to gravitate for their dissertation to the faculty that they've had in class. So, one thing that I started, which I believe has been helpful, is to actually bring in faculty every weekend to talk for an hour during lunch about what he or she is doing; in this way some contact is established. Integrating the students into the rest of the university is very difficult. What has been very useful is computer conferencing that all the fellows participate in. That has been a unifying element. There is a lot of conversation going back and forth among the scholars and faculty. Different topics are discussed. The fellows also have their own encoded conference that the faculty cannot participate in. It is very important for the fellows to have this opportunity. The only people that understand the kind of hell they're going through are the people going through it with them. They support each other and we foster that.

    e)     *relationship between faculty and students?*

    f)     *completion rates (where applicable)?*

We learned that they are no different from other doctoral students. The overall completion rate is about 50 percent (statistics on this are not very good), depending on your denominator, and that is about what we have had. Despite all our efforts, we have not been able to improve on that very much, but we are not any worse than other programs, and ours is a tough program to pull off. Given the unique aspects (students holding full-time, highly responsible jobs while taking courses and working on a dissertation) we are doing OK.

**7a.** *To what extent do you think there were "programmatic" barriers to student completion?*

The main hurdle at Michigan is the fact that the students are working full-time outside the PhD program. That is built in. It may or may not be considered a "programmatic" barrier. Perhaps it is a structural barrier.

**7b.** *To what extent do you think the program was beneficial for those who did not finish the program?*

I have spoken with a number of alumni who did not finish but who still believe that they benefited tremendously from the course work. The difference between them and someone who finished is that they did not write or finish a dissertation and the others did. One could argue about how much learning goes into writing a dissertation. We would like to think that everything we teach is useful, but the students on their own account have confirmed the usefulness of the course work.

**7c.** *How can we measure success for those programs where completion rates do not apply (i.e., postdoctoral programs)?*

We have some people whose entire direction changed as a result of the Pew program. For instance there is one alumna who entered the program as a practicing pediatric neurosurgeon and the last time I spoke with her she was working as a health aid to one of the representatives on Capitol Hill. She would not be doing that if it were not for the Pew program. And, she has not written her dissertation.

There is another alumnus who is now the Deputy Director for Health in Texas who says that how he approaches problems has been greatly influenced by the 2 years of course work at Michigan.

With regard to measures, did they change direction from non-health policy to health policy? Do they do what they do differently now that they have knowledge that they didn't have previously? Those are basically the two reasons why someone would come here.

8. *How does the Pew fellowship approach differ from a traditional fellowship approach?*

We are different from everything. We are different from a traditional doctoral program, other Pew programs, etc.

*How have the major outcomes differed?*

People who would never have been able to go for their PhD can and have. Precious few would have pursued any kind of doctoral education were it not for this program. A traditional doctoral program would have been way beyond their reach financially and careerwise.

9. *If you were asked to give advice to another university attempting to initiate a similar program, what would you say?*

If you don't have any experience in dealing with this kind of population, you're in for a very difficult time. There is a substantial investment that must be made up front, and a continuing investment that must be made throughout.

## Telephone Interview with Postdoctoral Alumnus Mark Legnini

Thursday, August 24, 1995, 9:30 a.m.

**1a.** *Based on your experience and familiarity with the Pew program, what did the fellowship really accomplish? What are the most important contributions?*

It seems to me important to distinguish between the two kinds of Pew programs (postdoc versus predoc). In terms of the UCSF (University of California, San Francisco) postdoc, the biggest contribution is that it helps one to make the transition from training to a professional career. Most people in their doctoral programs are busy learning techniques and how to apply them and such, but that's very different than building a career.

Pew plugged its fellows into a network of people corresponding with their chosen areas and got them involved in things that one would expect to be involved in at the start of a career.

**1b.** *What is the Pew "legacy" in terms of:*

**a)** *health policy?*

I don't know if the Pew program has changed the health policy field. I have no idea about that.

**b)** *education?*

I would imagine that some of the predoc programs are a little different in structure than traditional predoc programs. But I wasn't directly involved in those.

**c)** *your future?*

It provided me with a good transition from being a doctoral student to being someone in the field.

**2.** *What was the most innovative or unique aspect of your program design and implementation?*

The emphasis on networking and getting involved in the politics and the art of doing things rather than just plugging people into existing research projects and making sure they have a job was the most innovative aspect.

**3.** *What was it about the curriculum that contributed or did not contribute to the program's success?*

The best thing was that there wasn't a curriculum.

I went there ostensibly to work with a particular person, and when I got there that person decided he was going to take a sabbatical that year. So the flexibility of the program and the fact that people involved in the program could individually work with people to put together something that they needed was to save the day for me, and I think that was a strong point of the program in general.

4. *How was the Pew approach different from the traditional teaching approach?*

There are all kinds of postdocs. There are postdocs where you don't have to do anything but work on your tennis game. And, then there are postdocs that are really apprenticeships where you go and become the co-Principal Investigator on someone's research grant, and that's all you do. Pew was a little different than both of those models.

5a. *How has your professional life changed as a result of the Pew program?*

Specifically, the job I got after finishing the program was the result of some of the work I had done during the fellowship, and a result of some of the connections I made and people I met during my time as a fellow.

*What value has Pew training added to your life?*

It's nice to be employed.

5b. *Has your career trajectory changed as a result of your time spent in the Pew program? If yes, how?*

That's a tough one to answer. I don't know what I would have done otherwise. I don't know how it would have turned out. I went back to school after working for about a dozen years. After that I went into the Pew program. My path was therefore a little different than that of other people who went from college to graduate school and then the Pew program.

6. *If you did not complete the program do you plan to? If yes, why? If no, why?*

Not applicable.

**Telephone Interview with Doctoral Alumna Patricia Butler**
Thursday, August 24, 1995, 11:00 a.m.

1a. *Based on your experience and familiarity with the Pew program, what did the fellowship really accomplish? What are the most important contributions?*

I had three objectives when I went into the program: (1) to learn a number of specific technical areas that I had not previously had formal training in; (2) to have a chance to think about the great health policy issues of the day in a more academic setting; and (3) to read the classic literature in the field, because my background is in law and although I've been in health policy for almost all of my career (about 25 years), I had no formal training in it, so I always felt that I might be missing some of the literature that everybody who has formal training had. Of the three objectives, two were very well met and another not so much met given the nonresidential nature of the Michigan program. The courses that I particularly wanted to have training in were epidemiology, research methods, biostatistics, health economics, and, to my surprise, health behavior, which turned out to be one of the most useful and interesting subjects that we studied. I really got my money's worth there. In terms of reading the classics in the field, I now feel that I have that under my belt. In some cases I was pleasantly surprised that I had read a lot of the material but I need a confirmation of that.

Because the program was nonresidential, we went to classes for a long weekend every month. That meant 30 hours of classes virtually nonstop. Unlike a residential program, where you might have a couple of hours of classes a day and then you could perhaps go off to have a beer or coffee with your classmates and maybe even your faculty members in the great old tradition of graduate school, that opportunity for us was rare. People were so busy, and by the time we were done with class at 5:30 p.m. on a Friday or Saturday night, the last thing we wanted to do was spend any more time with one another. Although we always did go out together at least once. I had hoped, perhaps unrealistically, that we would have had a chance to process what we had learned together, but we were always too shot.

The fact that we were connected by a computer system did allow us to communicate actively, even though we came from all over the country. We were able to talk about current issues through this medium, and that was helpful. Some people participated more actively than others, and the faculty got involved as well. So, interaction was not completely unattainable, but it was a limitation of the program that Michigan offered.

On the other hand, for most of us who were midcareer and for many of us who live in places where there isn't even a graduate-level health policy program offered, this was the only way we could do this. That's why I am so grateful to the Pew Charitable Trusts for supporting this kind of program. I am disappointed and concerned about what happens when the money goes away, as it has basically begun to do. I think it is a unique and extraordinary opportunity and one that I think should be available to others in the future. I am particularly concerned that as Michigan turns and tries to make its programs self-supporting, as they need to do without an outside source of revenue, then they are going to get mostly people who have deep-pocket employers who can send them, and that will tend to be more people in the private sector, more health services administrators, as opposed to health policy folks from public agencies. Several people from my class were from public agencies, and the public just does not have the ability to do that. Most people cannot afford what is about $50,000 over the course of the 2-plus years. I think that's a shame. The kinds of people who have been trained in the past will change to people who have the means either personally or through their workplace and more residents of Michigan who don't have to pay the out-of-state tuition. I think it's fine that Michigan gets to take advantage of this thing, but it was such a unique national resource that I am sorry to see the dollars go away.

**1b.** *What is the Pew "legacy" in terms of:*

I think these are good questions that I hope someone who has a broader perspective can answer. It seems to me that there is great advantage to nonresidential programs. As I mentioned, they are not perfect, but nothing is. The notion of being able to go to a school with the reputation of Michigan when you don't live there is important. There are a lot of programs that are midcareer that are more mail order or you meet less frequently. Many of those are MBA-type programs and others are at the master's level. I don't think there are any in health policy at the doctoral level, if any at all. I would hope that someone would examine whether this is a good model for midcareer education in this field. It seems to me that it is, but I speak for myself and am grateful for the opportunity to do this, which I wouldn't have been able to do otherwise.

a)   *health policy?*

I certainly know the names of some former Pew folks of the various campuses, and I know that they are contributing to the policy world. I haven't been trying to figure that out. In terms of my own personal experience, although I had been working in the field a very long time, I still felt that I got something out of it. People asked me why are you doing that, you could be teaching that program? I guess I always feel a certain humility about that. One can always learn more. I feel that I am a better health policy analyst as a result of the program, even though I came at it with quite a bit of experience. Some of what I got personally was a sense of self-confidence in the field that I actually knew something about, but I wasn't sure I knew as much as I knew. Health economics was a good example of that. I always felt fairly intimidated by the subject, owing to a bad experience in college, and it was demystified for me. It was made very clear. We had a very fine economics teacher, and although I would never claim to be an expert, I now feel that I can talk knowledgeably and with a sense of self-confidence to people who are health economics experts. Some of that was just breaking down some barriers. For the younger people who may not have had the same exposure to some of the subjects, I think it also offered a real opportunity for a lot of new knowledge. My impression is that people who took the program seriously and worked hard at it should have not only learned a lot but should have also been able to be better policy analysts.

b)   *education?*

In terms of education, there are probably some lessons to be learned. I personally feel that way, but I also feel that it would be useful for educators to evaluate this and if it's a good model to try to promote it. It's a shame to think that there is only one such location in the country.

c)   *your future?*

Discussed above.

2.   *What was the most innovative or unique aspect of your program design and implementation?*

It was the nonresidential aspect.

3.   *What was it about the curriculum that contributed or did not contribute to the program's success?*

THE LESSONS AND THE LEGACY

I personally have a strong philosophical orientation toward public health. To me it was very valuable that we were housed in a school of public health. Some people who are more interested in health services research or health systems management may not care as much about that. To me, public health is a fundamental set of disciplines whose influence is often lacking in our current national debate. The neat thing about public health is that it is so interdisciplinary. Our degree was a DrPH, not a PhD, and we met requirements from the School of Public Health specifically, rather than just the graduate school at Michigan, and that meant that we got courses that even the master's students in our department don't get, like epidemiology and health behavior. Those were extremely valuable because they are or should be critical aspects of health policy in general. They are fundamental to an understanding to public health. When we talk about health policy we often think of financing and delivery systems, but at the core should be some of the public health disciplines. Michigan offered that interdisciplinary focus, and I think that's unusual at this point among the other programs. I found that very valuable.

4. *How was the Pew approach different from the traditional teaching approach?*

It was different at Michigan because of the location in the school of public health. It was also very small; our class had 9 people, 1 of whom dropped out, and I think other classes have had up to12. The current class, because they are trying to figure out ways to finance it and break even, started with 18 people and still has16. And, that's still pretty small. It is very intimate. We all got to be extremely close friends. We really needed one another for moral support. Perhaps this is more true here because of the nonresidential aspect. I was surprised at how important that is, because I am self-employed and very self-motivated. I work quite independently without needing to be around people at all, and yet the pressures were so extreme that we often turned to each other for support on both personal and school matters. We will all remain good friends.

Something else that the Pew funds offered Michigan, even though they have an excellent faculty, was the ability to bring in some of the best people nationwide to teach a course if they didn't feel that they had the capacity on their faculty. So we had the Dean of Public Health at the University of North Carolina, Michel Ibrahim, who is an MD/MPH to teach our epidemiology course. Rather than teaching it from a mathematical perspective, he taught more from a policy standpoint, drawing the principles from epidemiology but not getting hung up on how you estimate odds ratios. Michel was just exceptional. He is an internationally recognized expert on all sorts of things. We were taught how to use the epidemiological approach in health policy. I assume that's fairly unusual. We also had an exceptional methods professor who had been with the school, but then left and with Pew funds was brought back to teach. We also had a political science professor from Johns Hopkins. That was very valuable. We weren't constrained by the faculty and interests of people on the campus. That's something that a program that has to sustain itself internally cannot do.

By definition, the Michigan program drew from people from all over the country, and therefore, the diverse experience of the student body was very interesting to me. There were a couple of folks from state government, we had a state legislator, we had someone who worked in the foundation community, a hospital administrator, and a person in the insurance industry who also had physician assistant training: very interesting people who contributed to the very rich discussions that we would have. We weren't all of one mind. As long as you can keep an open mind, you can learn a lot from people like that. A few were people I might have encountered in my normal work with state governments, but at least half of them were not. I guess any midcareer program would attract diverse groups of people, but my sense is that at Michigan we were probably even more diverse, and that's a great benefit.

5a. *How has your professional life changed as a result of the Pew program? What value has Pew training added to your life?*

I didn't expect to change my career from the work I had been doing and I still don't. The one area substantively that I find very interesting was opened up to me during our research and methods class. I now know that if I were 25 again and starting a career I would be very suited for an applied methods career where I did evaluations. It is my hope that once I finish the degree to look around for those kinds of opportunities and see if I can do any of that kind of work.

In a way the value may not be measurable. The program has given me more self-confidence in a few areas, and it has made me more aware of the diverse sets of perspectives that I should bring to the policy work that I do. It's made me a better analyst, but it might be difficult to measure. People who I work with have commented on changes in my methodological approach. They have been pleased. There are opportunities for me to integrate what I've learned into my work.

5b. *Has your career trajectory changed as a result of your time spent in the Pew program? If yes, how?*

Answered above.

6. *If you did not complete the program, do you plan to? If yes, why? If no, why?*

Because of my age and because of my existing experience I don't happen to think that the degree is that important. But, I do plan to get it because I've come this far and because I feel that it is an indication of successfully completing something. The dissertation is a wholly different experience making me understand just how laborious the research experience is. I'm doing something with original data, and I've been at it for a year and a half. Prior to this I had no true appreciation of what it was like to start from an idea and think about data sources and take it all the way. That understanding of the research project is so valuable to me because I find it interesting. However, I'm pretty sure I won't do anything at quite that level again. Our degree program is not training us to be researchers per se; it's training us to be policy analysts, but we'll need to be able to know how to use secondary data, etc. (Patricia Butler finished her dissertation in February 1996 and graduated in May 1996 with her DrPH.).

Telephone Interview with Doctoral Alumna
Pamela Paul-Shaheen
Thursday, August 31, 1995, 9 a.m.

1a. *Based on your experience and familiarity with the Pew program, what did the fellowship really accomplish? What are the most important contributions?*

In the aggregate, in terms of the totality of the program, the jury is still out. But clearly the program has put a number of people into key policy positions. You can see the success of the program as you look across the spectrum of alumni and the roles that they are playing across the nation, regardless of whether they completed the program totally or not; many have moved into reasonably influential positions. I think what will happen over the course of the next 10 years is that people participating in this program will become part of the core policy network for states and the federal initiative that probably will be taken (post-Republicanism). In that sense if the intent of the program was to train a group of gifted people and allow them an opportunity to develop and move into positions that have key influence over policy, it has accomplished that.

Clearly, for the individuals involved, Pew has created both learning opportunities and incredible networking opportunities. I use many of the people in the Pew network continually, and I'm always amazed as I go through my professional life the people I run into and find out we share the common framework of having gone through the Pew program.

Creating a group of thoughtful individuals who can influence policy has been one of its most important contributions. The proof of that will be even more noticeable in the next 20 years, because, for the most part, its people in their 40s, 50s, and 60s who end up in policy-elite positions, and clearly, if you start with people in their 20s, 30s, and 40s you've got to give them time to move through the system.

1b. *What is the Pew "legacy" in terms of:*

a) *health policy?*

The program has successfully put people in the field who have made a contribution to the literature, who have moved into positions of administration, and who have created a more thoughtful environment in terms of decision making. Pew has, at least, expanded the level of talent that's available with good credentials. Look at someone like Larry Patton who has been through the program and is now one of the key advisers to AHCPR (Agency for Health Care Policy and Research). There is a sprinkling of Pew alumni all over in research consortiums, running hospitals, in consulting firms, etc. Can I tell you directly what it's done, like has it resulted in the expansion of health care or reduced costs? No. I don't think the "legacy" diffuses that way. It diffuses through the individuals who were involved.

b)    *education?*

It was a wonderful educational experience. My program was unique, and I would not have even been a participant had it not been for the fact that I could move into an on-job/on-campus (OJ/OC) program. I am a very strong advocate for the approach that Michigan took, because it offered people who were in high-visibility positions the opportunity to complete the program while continuing to manage professional work schedules and personal demands. It would never have been of interest to me to resign my position to go to school because the program would not have benefited me financially. It rounded out my education and gave me a credential I wanted, but I didn't go into the program because I knew it was going to move me up the ladder an additional $20,000 a year in income. From that perspective I feel that the educational experience was extremely unique. I would encourage other institutions to look at the OJ/OC model. If you recruit individuals who are in mid- or upper-level positions and bring them into a university setting, you have a class with a diversity of interest, expertise, and ability—it just creates an incredibly rich and interesting learning environment. Secondly, when you combine that, as the Michigan program did, with people who are actively engaged in policy activities in their work, a symbiotic relationships occurs between problems from work and techniques learned from class, adding an interesting dynamic into the program. The program empowered these individuals in their own workplaces.

c)    *your future?*

I wanted the professional credential as a way of rounding out my career. It also has given me access to a vast network of individuals who I have drawn on over and over both for work-related issues, to bounce ideas off of, and to do papers with. That part has been very good.

2.    *What was the most innovative or unique aspect of your program design and implementation?*

The OJ/OC approach was the most unique. Without it I never would have ended up as a Pew fellow. That's the one overriding feature. I would really like to see in today's demanding world more universities look at developing that kind of approach to attract mid- and upper-level career people back into a university setting. I think it benefits both.

3. *What was it about the curriculum that contributed or did not contribute to the program's success?*

There are a couple of parallels here that are interesting. On the one hand, one of the things that contributed to the program's success at Michigan was the fact that the administration had experience in dealing with off-campus students. Therefore, the supporting infrastructure was in place, allowing the program to run smoothly. On the other hand, I was in the first Pew class, so it was a situation where we were kind of learning by doing and also they were really creating the program around learning by doing because they had never really had any of these challenges at the doctoral degree level. Since we were the first "guinea pigs" there were more barriers in terms of people not knowing how things were going to operate. There were still faculty discussions of what was going to be demanded of students and were these really doctoral students, etc. By the second and third years of the program, those things were all resolved. The only downside was that we were the first class, there was a high degree of uncertainty about how the program was to be run, and what the protocols would be, but that's just part of getting something off the ground.

4. *How was the Pew approach different from the traditional teaching approach?*

Most of it was around the OJ/OC approach. I didn't find anything else different. I think we were held to exactly the same standards, if not higher ones! Higher perhaps because there were people coming into the program who were very experienced in some aspect of the health field; thus, the expectations extended even higher.

5a. *How has your professional life changed as a result of the Pew program? What value has Pew training added to your life?*

The most value has been the networking that has resulted. It has offered me an opportunity to link up, work with, and collaborate with a whole range of people across the nation. That has been invaluable.

**5b.** *Has your career trajectory changed as a result of your time spent in the Pew program? If yes, how?*

I did not look at the program as a way to make a major life change. I followed the same career trajectory for the last 20 years. My whole focus has been on health policy and analysis, planning, and research. That has not changed one iota. What the program has done for me is that it has given me additional credibility, some additional options for choices of work than I would have had without it, but it has not made a major change in my professional life at all. It has just augmented and supplemented it.

**6.** *If you did not complete the program, do you plan to? If yes, why? If no, why?*

Well, I got through finally! This past June I defended my dissertation and now can add the DrPH to my name! I'm done. Why did I finish? First of all because if I start something unless there are things in life that I cannot change I will finish. Also, because people made a commitment to funding my education; had I not finished I would have reneged on a commitment I made. It was important for me to complete it. Also, because I was the first woman to come on board at Michigan. I was the only woman in the class. I said come hell or high water I would finish the program. What I didn't want to do, but what I found I needed to do, was take a long time in order to balance my life. I didn't want to get a divorce or give up raising my child. I said I would finish, but it will be on my own time. I'm very proud of the job I did and how everything turned out.

**Face-to-Face Interview with Stuart Altman**
Friday, September 1, 1995, 10 a.m.

1.    *What was your role in the development of the Pew Health Policy Program?*

If you go back to the very beginning, one of the things that was very impressive and very unique about the original solicitation that I had never seen before and have never seen since was the fact that a small group of advisers to Pew said there are important issues that are likely to develop in health care over the next few years, rather than the foundation saying what they are. Therefore, the small group of institutions that were selected to train people were allowed to (1) indicate what they believe are going to be some of the major health care problems that this country will face over the next decade and (2) how they could design a training program to help individuals meet those needs. The foundation didn't dictate what the problems were or how to do it. I have never seen that before.

Stan Wallack and I put our heads together (I give most of the credit to Stan) and worked on developing an application. We were the little kid on the block as a school. We were up against the biggest and the best. But we really focused on what the issues were and what needed to happen. We put together a program that took individuals from the social sciences and provided a more focused training in health care.

2.    *How did the Pew Health Policy Program start? Who are the key people involved?*

The next question was how we were going to make it work and we had several issues. One was how to divvy things up between Boston University and Brandeis. Even while there were different programs between us and Michigan and between Michigan and UCSF (University of California, San Francisco), there also was a very different orientation between Boston University and Brandeis. Our students were integrated into the traditional PhD program here at Brandeis while taking certain special courses that were provided. We required that every student meet all the requirements. Boston University (BU)created a very special program. The advantages for Boston University was that they could really focus directly in on what they thought was needed, but the disadvantage that the students felt was that it was very unstructured. The students were free to pick and choose; they were sort of left alone. They focused much more on health providers: physicians, etc. Our program was much more social scientists getting more of a background in health care. BU added one dimension which I believe was the most critical component to the program's success and that was a person by the name of Steve Crane. Steve Crane really was the father/mother of the Pew program for many years both at BU and Brandeis. We worked well together. We got a lot of good credits for that. That also had to do with the good relationship I had with Dick Egdahl and other people here who did similar things as Steve but not to the extent that Steve did.

I was the dean through the whole program, so I played a reasonably important role in making sure the resources were there and that the program ran smoothly. There were some tricky spots, for instance, funding issues. There was somewhat a feeling of elitism on the part of the Pew fellows. There was some jealousy around the school that I had to deal with, but it was not overwhelming at all. I think most people, outside health, were very appreciative of having gotten into the school. But there are always, on the margin, individual students who don't get a Pew fellowship. I pretty much left the running of the program to Stan Wallack.

When Steve Crane left BU, we moved the whole program [to Brandeis University]. We were then forced to deal with the fact that we had the whole program and that Steve was gone. Mary Henderson ran it for awhile and then we were very fortunate to get Jon Chilingerian to run it. He added a different, more of an intellectual force.

3. *What was the environmental need at the time of the program's inception?*

Our main thrust was that we could take individuals who had been working tangentially in the health field (mental health, nursing, child health, etc.) and provide them with a more fundamental understanding of the core problems in our health care system so that they could function as a policy analyst or researcher.

We were also trying to recruit, and we did recruit people who had worked for governments either at the state or federal level, but who had started out without a lot of formal training and needed a deeper understanding.

*Has that need been met by the Pew Health Policy Program?*

We did attract a number of individuals who had been working in the health policy arena at the government level but who had come in as pretty junior people. We added a conceptual framework to what they were doing. They then reasserted themselves back into the policy process, often at higher levels.

We also had the relationship between what we were doing in the health policy center and the work that was going on here with the Pew program. That was a very valuable synergy. It allowed the students to often participate in direct research and in a policy environment. Most of the research going on here is a very policy-related research that they could be a part of. It helped us too, it gave us the benefit of these individuals, and a lot of them stayed with us and became part of our staff for a period of time.

*Will there be a future need?*

The answer is definitely yes. There is always a need for individuals who have both a broad sense of what the issues are and do not come from a narrowly based discipline and yet have analytical training that allows them to think clearly and to do research. The problems in health care are truly interdisciplinary with multiple dimensions and require individuals like that. There are relatively few places in the county that provide such training.

4.    *What is the Pew "legacy?"*

It's hard to say. I think it's demonstrated that these programs are important, that they can produce value added. I know that the most difficult aspects of evaluating a program, Pew or any other program, is determining what is the "value added"? What's the value added to the individual, and what's the value added to the system? Now, it's a little presumptuous to think or to attribute to any one program, even one that has trained a couple of hundred people, what impact it has had on a $1 trillion industry that affects every American, that employs one out of seven people; let's face it, we are dealing with a gigantic industry. We have to evaluate its impact on the margin.

Clearly, the Pew program did demonstrate the importance of interdisciplinary research. It was also terribly valuable to the Heller School [at Brandeis].

### Telephone Interview with Doctoral Alumna Sarita Bhalotra
Thursday, August 31, 1995, 1:30 p.m.

1a. *Based on your experience and familiarity with the Pew program, what did the fellowship really accomplish? What are the most important contributions?*

The most important thing that the Pew program accomplished for me was the opportunity to network with a lot of important players in the health policy field, including the other Pew fellows, as well as the people that they worked with. The Pew conferences were very important; we got to meet other Pew fellows and the senior persons they worked with.

1b. *What is the Pew "legacy" in terms of:*

a) *health policy?*

The Brandeis program is a good program, built as it were around the Heller School. The PhD could have been a little more in depth as far as health policy is concerned. I felt that I got a lot more familiar with health policy with the work that I've done beyond what the PhD program had to offer.

b) *education?*

In terms of my education, it's been priceless. Frankly, without the Pew stipend I wouldn't have entered this program. It was just enough to get me to stop working. It provided the catalyst.

c) *your future?*

I think it has changed my direction in terms of health services and health policy research. When I entered the program I didn't think it would have had that effect. I thought it would be a stepping stone for health care settings, which I am not ruling out right now, but at this point at least I am more interested in research.

2. *What was the most innovative or unique aspect of your program design and implementation?*

Jon Chilingerian's seminar, which he implemented the second year that I was a Pew fellow, was not just innovative and unique but was also very influential. It filled a spot that needed to be filled. I'm sorry that we did not have it that first year. He introduced us to different theoretical ways of looking at things and to readings that were important regarding health policy and other more general issues.

3. *What was it about the curriculum that contributed or did not contribute to the program's success?*

I think the dissertation seminars were good. They have a lot of potential. I think that the way that Jon had structured it was something that I really liked. He provided materials for us to discuss. He provided an opportunity for us to present our material. It was structured just enough to lend a good framework. It was unstructured just enough that students had an opportunity to share, develop, and exchange ideas. When it was too unstructured, frankly it was a waste of time. Sometimes it just became an opportunity for one student to speak his or her mind or his or her pet peeve. That was not a useful exercise. Making it too structured is also too restrictive because it is different from a class.

4. *How was the Pew approach different from the traditional teaching approach?*

The only thing different about the Pew program was that we did have the dissertation seminar. The first year it was a little scattered and that was partly circumstantial. Then there was a change of guard: Steve Crane left, Mary Henderson left, and there really wasn't anyone to pick up the slack. So, it was a little fragmented. However, the second year was a little more concrete, not just Jon's seminar but even at [Boston University].

5a. *How has your professional life changed as a result of the Pew program?*

The PhD, this particular PhD program, and the way that the Pew program was structured in a way that I was doing projects that seemed to involve more of the senior people. I'm not sure how it came about, but I think my professional life has changed direction because of the Pew program. I have gotten more interested in health policy and health services research than I was before.

*What value has Pew training added to your life?*

There really wasn't a separate entity called Pew training that so much influenced me; rather it was the whole PhD program that influenced me. Overall, the program enriched my knowledge.

**5b.** *Has your career trajectory changed as a result of your time spent in the Pew program? If yes, how?*

I was working in a hospital, so I would have expected that I would have continued to work in health care organizations. I am not ruling that out in the future, but at this point it seems like I'll pretty much stay in health services research for the foreseeable future.

**6.** *If you did not complete the program, do you plan to? If yes, why? If no, why?*

I am ABD (all but dissertation). I haven't finished my PhD but yes, I plan to finish it. I got too caught up in working here. The dissertation was put on the back burner. It became so much more interesting to do these research projects and be part of a research team. Thus, the dissertation kept receding further into the background. However, I do intend to finish it.

**Telephone Interview with Stan Wallack**
Wednesday, August 23, 1995, 10 a.m.

1a.   *Based on your experience and familiarity with the fellows and the pro-*
      *grams, what did we really accomplish? What were the most important*
      *contributions?*

If we looked at this from the perspective of individual programs, the answers would be very different; after all, they are all very different programs. The orientation, philosophy, and politics at Brandeis are very different from those at the other schools. Michigan was very concerned with public health and methodological issues in terms of evaluating different programs. San Francisco had a very different focus because they were training postdocs who already had good theoretical skills in research. Also, each institution had a very different leadership, with very different people with very different interests. The individuals played very important roles. Looking at each institution individually gives only small parts of the program. It is very important to look at all the programs collectively and say that this was more than any one individual program; it was a set of programs that did different things. The institutions very much dictated how you looked at your program. If you were coming from a medical school, you were looking at the focus from a delivery perspective. Schools of public health look at things from a methodological perspective. We looked at things from policy perspectives. But we were all looking at solutions to problems rather than analyzing problems through our varied focuses.

Most traditional PhD programs are teaching methods and theory. Schools of public health teach a lot of statistics, etc. Health is a problem area. Health policy programs are different in the sense that they focus on the problems trying to find solutions. It is a different niche. The Pew program did do something different in developing people who were in that niche in the 1980s when we all focused on problems and their solutions. It was really appropriate for the time.

1b.   *What is the Pew "legacy" in terms of:*

      a)   *health policy?*

For all these programs the legacy is the people. We have gotten some really committed, interesting people into the program. That's the nice thing about these fellowship programs: people stay around for a long time, and they have real careers and real interests. The issues will change, and the policies will change, certainly they have changed in the last few years with the rapid changes in health care. So, it won't be as much the content as it is the people.

b)    *education (doctoral, postdoctoral, or midcareer programs)?*

Each institution probably got very different things out of it. The Michigan model was a very innovative model: to try to take practitioners who are out there doing it and give them skills. I think we are going to find more and more that it is a way of educating people through other kinds of media, probably. It's just the beginning of a way of educating people on the job in effective ways. It will continue to be very exciting into the future. I think in terms of Brandeis, Pew has allowed us to have depth. It has and will continue to affect us on the institutional level. Each institution will have had its own impacts on its individual programs and faculty.

c)    *your institution?*

It certainly changed us at Brandeis. We had a very broad curriculum that had a lot of contexts, historical contexts and values, and looked at the vulnerable populations and how they were doing. What it did not have was a deep and sound policy framework. It did not look at public- and private-sector policies that make outcomes possible. So, we have added a real depth and focus on policy, and I think we are still building, but we have filled a missing link in the school. We went from social welfare to social policy.

2.    *How and why did your specific program develop? To what extent will your program continue now that Pew funding has ceased?*

We did not have a training program. We didn't start off trying to support something in existence. We were invited to participate and asked, "What would you do with a health policy training program in the future?" We saw a world with a delivery system and a passive payment system driven by the providers. We saw a lot of frustration, particularly with costs going up. We thought there was a need to get payers involved, to have a better balance between payers and providers, so we said we should work with payers, and the initial proposal defined those payers as business groups within the community. And then we asked, "How do we get cities involved?" That was a forerunner to getting many cities involved. We were involved with Denver and Cleveland. We developed very strong coalitions, I think we had something to do with those. We had a major symposium for the major corporate sponsors at Boston University (BU). Business firms could become better purchasers of health care managers. We really had a public policy perspective, in that the financiers in states and governments needed to get more involved in managing and running the system, and clearly, over the past 15 years we have had the government move to being a more aggressive payer and policy maker. So, really it was an attempt to get the payers into the equation of health care. We saw a number of different ways of doing it. One way was to get people into Brandeis and educate them about payment and the effects of payment on cost and the delivery system.

We now have courses and a faculty. We know what we're doing. We have a much better handle on how to develop productive people who are going to be problem solvers. We have already institutionalized the curriculum here and the processes.

3. *What was the need in the health policy community when your program started, and how have those needs changed today? Is the job done?*

We started off in the 1980s with this notion of payers. Just when the private sector began getting involved, together with the HMOs (health maintenance organizations), moving the delivery system. It was early into the era of managed care. We did a lot of projects in this area. Clearly, this has changed over the last 10 to 12 years. When the program switched from BU and Brandeis to Brandeis alone, we became more concentrated on the vulnerable populations that we are most concerned with at Brandeis. We integrated more with the Heller School. We started to be more focused upon disenfranchised populations. We accepted students who were more interested in broad social change. These people did OK, but we probably didn't do as good a job as we should have in terms of focusing them on the health care of the vulnerable populations. Some of our students did, however. We focused on women, poor kids, and inner-city dwellers. However, we may have lost some of the focus that we had had initially as we moved from health care cost and utilization to vulnerable populations.

One particular area in which I believe we can play a major role in the future is organizational behavior and organizational change. Policy research in this area is just starting. We don't know who will be successful and who will not be successful. We don't know how well disabled people are going to perform in these systems. We've gone from a fragmented delivery system to a horizontally and vertically integrated system. It's interesting, but what are the implications of all that? I think policy makers don't understand how they have affected this change and I don't think the people running organizations understand how they affect policy and how policy affects them. I think the link between policy and organizations is really key. We have to figure out how to regulate organizations as they continue to grow larger.

4.   *What was it about your curriculum that contributed or did not contribute to your program's success?*

Both the weakness and the strength was being in the Heller School. The health policy curriculum is multidimensional in terms of political science, economics, and sociology. We tried to build in a specialization in health after that, and in that we tried to put different lenses on it: lenses of the economist, the political scientist, the sociologist, and the medical system. We looked at policy from different paradigms and different perspectives. I think that is critical if you want to do "health policy."

5a.   *What was the most innovative or unique aspect of:*

a)   *your program design?*

Our initial program was very innovative in terms of bringing in business leaders from the community and really working with them and working with their problems and also working with communities.

b)   *methods of implementation?*

c)   *educational process?*

Educationally, the most innovative was the building of a series of policy courses from different perspectives. Health policy is about problems and solutions. How do you get to the solutions? How do you look at a problem? How do you solve it? It is a very doable kind of thing, driving home the need to link a solution with a problem and its analysis. The dissertations therefore have this mix of looking at a problem from a multidisciplinary perspective, although we always stress having a theoretical perspective as well.

5b.   *What were the biggest challenges or barriers to overcome of:*

a)   *your program design?*

b)   *methods of implementation?*

c)    *educational process?*

I think the biggest challenges stemmed from the fact that the Heller School curriculum was so broad. It tried to cover social welfare, different methods, and different theoretical disciplines. How do you then add a specialization on top of all that? It would be a lot easier to just be a health research or health policy school rather then a school of social welfare. The educational curriculum was driving our program, and yet we had students who needed certain skills and needed to take certain courses, and yet there were many other courses to take under our program. So, placing the Pew program within the Heller School's curriculum was a very big challenge.

6.    *Based on your experience, what lessons were learned about the educational process in terms of:*

a)    *recruitment?*

One of the reasons that we wanted to do this program is because we saw it as an opportunity to attract students because of the stipend level and the national reputation that Brandeis would now have. We were competing against top schools: Michigan, RAND, California, the Massachusetts Instituteof Technology, and Harvard. All had applied. That we were one of the schools that won gave us an opportunity to attract a different quality of student with a different set of interests. That was very important. Having said that and given that we were doing an awful lot in policy research that was being recognized, it still did not mean that the best students naturally came to Brandeis. Harvard still attracts very good students; it wouldn't matter if it had nobody in policy, because it's Harvard. We found ourselves still needing to get out there and do a lot of recruitment. We had one person here at the program who did a great job at recruitment. The program really did very well when he was here. Steve Crane really took this program on as his mission. He was a key force. He tried to work with both institutions (BU and Brandeis), and he took a real interest in getting out there and selling the program. You need a champion. Steve Crane was our champion in terms of recruitment, but I think you need someone who can link up recruitment and content. I think we found ourselves both here and at BU more interested in policy. Steve was more interested in organizations. He may have been right. There was a little conflict there. But the success of this program had a lot to do with Steve running this program. Going out there, really identifying people, working hard, writing to people, and going to the right kinds of meetings were very important for us. I don't know about the other institutions, but we certainly found that we got many more applicants and much higher-quality applicants. That was a big positive for us.

b)   *degree requirements?*

I talked a little bit about the breadth of the program. I really think we are trying to get people prepared to have very good methodological and statistical tools because of the quantitative nature of policy work today and to have a solid theoretical background. It is very difficult to do it in three different paradigms. I think one of the things that we have learned along the way is that although people need to be exposed to many disciplines, it is important that to understand that they still need a specialization. It's important to understand, yet they really do have to get this notion of specialization. It's important to have one discipline you can really think in terms of so, regardless of the problem, you have a way of thinking about it. You don't just look at a problem and try to find a solution; you really need to have a theoretical paradigm driving you to understand the problem. That would be something that I think is very important in a PhD program. I think the people at San Francisco brought in people who already had PhDs in disciplines, and I think that is important for the kinds of research and publications we need to do. We need to do a lot in a couple of years. One of the things we did was try to do everything in 2 years. I think for learning just a policy framework that would be fine. But if you want to have your trainees do policy writing and research, you need to give them a stronger base in one or more of the disciplines. We train people for the policy world. But we probably train them better as users than doers. We needed more users out there because the world was changing, but now we need more doers with greater theoretical training.

c)   *curriculum and content?*

The other thing that was key in terms of our 2-year curriculum and our very high success rate was the focus on problem solving and learning how to get to an answer. The seminar led by Jon Chilingerian was very critical. We've always had very strong cohorts. Jon got them to see studies of successes. How does someone who is in political science move ahead and complete a project? How does an economist go ahead and do it? Our educational process or approach was pragmatic in that we used the procedures any business or person would adopt in solving a problem. Being exposed to this process from the beginning of the program to its end is very important. It is very difficult, but very important for students to see at the outset how they get from where they are starting to the end. This road map became a backdrop for students—one they could put their hooks into as they moved along.

d) *integration of fellows with other students, the rest of the university, and the program in general?*

I think we had a problem initially because the Pew students identified with the BU Pew students only. This problem became different once all the Pew students came over to Brandeis. I think there was a little bickering about the stipend. I think the Pew students got a little more; a lot of government stipends are about $10,000, and they were getting $12,000. But in those years they were the best students we were getting. I think some of them found the work less challenging than other students in the school, but I think over time, as we developed our own program, that concern dwindled. Also, we opened the Pew program to all the Heller School students by not making our new courses restricted to Pew fellows. We started off with just having Pew fellows in the courses, but we realized that while the Pew students were very good, there were some other students who were very good who didn't get a Pew stipend. So we broadened these classes, and I think that by changing the educational process we helped to break down those barriers that we had in effect created by saying it was such a special program. So, the Pew program came in and we developed a new curriculum. When we opened up the program it integrated students. Currently, the seminars we have are open to everybody.

e) *relationship between faculty and students?*

It's probably a little closer for those in the Institute for Health Policy. The institute has housed the Pew program, and therefore, we have really developed strong relationships. To the extent that students wanted to identify with one or more researchers, it has worked out quite well. When Pew fellows went outside the institute faculty, some developed strong relationships as well. Debra Stone is a good example of someone outside the institute faculty but with whom some of our students developed a relationship, and they kept working with her, particularly the lawyers we've had in this program. Students basically found their way. The institute has some excellent economists, political scientists, and policy analysts, but outside the institute there are other interesting faculty with whom the students may choose to work.

*f)* *completion rates (where applicable)?*

I think our high success rate is pretty amazing given the brief time that people are here at Brandeis. They have done very well. We have had them start thinking about their dissertations right away so as not to make it an overwhelming task. They try to spend that first summer developing a topic. These people are highly motivated. We have been successful because by the time the students leave here they are pretty far along knowing what they're doing. We can help students choose doable studies and make sure their approach has both a sound basis and a sound method so that they can get it done. Doctoral students can get lost in a place like this or in any place. Being in a training program ensures that they don't get lost. The greater intensity of the Pew program probably helped as well. The focus, the intensity, and the caring all worked together.

*7a.* *To what extent do you think there were "programmatic" barriers to student completion?*

Not having student support for that third year was a barrier. I think some people needed it. I think we assumed going in that people came knowing a lot about health care, some came with backgrounds in various disciplines, and some had very strong analytical skills. To the extent that someone comes here with no analytical skills and hasn't done quantitative work can be a real problem. I guess they could go off and do a qualitative thesis, but they really should have a quantitative understanding both to get through the program and to move on in their careers. So, the time they may have needed to make up for their deficiencies may be considered a programmatic barrier. We really were not prepared for people who did not have some sound quantitative and analytical skills.

Another thing, related to recruitment, is that there were individuals out there who, when we first started the program, were ideally suited. They were seasoned people who were working in the real world for a long time. They didn't want to spend a lot of years in graduate school. I certainly didn't when I went to graduate school. Enough is enough. Ready to get out because the work is to be done afterward. They just wanted to pick up some tools. The 2-year program was appealing to some students, even if they struggled a little when they got here. But it is unrealistic to expect students to have completed all requirements in 2 years. We expect them to be done with their course work in 2 years and to have a dissertation subject and be pretty well along when they leave. Then they could be expected to finish their dissertation within the third year. We wanted to make it a very fast-paced program that would distinguish us. And some students have come pretty close to completing everything in 2 years. But then looking back to those who have, I think they paid a price. They had such a drive to get out of here that they didn't do enough reflection. Where they had a weakness, they skirted around it rather than dealing with it.

7b. *To what extent do you think the program was beneficial for those who did not finish the program?*

Either way the program is pretty important. After all, we are getting people to take a problem and solve it. Still, getting through the entire process is important. The courses themselves help, but I think doing a dissertation really forces people to take a problem and analyze it.

7c. *How can we measure success for those programs where completion rates do not apply (i.e. postdoctoral programs)?*

You can look at the positions people are holding, what roles they're filling, what they are writing. There are a lot of different measures; probably in the postdoc programs they were trying to get people in health and redirect them out of the traditional academic fields. Therefore, the areas they are working in, the problems they are working on, and the positions they are holding would be key indicators. They had a real emphasis on producing research and writing articles. That is an important part of postdoc programs: getting people to hone their skills and start writing articles.

8. *How does the Pew fellowship approach differ from a traditional fellowship approach? How have the major outcomes differed?*

It's the policy focus. It's the solution focus. Students are focused on critiquing and understanding an issue. We are really focused on solving problems. We are focused on looking at a problem and figuring out how to solve it. We go beyond teaching understanding; we evaluate and teach how to formulate solutions. And the compromises one has to make are very different. We are not looking for the ideal solution; we are looking to make things better.

Major outcomes? The people we put out. The places they've gone, the things they've done. How they are taking on and dealing with real-world problems. I think the real world is finished analyzing the health care problem; we have pretty much analyzed the health care problem as much as we can. Now the world is looking for solutions. Learning by doing. I think our people probably find themselves in a lot of those kinds of positions. Hopefully, they will be able to contribute.

9. *If you were asked to give advice to another university attempting to initiate a similar program, what would you say?*

So much of what was successful in this program, in terms of a policy curriculum, was really responding to what was needed in the last 10 to 15 years. I don't think starting that same program today would work. It would have to look different. But, let's say you wanted to put together a new, innovative program within a university. Critical mass is important. You have to really identify with a program. You have to have real expectations. You have to have faculty who are committed to it. I think you really need someone who spends a lot of time doing it. One of the problems that we have here is that once Steve left we had people committed, but we didn't have anybody whose major focus was the program. A lot of us teach in the program but have many other things going on. The other thing is that you need time to work out what the right courses are and what the right procedures are. Another thing is that if you are training people to do policy in the real world, you must be flexible.

Telephone Interview with Marion Ein Lewin
Tuesday, November 7, 1995, 10 a.m.

**1a.** *Explain the role of the Institute of Medicine (IOM) in administering the Pew Health Policy Fellowship Programs.*

This program was brought to the IOM from the American Enterprise Institute (AEI) (1987). The interesting footnote about that move is that when the Pew Health Policy Program was first thought about at the Pew Charitable Trusts and they were looking for an organization to direct it, IOM had responded to the proposal. IOM didn't win the competition; AEI won. IOM at a very early stage had an interest in this program. Until 1988, IOM was not even called officially the program office because most of the national programs until that time were directed out of Philadelphia. However, at the recommendation of Bill Richardson, after he did an evaluation of the program prior to the last refunding, he recommended that IOM officially be the program office.

Since the beginning, the role of our office has been to develop the joint activities of all the programs: to plan the annual meetings, to plan the meetings each year for new fellows, to develop the annual directory and the semiannual newsletters, and to be responsible for the network and really be responsible for the family of Pew fellows over and above their connection to the individual programs and institutions. Also, aside from the whole idea of the networking and the overarching activities, another role that we've had all along was to provide the interface of the programs to the Washington health policy scene, and the meetings each year for new fellows were specially directed to acquainting fellows with what's happening in Washington. Aside from that, we have a role in monitoring the budgets and making sure that all the programs are performing according to the requirements of the program.

**1b.** *How did program variation between sites affect your administration?*

I think one of the really wonderful aspects of the program has been the learning curve at every stage. Another important aspect was the evolution of four different programs and the IOM program thinking of themselves mostly as individual fiefdoms all a little bit in competition with each other to a point where everyone now is working toward a common goal. The program has many more synergisms and mutual interests than issues of conflict and divisiveness. In the beginning everyone was trying to understand what the program was all about, what kind of training program they wanted to pursue, what kind of fellows they wanted to have, etc. So, everybody was very much involved in deciding what they really wanted their programs to represent. In the beginning, when I was still at AEI, we very often felt like we were the umpires or facilitators because the programs were all looking over each other's shoulders and being a little judgmental about other programs. RAND thought that they were much more substantive and analytic than the Brandeis program, and the Michigan people felt that they were much more real world than the people at UCSF or RAND and thought the Brandeis people were touchy-feely community organizer types. So, in the first few years we spent a lot of time just promoting a mutual understanding and linkages across the programs, and I think what started off as a challenge became really very much a reason for the success of this program. The programs now have common objectives, and there is much more commonality among the fellows than there was in the beginning. They are all working toward mutual goals. From my perspective, Pew fellows are not differentiated by where they come from; I am just concerned with making sure that the network continues, that the interface with Washington continues, and that the legacy and the next generation of this program are given every opportunity to succeed.

2a. *Based on your experience and familiarity with the fellows and the programs, what did the Pew Health Policy Fellowship Program accomplish?*

Above all I think the fellowships enriched in a remarkable and significant way the field of health policy research both in the quality and in the level of people that they were able to attract. This program came along at a time when health policy research was becoming increasingly recognized as an important discipline, and health care programs and budgets were becoming such a significant aspect of public, federal, state, community, and private-sector budgets. Until the Pew Health Policy Program came along there were not many people who were good at policy but who also had the analytic skills to really understand what these dynamics were all about, how to develop a changed agenda. My feeling is that this program really enriched the field. To the degree that it was multidisciplinary and to the degree that there were individual programs, these were also very significant and valuable accomplishments. Even though everyone who was a Pew Health Policy Program fellow has a grounding in the statistics and the analytic skills and a knowledge base in policy research, they all have different expertise to bear on an issue, and so I think that was certainly another wonderful idea that the originators of this program may not have even really thought about. What resulted was that each program has specific expertise, but they all complement one another. The feeling is that the Pew Health Policy Program really enriched the field of health policy research and informed the debate. When you look through the literature at how the Pew fellows are represented, in what areas, and with what activities they've been active, it reflects the world of health policy and health care reform in the last dozen years.

2b.  *What are the most important contributions? What is the Pew "legacy?"*

The legacy is really even more valuable today than it was several years ago, because funding for these types of activities are going to be ever scarcer, and even the recognition of solid, objective, nonpartisan health policy research is going to be more difficult to come by. The legacy is that these programs have developed the infrastructure, they have developed the institutional memory, and they have developed the potential mentors who are not only the incredible people who led the various programs but also all the alumni. Now all these things are in place, and these people are at the peaks of their careers. The state of health policy research, I think, is not as endangered today, even given the budget constraints and political constraints. These are all issues we need to be concerned about; however, our people are off and running and are ready to do the job. We are much better prepared; it's like saving for a rainy day. We're better prepared to face a future where the funding of these efforts or the capacity building may not be as readily available.

3.  *What was the need in the health policy community when the programs began, and how have those needs changed today? Is the job done?*

When you look in the original brochures that announced the program there were two issues that were emphasized; one was that health care was becoming ever more complex, ever more prominent in the social, physical, and economic fabric of America and did we really have the leadership and the caliber of people who could steer this ever larger and significant shift? One major purpose was to enhance and improve the state of the art in health policy research. Also important was developing a multidisciplinary program and looking at different fields that affect health policy issues: economics, political science, and sociology, not to mention research methods and all the analytic tools. This program was dedicated to training people who could look at health care in this multidisciplinary way, which was very important.

Have those needs changed today? I don't think so, not at all. They may be even more important. When you look at the demographics and social fabric of this country, when you look at the determinants of health, we realize now that health care encompasses so much more than just purely medical care or health care services. The need is there and may even be greater.

Is the job done? Clearly, it is not done. Health care now is moving from the federal level to the states, the private sector, and to local communities, representing an even bigger challenge because these people, to a more significant degree, haven't had the resources to build that infrastructure of expertise. I don't think the job is done, but what I think the Pew program has done, as I said before, is that it has developed an infrastructure for this type of training. It has people who are now in the field who can be applied to these new challenges and who are extremely well trained and can serve as mentors to people who follow after them.

4.  *Based on your experience, what lessons were learned about the educational process in terms of:*

   a)   *recruitment?*

There has been tremendous improvements in terms of thinking about the kinds of people you want to recruit to these programs, the kind of people who could succeed in these kinds of programs. It couldn't be only the desire to get a doctoral degree or a postdoctoral degree and an interest in health policy. You really needed people who had the motivation, organizational skills, and discipline to do this particular kind of fast-track program. Everyone realized after the first few years that this was an exceedingly demanding task to do these fast-track programs. In the beginning, at schools like Michigan, more than half of the people they had recruited were not able to complete the course of studies, not because these people weren't smart, but because it took a certain type of person to really succeed in this kind of program.

   b)   *curriculum and content?*

Even though the schools had different emphases (i.e., RAND was more analytic; Brandeis was more involved with community change agents and looking at the broader issues like public health and environmental health; UCSF became a postdoc program; and Michigan is a weekend program where people stayed in their jobs), all the programs realized that everyone needed to have a confident knowledge of basic skills of analysis, statistics, evaluation, etc. All of these skills are so important if you're going to stay in this field. For some people, the technical aspects of the health policy research was going to be the mainstay of their program, but even at schools where that was not the mainstay, people realized that the fellows still needed to have rigorous training in basic skills development. Also, the schools realized that the people who were in these programs were very much experts in and of themselves. These were people who were not the traditional students who came in with a blank slate. In many respects these people could teach the course. So, over the years there was a much greater respect and recognition that you had to develop a curriculum that was responsive to people who knew a lot about various aspects of this field and tailor some of the curriculum so that it would still be challenging for them and to make it really nonacademic but rather relevant to today's issues and today's policies. That was another uniform advancement of the curriculum and the content. The programs contributed a great deal in their recognition that you wanted to pay attention to what was important to people who were going to be on the front lines as decision makers and that you also wanted to pay some attention to how to write for decision makers, the politics of research, how to communicate research, and how to interact with politicians. How do you marry the worlds of health policy and health services research with decision makers who have very different requirements and timelines? So it was not only being very aware of the quality content of the curriculum but also being very much aware of how this content needed to be applicable to people who were not going to wind up in an ivory tower but who were going to be on the front lines of change.

 c)  *integration of fellows with other students, the rest of the university and the program in general?*

 When I did my first site visits to the schools early on, all the schools (with the exception maybe of UCSF) were struggling about how they were going to be accepted in the larger university. In the beginning these programs were looked at with a lot of mixed feelings and suspicions and almost like this was a second-class degree, questioning this method of training academics. So, another very large challenge for all these programs was that they had to prove themselves, and they were in many ways the pioneers of making health policy research more applicable and more relevant to the health policy debate. The schools felt very confident that this was needed, and the Pew Health Policy Program funders felt very confident that this was needed, but it was an uphill battle: the blending of the old world and the new world. Because this program was multidisciplinary there was the question of whether the fellows would gain any thorough expertise in any one discipline as one does when pursuing a traditional PhD. That's not what this program required, and I don't think anyone would change that, but in the university this was sacrosanct and something that raised a lot of skeptical eyebrows. So, I give the programs a lot of credit for holding together all the aspects of putting together and developing the content and curriculum, working on recruitment, and all the while fighting this other larger battle about how to gain respect. It's like primary care physicians in an academic health center. So, they were the vanguard of change, and I think that's always difficult.

One of the immediate proofs of success of this program is how these programs now are valued at their universities, how they are now an established part of their universities, and how the fellows and the alumni of these programs are every bit as prominent as other more traditional alumni of these universities.

Another interesting issue for me was, in the beginning, when we used to have these annual meetings, that no one ever thought of themselves as Pew fellows. People thought, "I am getting a degree at the University of Michigan or at Brandeis or UCSF or at UCLA." Everyone at these different programs was so intense and wrapped up at developing and establishing the individual programs at the individual universities that they looked at the Pew Charitable Trusts as only a financier and that's all we have to do with them. I remember what was for me one of the low moments but also one of the high moments of this program was when we had our annual meeting in Texas (this was the first annual meeting of the Pew program that I ran out of IOM). At that time there were a lot of fellows who were community activists and who wanted to be change agents but who were change agents in a way that said, "We have our values, we have our agenda, we know what we want to accomplish, and we don't care what the rest of the world says. We don't have to communicate with the rest of the world." I remember the year before, Reagan had just won his first election and we had a reception for the fellows where we were lucky to get the new hierarchy at the U.S. Department of Health and Human Services, the Undersecretary, the Assistant Secretary for Planning and Evaluation, etc., and the Pew fellows refused to even talk to these people. The fellows said, "We don't understand their policies, we don't agree with them, we don't need to talk to them." I remember that I felt that we really had our job cut out for us. If you're going to be a change agent, I think the first lesson is that you have to able to dialogue with the people who are in power, even if you disagree with them. If you're just going to wall yourself up as the strong opposition and you're not going to understand where these other people are coming from, you're never going to be an effective change agent. And so at the next meeting at Houston we really carried that out. Some of the fellows didn't like some of the panelists because they didn't share their views, and I remember that some of the program directors felt that it was really time to call the fellows together to talk about this hostility that was being expressed either explicitly or implicitly through sign language, etc. Leon Wyszewianski from the Michigan program got up and said that the purpose of being a Pew fellow is that you gain an understanding about how to be an effective change agent in the world of health policy and that the purpose of the Pew Health Policy Fellowship Program is for people to become good communicators and to work in the real world, not in some ideological world. Several people got up and said, what's a Pew fellow? They said all they knew was that these people paid their checks so that they could get an education. It was really an epiphany for this program, because for the first time we had a very interesting discussion about what it meant to be Pew Health Policy Program fellow; that there is something over and above people paying for you to get your degree, and that the program had a purpose and wanted people to be able to work effectively in the real world. You couldn't work effectively in the world of health policy unless you were willing to listen to people who had other perspectives, and only after listening could you respond in a professional, thoughtful way. There were certain people who were so key in trying to imbue that culture: Steve Crane at Brandeis/Boston was very interesting, as were Leon Wyszewianski at Michigan and Phil Lee and Hal Luft (later on). People really took this upon themselves as something that was very important to do. and it was really only after that meeting that there was a new identity of what it was to be a Pew fellow and a much greater tolerance. The interesting thing is that the recruitment process has changed. We no longer get people who just want to be ideologues. We get people who certainly have strong passions, strong feelings, and strong beliefs, but who also want to think about some of these things rationally.

The whole integration among the fellows across programs and integration with the mission of the Pew Health Policy Program were other very important contributions, as was evolution, which I think is really to be applauded. The credit for this goes to alot of the people at the various universities. They took this challenge of "what is a Pew fellow?" very seriously and wanted to develop a cadre of people who had some important commonalities.

When the program office was at AEI and I was brought in to cool some of those waters, early on there was a lot of hostility. If you looked at the fellows across the programs, you would have to describe them as liberal people who thought more expansively and positively about the role of the federal government, and the program office was run out of what was then perceived as a very conservative think tank. The marriage was not a great marriage, even though people like Jack Meyer were very thoughtful and made enormous contributions. Still, there was this gut reaction. In retrospect that hampered the feeling of commonality with the program office. It was almost a little bit of them versus us. I was there in the early years; I came aboard a year after the program started at AEI. I remember that time after time we would ask the programs to give us topics and ideas for the annual meetings and nobody would respond. Finally, we developed our own agenda, and of course people didn't like it. But that was all part of the growing process. People were so involved in the beginning. Very few people were completing the program. The programs were just getting started, so that people didn't think of themselves as a "family" of Pew fellows. They just thought of themselves very much more as individuals and one school as opposed to another school.

d)   *relationship between faculty and students?*

Although my knowledge is secondhand, my feeling all along has been that one of the stellar jewels of this program has been the quality of the mentors. The Phil Lees, the Stuart Altmans, the Steve Cranes, the Hal Lufts, the people at Michigan, and the people at RAND really were terrific role models and mentors. I don't think you could have selected a lot of other universities where you would have had people who were so nationally recognized and still willing to be role models and mentors. The faculty was one of the aspects of this program that was responsible for so much of its success. And, even though students would sometimes gripe that the faculty were never around or didn't have time for them, others would say if Phil Lee spent 3 minutes with you it was worth 3 hours of someone else's time. And even for these people to tell the students to call up someone and tell them I sent you, that was already an advantage.

The universities where the programs were based were already the leaders in the field of health policy. I thought about whether we would have had more "value added" if we started this program at schools that were still a little bit behind but with some resources that could get them into the first rank. I think it is a shame that we were never able to get some funding to expand these programs to schools (e.g., the LBJ School) that are almost right up there but not quite there. The Pew program and its financial support maybe would have allowed them to have entered this exalted field of top health policy research training institutions. But, I do believe that the quality of the mentors and the fact that they were national leaders was a great bone to the students. You wouldn't be a student unless you had some gripes, and they felt that this was a very demanding program. I've heard students say that sometimes faculty were not that readily available and also that in a program like this what you really need are faculty who really are both facilitators and mentors to the students. But that doesn't get you tenure. It doesn't get you published in the literature. It's not the kind of things that are awarded in an academic institution and my feeling is that the schools were lucky that they always had someone who, just because this was important to them, played that role. But in these kinds of training programs some of the things that are most important on the part of faculty are not awarded in the general structure of academia. Generally, however, the students have really respected the faculty, and both have been willing to learn.

In the beginning, when I went out to Michigan for a site visit, it was clear that the faculty were initially resentful: who are these fellows; are they going to measure up to the other people we have at this school; do I want to teach Friday nights or Saturday morning or Sunday morning; do I want to change my lecture to fit these real-world people? There were these tensions, but what is remarkable is that both sides were able and really wanted, in the end, to roll up their sleeves and do the best that they could do. There was very much an interest and commitment by both the students and the faculty to try to accommodate one another, and in general people are pretty happy with those relationships. There may be some more specific stories either on the pro or con side that I don't know about.

e) *completion rates (where applicable)?*

We were always concerned about completion rates in the beginning. People were distressed that people didn't complete the program in the time that was originally estimated. I think people were overoptimistic in terms of the ability of the fellows to complete this kind of program considering that students had families and outside responsibilities, etc. But it has improved, and it is all very much a part of the improvement in recruitment and the improvement in curriculum and content. For example, in the beginning at Brandeis and Michigan there was a recognition that you have to start people in a very productive way looking at the degree requirements. So, as Jon Chilingerian indicated, the completion rates are admirable and compare very favorably to the completion rates for other training programs.

5. *What are the critical success factors?*

The schools learned to recruit people who had the initiative, discipline, and interest to pursue this kind of program and who had what it would take to be a successful Pew fellow once they completed the program. My feeling is that the *recruitment* really was very much improved to ensure the success of the alumni.

There was a tremendous learning curve. The people from various schools devoted a lot of time and effort to changing the *curriculum and the content* to make it relevant, to make it constructive, and to make it so that when people finished this course of study they were very much prepared to take on very senior responsibilities in the world of health policy research or health policy administration.

I think the *mentorship*, hopefully from the program office, but certainly from the individual schools, was a very important component.

I think, not blowing the horn of the national program office, that the *network* has contributed very much to the identity of the Pew Health Policy Program fellows as a group, and the vanguard of change certainly enhanced the visibility of the program in the larger world of health policy and in Washington. It always amazes me when I go on the Hill and I say that I run the Robert Wood Johnson Health Policy Fellowships Program and also the Pew program that everyone knows the Pew program. It's quite remarkable. The individual Pew programs are not in Washington, but there are a lot of alumni. These people now are at the vanguard. If anyone is looking for a job, all they have to do is get the list of Washington-based Pew fellows and they are in very good shape.

Another critical success factor is the *leadership* of the program. One has to give credit to the Pew Charitable Trusts because this did not end up being one of their major interests, but they continued to have faith in the program, they continued to fund the program, and they were open-minded about it. People like Carolyn Asbury had an uphill battle because foundations don't inherently like to fund programs for the long term. Their willingness to just hang in there was very important. Among the early board members, certainly Bill Richardson was a guiding light of this program from the beginning and until recently. The people who were the original thinkers behind this program—Robert Blendon, Walter McNearny, and Bill Richardson—should be given alot of credit.

6. *To what extent do you think the program was beneficial for those who did not finish the program?*

My feeling is that programs like this have a halo effect. Even if you didn't finish you participated at least for a time in a very exciting, learning activity, you met the people, and you got alot of value even if you didn't actually get the degree. Those who went through the whole 2 years or so of course work and then didn't get their degree are still considered Pew fellows in discussion and in the directory. So, my feeling is that for the most part there isn't that distinction, even though clearly the purpose of the program is for people to get their degree and to complete the program. Still, it was beneficial for those who didn't complete the program. If you look through the list in an analytic way, there are a lot of people who haven't gotten their degrees who are playing very important roles. We accept them in the "family."

7a. *How does the Pew fellowship approach differ from a traditional fellowship approach? How have the major outcomes differed?*

My feeling was that this program had all the ingredients to be uniquely successful because it had the rigorous academic training. That was one important element. It had the very exceptional faculty and mentors, and that was another element. It had a built-in network and family and these common interests. Everybody wanted to get advanced training in health policy research, but there was a partnership with other programs that had different levels of expertise and other people who had different career objectives. It was the enrichment of a broader environment and of other programs that added another layer of enormous value. Also, it had the exposure to Washington, which at least until recently was the central focus of some of the major activities in the national health policy debate and in the financing and organization of health care delivery. So, it really was a comprehensive attempt at leadership training. It didn't miss a beat at any score. You look at other fellowships where you get a wonderful training and you see a great curriculum, but where is the network, where are you counterparts in the rest of the country? You may know, them but do you really have a chance to interact with them several times a year through newsletters, through directories, and through meetings? Such an important cadre of alumni are now in Washington at the vanguard of change. They are also at the state and foundation levels. So, what was unique about this program was just that it had a critical mass. You weren't talking about four or five graduates from prestigious organizations; you were talking about hundreds of people, and that makes a difference.

Major outcomes were clearly that these people were trained to be effective change agents in the real world, and to that degree I think that this fellowship was so much ahead of its time. I don't think that when the Pew Charitable Trusts thought about this program many years ago that they even realized how on target this program would be for the world today. You just can't train people in an ivory tower environment and have them be effective change agents in the real world where decisions have to be made under pressure and, within budget constraints, where you have to dialogue with people with very different policy and political outlooks and perspectives. So much of the purpose of this program was to train people to play a leadership role. You can see that now from the number of people who, after they go through this program, are working in the private sector and for some of the major think tanks and consulting firms, whereas in the early years a lot of these people went into academia and into the foundation world. As the responsibility for health policy research falls more to the private sector and to states and localities, the Pew fellows are a wonderful match and are a wonderful addition to the field at every level.

## Telephone Interview with John Griffith
Short version phone interview, June 27, 1996

1. *Based on your experience and familiarity with the fellows and the programs, what did the Pew Health Policy Program accomplish?*

The Pew Health Policy Program raised the sensitivity to policy issues and the ability to handle policy issues. Everyone who entered and completed the course work (not just those who completed the degree) were trained to handle policy issues.

Those fellows that finished the degree at Michigan all went on to positions with considerable influence. (many fellows came into the program in positions that already had considerable influence).

2. *What are the lessons learned?*

There is a market for the kind of a training program that Michigan developed, even with limited support. There is a very responsive market for this kind of a training program with adequate support.

It is possible and productive to explore policy issues in a seminar-style course with nontraditional students.

It is important to remember that Michigan had already experimented with a nontraditional training program; the challenge was to transfer it to a doctoral level.

3. *What is the Pew legacy?*

The health policy community is so big and so diverse that it is difficult to speculate about the value added by training a small cohort of people. The community is many times bigger than the output stream.

Nonetheless, since we started the program approximately 15 years ago, there has been a noticeable increase in willingness to use factual analysis and careful empirical data as a basis for conclusions.

4. *If you were going to give advice to another university attempting to initiate a similar program, what would you say?*

There is a small market for this type of training. It will never be a large market. There is an immense burden placed upon students in this type of program.

One needs to look for benefits in the context where a few can make a difference.

## Telephone Interview with Dan Rubin
Tuesday July 2, 1996 4:30 pm

1. *Based on your experience and familiarity with the Pew program, what did the fellowship really accomplish? What were the most important contributions?*

At the Pew program breakfast during the Association for Health Services Research Conference, I thought about the Pew program as a whole. I hadn't thought about that for awhile; it was sort of fun. I think probably that the contribution to interdisciplinary doctoral education in the health policy field rather than the specific training of some number of people is the biggest accomplishment. Because of the prestige of the schools that were involved, it speeded up and added prestige to the field of health policy education. At the breakfast I realized that I had probably underestimated how big a change it was for doctoral health policy studies to move toward a policy analytic framework. My own background is in policy analysis. I have a master's from Berkeley in public policy from 1976 and that was always very interdisciplinary. At that point it was very new to have professionally excellent policy analysis training at the graduate level. I think the first programs started in the late 1960s and Berkeley was one of the first. Frankly, I think there is more interdisciplinary work at the master's level than at the doctoral level. I knew that the Berkeley program went on to doctoral studies. At the time I was there there was no health concentration. Later on a dual program with the school of public health was developed. I probably would have continued if it had existed when I was there. When I was there, there was a joint program with the law school, but that was intensifying the legal tools, not focusing on the substantive areas like health. The core curriculum was philosophically very similar to what you or I had, in that it took some rigor in thinking about major political events. Thus, I kind of have a blind spot as to whether or not this was innovative in the Pew program. I heard about the Pew program in the mid-1980s and seriously considered the Brandeis program but I wound up not being able to apply. Things were happening in my job and I found myself at a point in my career where it seemed less realistic to leave for 2 or more years to get the doctorate.

*And then you wound up at Michigan. How?*

Several years later I looked again, and the Michigan program at that point looked exciting.

Back to the first two questions. If it's true that the response of prestigious universities vying to offer the Pew programs caused a change in their behavior, then in terms of what's known about how innovations are disseminated, the first people to innovate are often in marginal status positions, so often innovative educational programs have low status. Typically, the next stage in the dissemination of innovation is high-status entities or people pick up the idea, and then the third stage is that, because of their status, what they do is taken seriously by others. It may be, in that dimension, that the Pew money and the high status of the schools that jumped for the opportunity pushed us to a point where that many other schools would want to emulate us. That's a speculation on my part. It will be interesting to hear what people who have been institutionally involved think about that—people who nurtured and developed the programs. This is, however, theory based because I happen to know a bit about the theory of innovations. It has nothing to do with higher education; it has to do with people. So, if that effect is real (i.e., speeding dissemination of interdisciplinary policy analysis into health policy programs), then I think that is the Pew program's biggest impact.

Certainly, churning out a number of graduates is a contribution, but I have some trouble seeing that as the main accomplishment. My sense of realism is that people do end up getting interdisciplinary orientations one way or another, for example, through rubbing shoulders on interdisciplinary teams or because of their own career paths. So, the average doctoral graduates in health services research may not have been as interdisciplinary before the Pew programs. That didn't mean, however, that there were no practitioners who combined fields, whether at the individual level or by being active participants in study centers or on interdisciplinary project teams where there was a good intellectual process. My sense of reality is that the Pew program didn't lead to there being interdisciplinary doctorally trained people for the first time; it's one path to do that. It probably did give those individuals more prestige, whatever that meant. I think there is always a tendency for those who have been through a particular path to exaggerate how special it was and to say that it may have been the only way to reach the same endpoint. We [Pew fellows] may be inclined to believe, because we were chosen to be in the Pew program, that we are completely special and that there would be nobody like us if not for this training. That is clearly exaggerated. This is the way that elitist feelings emerge. There is some truth, and there is some exaggeration.

I was very pleased to hear at the AHSR (Association for Health Services Research) meeting how the Agency for Health Care Policy and Research (AHCPR) money is stimulating more schools to do the same thing.

There can and should be concerns about how to judge the quality of an interdisciplinary product, but that is nothing new in academic training. The same good and bad stuff about reputation and judging the individuals that is always applied will continue to be applied. We can't expect this program to solve the problems of all higher education. I'm not sure which of these questions this belongs in, but I certainly was aware, at least in the Michigan program, of the difficulty in defining the dissertation. I think it will come up later.

2.   *What was the most innovative or unique aspect of your particular program design and implementation?*

Certainly the on job/on campus (OJ/OC) structure was one of the most unique aspects. It is not innovative in the sense that it wasn't done before, because Michigan had been doing it in the master's program for about 20 years. But, it certainly was innovative compared to any other high-quality doctoral option that I saw. There are other nonresidential doctoral options, but I was unaware of any that was focused and that had the quality of faculty and certainly an actual student body working on similar things. I think the experience level and the caliber of the fellows at Michigan also were exceptional. Just over the years, listening to comments and meeting the fellows from the schools, clearly, there is some distinction of who was in which program.

The Michigan program tended to have a higher percentage of real midcareer, senior-level professionals with considerable responsibilities as opposed to my perception that the Brandeis program tended to have a higher mix of earlier career people who were several years out of a master's program and on a track of considerable responsibility but not yet in senior positions. At Michigan, not everybody was in a truly senior position, but every cohort that I was aware of was peppered with people who had large impacts or major management responsibilities within organizations or major political roles. The intimacy among the fellows at Michigan, combined with that caliber, was very strong. I think a number of people in my cohort felt that the most important thing for them was watching how other students reacted and thought differently about the same topics. There was a very high ability to critique thoughts, based more on practical judgments than on being a master of the disciplines.

Going beyond common sense, though, in my group Pat Butler had done seminal work in her field, had been on Institute of Medicine study groups, and as a lawyer was often called upon to write for government audiences about what the legal framework of ERISA (Employer Retirement Insurance Security Act) means. So, classmates really were in cutting-edge policy roles. There were others, like Bill Lubin, whose experience in senior insurance positions was priceless. How often, in a position like mine, do you get to have extended discussions with somebody who has been living in that corporate environment? It's less true now, but for a long time the exchange between insurance types and clinical or public policy types was very limited.

Another thing that was notable in my cohort, but that wasn't really about program design, was the strength that the external faculty brought in. The way that happened, though, was due to problems finding internal faculty to give the right course at the right time. It was sort of ironic. Michel Ibrahim was there because the epidemiologists in the School of Public Health either were or were perceived to be fairly limited in perspective, most of them doing highly technical as opposed to policy work. Past cohorts had probably found that a typical introductory technical course was very unsatisfactory. With the audience of the Pew fellows, the faculty were challenged to deal with relevance to policy issues. This surprised me. It's hard for me to believe that in truth that there aren't epidemiology faculty who are involved all the time in policy debates. I don't know what to make of it. But that was the story I heard. I don't know how much was a matter of specialization in the epidemiologists, as opposed to the availability of people to work Thursday, Friday, Saturday, and Sunday shifts. Michel liked it; he liked the stimulation. He actually didn't do a very in-depth introductory course at all, but he led us through some very good discussions using epidemiological concerns in policy. We got this benefit because of things that didn't work well in previous cohorts.

3. *What was it about the curriculum that contributed or did not contribute to the program's success?*

The general fact that the curriculum was interdisciplinary certainly was important. I don't want to dwell on that, but it needs to be said because I would never have applied if it wasn't. I think that the way that the dissertation seminar (and this started with my cohort) was structured was very good. It really focused on producing a draft of a prospectus as the course material. The discipline of doing that step by step was fabulous, integrating things we had thought about before while pushing for production. Those of us who didn't think we were going to go on to do work as principal investigators on major grants thought that the focus may have been too narrow, but the emphasis on getting organized was very helpful. The dissertation was demystified for us.

Some of the lead-in courses that Bill Weissert put in place with policy analysis and quantitative analysis methods were very strong. They built a lot of competence through doing typical steps in a quantitative analytic process. Having senior faculty teaching the courses certainly helped strengthen the curriculum.

One of the things that attracted me to the Michigan program was that it was housed in the School of Public Health. Although I was warned by Leon Wyszewianski that I may not get the rigor in public health policy topics that I wanted, I thought they could have done a better job. The Health Services, Management and Policy Department had very little interest in issues of governmental population-based public health. It was almost entirely health care system. The required courses for a public health degree which the school demanded were not always taken seriously. There are four core requirements to get any public health degree at Michigan: epidemiology, biostatistics, environmental health, and health behavior and psychology. Biostatistics was treated very seriously, that was a core tool whether you put the "bio" prefix on or not. Any good program would have intermediate statistical work. The environmental health part was not taken seriously. We had senior faculty doing a class with us, but they never successfully found a way to apply policy thought to environmental health problems. The course was a modification of a survey course on topics in environmental health, and what happened was that the students essentially took control of the course. We were presided over in a very friendly manner by a very nice person, but we did the presentations. It was a great learning experience, though unfocused. The reason we did that was because the structure was failing to give us what we needed. Lectures would go off into digressions about the chemical basis for air pollution. What we got out of the course was valuable, but it did not get into the questions that we had hoped to address, such as: How do you approach environmental policy using tools of policy analysis? How do you interact with scientific issues?

How do you interact with science politics and the limited ability of governments to act together? That is profound in health policy. Environmental health is a classic example, because the science tends to be hard science, but setting science-based policy continues to be very difficult. I am critical of the fact that after a number of years had gone on the program was unable to find a way to combine environmental health and policy.

Health behavior and psychology was well taught, and that worked as a basic skill, as a discipline that we needed to be aware of. The fourth, epidemiology, we talked about already. Because the methods of epidemiology are extensively used in research, we got the skills that we needed, but if it hadn't been for Michel Ibrahim we might have gotten an inadequate course.

I thought that the program could have done alot better working across disciplinary lines or across interests with people who were involved in public health policy. To my mind the lack of rigor in public health policy is something that needs to be addressed, rather than a reason to continue separating public health from health services research along traditional lines. While my cohort was in progress, the School of Public Health reorganized and a formerly separate department of public health policy was combined with the Department of Health Services Management and Policy (HSMP). The scuttlebutt at the time was how HSMP faculty disliked the combination. I sensed a disrespect of the caliber of work done by most, or some, of the faculty in public health policy, although that was not true across the board. The bottom line was that the chance to work on public health projects with equal rigor was not taken up. In theory, a dissertation could go into those areas. Some dissertations have.

4. *How, if at all, was the Pew approach different from the traditional teaching approach?*

It's more interdisciplinary and analytic. The students have more to offer; that's my impression. What I heard about the doctoral students that weren't in the Pew program was that there was more of a possibility of drifting and not coming to grips with the need to choose a research topic. Not much of a peer network existed among the non-Pew doctoral students, especially if they came in post-master's. The master's program is more professionally oriented; thus, there is a gap between most master's students and the doctoral students.

5. *Has your career trajectory changed as a result of your time spent in the Pew program? If yes, how?*

I'm not sure. I don't have a good sense of this. I think part of that is unique in my life in that I was interrupted in other ways while I was in training—my daughter became sick and ultimately died. I can answer the value to my life. My reason for going into the program was not a clear career goal. I heard that the [Pew Charitable Trusts] wanted to avoid taking students whose career goal was to shift gears toward teaching. I have taught in the past. I would be interested in doing some teaching in the future, and so it's likely that the degree will help me do that. But, I'm not that interested in moving into academia. In that sense what I want is consistent with the Pew program goals. Whether my career speeds up or changes, I think that I can talk the language of health services research better. I know the technical, methodological issues a lot better. That helps my relationship with peer researchers. But I didn't experience a problem in that area before. I simply am sharper. Going back some years, I never had trouble talking to researchers or academics, engaging in dialogue, and talking about both policy issues and technical issues. My master's training sensitized me to the kinds of things that come up, although I learned a great deal technically in the doctoral courses. I knew the generalities but I didn't know that much particularly about statistics. It's too early to say if my career trajectory has changed. I don't know whether it will or not. The more I have to offer, the more value I have. My skills tend to be used in the area of consulting and forming marriages among activities that are more connected than their party's parts may realize. That is a continuation of the kind of role I played in the past. I do think, however, that I do it better now. Right now my work has to do with connecting government roles that relate to health care quality and information use. It calls for judgment about what needs to be related to what, more than judgment about how to assemble the research plan for a study.

> *Do you think that the people who did not come in with the same interdisciplinary background that you did, can, as a result of the program, better see these "connections" that you're referring to?*

Yes.

6. *If you did not complete the program, do you plan to? If yes, why? If no, why?*

I do intend to complete the program. I am still predissertation. Life delayed my progress; however, I do intend on completing.

*So, you are in a position to do much of what you have always wanted to do and you are called upon to consult, why finish?*

The intellectual closure of doing extended work will cause me to finish. One of my personal reasons to do the program was for me to see what it really took for me to do extended work. The bread and butter of government work is not extended, analytic ventures. Sometimes there is extended writing and certainly extended thinking about a topic. But, the kind of thing involved in writing a dissertation is very important for me to learn from and to learn about myself. One of the things I said in my application was that I want to find out whether I would like to shift the mix of work I do into more extended products, and that is still true. I learned a lot through writing the papers in the program, but most of the papers were all short products, more similar to the kind of thing that I've been doing for years.

Once I get the degree it will probably make me a candidate for different things, for good or for bad. I think that perception is very important in who gets screened in and out of job searches. The last few years I haven't been looking to change jobs; I've been looking for stability so that I could be in school and so that my personal life could normalize. I may enter a period in the next few years where I'm beginning to look around more.

*Could you speculate about the value of a program like this to people who do not complete it?*

If it's a new interdisciplinary perspective, it could be a very high value. In my case, if I decided to stop after the classes, I would have learned a great deal, in an expensive way for the foundation.

7. *What is the Pew "legacy" in terms of:*

a) *health policy?*

"Impact on health policy" is the impact of what evolves in the health policies of the United States. I think it's unclear, but the network of people trained by Pew is a well-trained and mutually credible group of health policy pros, and they may make a real contribution to good exchange among sectors. There always has been exchange among the university and private research groups and some areas of government. The interchange with the private sector has been less common. One has to ask, though, in how many of the cohorts in all the schools was there a substantial stretch in dealing with people from other perspectives and, particularly, from senior private-sector roles, especially other than hospital administration, which is the area that has had the most interchange traditionally? Mutual credibility at a sophisticated level would be a contribution to policy.

Research analysis being done that affects health policy could have been accelerated by Pew. Yet, I don't think there is anything fundamentally new about interdisciplinary project teams in health policy. Look at RAND studies or General Accounting Office work. This is not unidimensional.

b) *education?*

This I spoke to earlier when I answered the questions of what is the biggest contribution.

c) *your future?*

I've addressed this too.

8. *Are there any important issues that this interview does not address? If so, please feel free to add comments and/or concerns.*

The issue of the dissertation. What is the dissertation in doctoral health policy studies/policy analysis? The interesting thought that I heard from senior faculty at Michigan was that interdisciplinary things happen through teams of people primarily, not through an individual. So, in the health services research or health policy research side of things, the question is, "Is an interdisciplinary dissertation real, or is interdisciplinarity something that happens in groups of people and a dissertation would become too big if you tried to do it with multiple disciplines to a standard of excellence?" I personally think it is possible to do a multidisciplinary dissertation. Is there such a thing as a policy analysis doctoral dissertation, or is excellence and competence supposed to be judged by the part that really is research? The distinctions aren't complete. In real-life, practical policy analysis, the closest you get to it is probably modeling, where you take a policy problem, model it, deal explicitly with policy options and environmental variables, and get your model to try to speak to various dimensions of outcomes. I think it is very hard to weigh things toward "what is the correct policy?" as opposed to "what is the right answer to a research question?" and come up with a dissertation that you can negotiate with your committee. I've shied away from that because I don't want the hassle. The general question is, "What is meant by a dissertation in this field?" To what extent can the dissertation as well as the instruction be interdisciplinary?

Another thing, to follow up what I said at the AHSR meeting, it might be interesting to look at how people came to the programs. For me, the structure of the Michigan program and being in the School of Public Health were very attractive. The Heller School had other aspects that were attractive.

## Telephone Interview with Doctoral Alumna Joan DaVanzo
Wednesday July 17, 1996, 2 p.m.

1. *Based on your experience and familiarity with the Pew program, what did the fellowship really accomplish? What were the most important contributions?*

I thought there were three very different accomplishments that I saw in a production modality. The program produced doctoral- and midcareer-level students who had a very particular expertise. It produced a network of these folks who were involved in different policy work around the country, and it contributed and expanded the real construct of health policy to sort of produce a certain model of how you think about and how you might do an analysis. I think the most important contribution is that it created this multidisciplinarily trained cohort of individuals who are all working in big ways to influence policy.

Doctoral programs are usually very hard to finish, and there are a whole bunch of ABDs (students who have completed all of their doctoral requirements except for the dissertation) around. At RAND/UCLA (University of California, San Francisco) the motivation to finish was very strong. The Pew programs created a strong motivation to finish, and they did that in a variety of ways. Some of it was networking with alumni. It was seeing the people that you knew in these neat jobs and writing these great papers, and you wanted to finish and join them. My class at RAND had four students, and all finished in a very timely fashion. A lot of that motivation is created by the program. I don't know how much is the selection of people or what you did along the way or being associated with RAND/UCLA, etc. But it seemed to be that the support of the Pew programs distinguished them from other doctoral programs in university settings.

*What about your particular program?*

Well I have to backtrack and tell you that I started in 1989 at RAND, and then in 1991, when I heard Ron Andersen was coming to UCLA, I switched to UCLA. I don't think I could have had a better program if I set out to make a perfect program. The RAND program was heavily quantitative, I had microeconomics 1 and 2, macroeconomics 1 and 2, microeconomics for regulatory policy, econometrics, and calculus, which I had never even taken before. Then I took four statistics classes to get credit for two and more. The culture in RAND is such that the hierarchy is the economist, the statisticians, the operations research folks, and then the behavioral scientists. You get this sort of skewed perception of the world, where the economics is king, and it sort of shaped your perception and the analysis you do. I'm a psychotherapist, and this route was difficult for me, but I picked it because I knew that's where I needed to go. Then I realized I knew nothing about health, epidemiology, public health, the broader picture. So when I switched to UCLA I got all that. I got the public health stuff, the underserved population stuff; we talked about access and equity and all these important issues that you might have to know about if you wanted to work in an advocacy sense. It was a whole different spin on health policy. So that's the good news and the bad news. Because RAND was so influential in the 1970s and 1980s and had all these great people there, it was good to be exposed to that. However, it was limiting. There was not enough breadth. I got the breadth by going over to UCLA. RAND didn't encourage students to go to UCLA for classes, although they said you could take classes there. I had the best of both worlds. There is a sequence element also. I really had to do the quantitative work up front because then when I went to UCLA I was prepared. I would not only say to someone "do both," I would say "do both in that order." The combination is very valuable.

2.  *What was the most innovative or unique aspect of your particular program design and implementation?*

I would say the flexibility among the programs. I was able to do RAND and then UCLA. Others did RAND and then UCSF. That was a real important aspect of the program.

3.  *What was it about the curriculum that contributed or did not contribute to the program's success?*

What I thought did not work as well was this devaluation of behavioral research, and at UCLA health behavior was really important. Because RAND was so economics focused you did not get a sense that the behavioral aspects were as important as they really are. You also did not get any kind of clinical exposure at RAND. At UCLA there were people doing cancer research and you could go to where the medical students were taught and you could go to seminars where they talked about clinical research, and things were framed clinically, with clinical examples. When they talked about outcomes research there was a clinical realness to it. That wasn't part of the RAND curriculum. RAND was great at what it did; it was fantastic to have had it, and I wouldn't trade it for the world but it was limiting.

*What about the dissertation process?*

I experienced that at UCLA. My initial idea was to look at depression, autonomy, and Medicare expenditures. The relationship between depression and autonomy was something I was interested in and working with a lot clinically in my private practice (I kept a private practice throughout). Everybody liked my preliminary proposals, but when I got it down to the wire this one professor said I couldn't do depression because it was his research area. I was so steamed, but then another principal investigator said, "Well, you can get mad or you can get a dissertation." So I swallowed it and did autonomy alone and got great results. I never went back to the mental health stuff while I was there. I know everyone has that experience. It seems to be very critical to doctoral programs in general. But I had a fabulous committee. There were six members, and each had their own spin on things. I was lucky because I was working on a project where there were data I could analyze.

*What about the Pew conferences?*

They were great. The first year was hard because I didn't know what to expect. But I met a lot of people. Then the second one was in Toronto, and that was great. It was all on the Canadian health care systems. Then they had one in Savannah that I didn't go to.

*What about the interaction between non-Pew fellows and Pew fellows?*

Perhaps there was a tension here as in all other programs, but I think less so at RAND because if you were accepted to RAND, whether or not you were on a Pew fellowship, you had the same project opportunities. We were in lockstep for that first year. We all worked together in the same room, all day, every day just about. There really wasn't that great of a differentiation. The expectations were the same in terms of how people did, the distribution of students, etc. We had very little tension actually. We didn't have any closed seminars. The only thing we did differently was to be able to talk to Kate Korman. That was really it.

4.  *How, if at all, was the Pew approach different from the traditional teaching approach?*

The work projects were great. You learn about stuff conceptually in the classes and then you do it on the projects. The students have to interview and get hired on the projects. Students have to go around and talk to everybody about their projects; meanwhile, you know nothing and the project directors know that. After you've been there a while and you've developed certain skills and people know you have them, project directors come to you and ask for your participation. It flip flops, but on the front end it's tough. Overall, it was a really great experience. It forces you to learn how to ask the right questions. First you gravitate to what you know, where you strengths are, and then you learn to find projects that will help to strengthen your weaknesses. You learn where your holes are, and you seek out opportunities that will strengthen those holes. Initially, I wanted qualitative because I was getting my head handed to me in quantitative. So, initially I did some ethnographic work, which was so useful, and I did some of that when I got out. I got a job directly from working on the work projects at RAND. Then, at UCLA I was on a Medicare Demonstration Project, and that was working with a super data set. I was forced to learn SAS on a mainframe and learned to do these analyses. It was exactly what I needed. I came out with qualitative and quantitative experience.

The other part is the people. Working on the projects allows you to get to know the professors in a different way. As a student you know a professor is a professor and you are both locked into that role, and then you're thrown on a project with a professor and all of a sudden they are more collegial. You're not just one of the graduate students anymore. You have access to them in a different way. Being able to switch the role is very important when you are a student.

5a.  *How has your professional life changed as a result of the Pew program? What value has Pew training added to your life?*

5b.  *Has your career trajectory changed as a result of your time spent in the Pew program? If yes, how?*

My professional life has totally changed. I was a health care professional. Now I'm doing research. It gave me skills that have increased my flexibility. There are many things that I now have open to me that I didn't before with just a clinical background. My head has changed. I was told early on that as I learn more about statistics I'd become a better therapist and

I didn't believe that. But it was true. It was absolutely true. The process of cognitive development that I went through in this program was probably the most differentiating experience. It's like having a growth spurt in a three-dimensional way, driven by the cognitive development, akin to a baby having a growth spurt that's driven by physical maturation. It was just fabulous, and I would recommend it to anybody simply for the way my thinking changed. Does that happen in all doctoral programs? I just don't know. I don't think so.

6. *If you did not complete the program do you plan to? If yes, why? If no, why?*

Not applicable.

7. *What is the Pew "legacy" in terms of:*

a) *health policy?*

Pew brought a broader range of individuals to the field, so it's a thing about people. I don't know how much of the curriculum at the schools was the same, but the Pew model seemed to me to provide a pretty heavy dose of economics, a fair amount of stats, and then other stuff. I think we all had a fairly similar analytic strategy, if you will, across the set of programs. At least it seemed that way to me. I don't know the influence of having this bulk of people who have that same view of the world dropped into the health policy arena. I would think that it shapes the construct and enriches it and gives it more depth. On one hand it's a grandiose statement to make; on the other hand it's really not. If you think about the economics of the health policy field, it's really a small field, and if you get that many people (what about 200 or so?) with the same combination of classes yet with varied backgrounds and training, the scene is hit from many different levels.

b) *education?*

Between the network of alumni and the network of the other Pew fellows, it's the people and the stuff together that made the educational experience what it was. The combination of topics from economics, statistics, behavioral, public health, etc., to produce this gestalt is just revolutionary. It was such a great idea.

c) *your future?*

There are two parts to this. The real abstract part is that it has allowed me to synthesize all my experiences and provided a vehicle that is useful. I'm still doing work for people that I met in Pew. I moved from San Francisco to Washington, D.C., because I said to myself, "If you want to be in health policy Washington is the place to be." When I landed in Washington I found this whole community of Pew folks that I had access to. It was like being home. Not only people that you know but even people from the Pew Directory, you could just ring them up. Marion Ein Lewin and the Institute of Medicine do a really good job of keeping the network alive with the newsletter and having the functions and the updating of the Pew directory. I know that takes a lot to put that all together, but that's part of the Pew legacy, part of creating an entity and then calling it the Pew legacy. You have to devote time and space. I just think it's been great.

8.  *Are there any important issues that this interview does not address? If so, please feel free to add comments and/or concerns.*

A lot of what I experienced was tied into the fact that I was at both RAND and UCLA. I am a sample of one. I think many people you speak with will have something similar to say. There was something unique in the way that the program unfolds for each and every person. I don't know how you would analyze something like that, but it certainly speaks to the flexibility of the program, and that flexibility is one of its great strengths. Maybe the program instilled this feeling of ownership: every individual had their own piece. Maybe this is part of the Pew mold, the uniqueness, the individuality.

## Telephone Interview with Midcareer Alumnus Terry Hammons

Friday July 12, 1996, 8:30 a.m.

1. *Based on your experience and familiarity with the Pew program, what did the fellowship really accomplish? What were the most important contributions?*

My program's principle accomplishment was that it pulled a number of experienced people, so-called midcareer people, into an environment where they were enabled and helped to become valuable contributors to health care policy, both public and private. They were enabled to do this in a way that grounded policy making in experience and knowledge based on research, which I would say is a very high-quality way to approach policy. That does not mean that policy is not carried out in a political context, which it always is. Yet my experience is that there is a huge advantage in terms of the policy that ends up being made or implemented, grounding it in principle and knowledge, and the political context doesn't just drive it. My program took people who weren't just graduate students and gave them an opportunity to contribute in that way, for example, my participation with the U.S. Congress and also private or quasipublic things like the Kaiser Family Foundation, the University of Virginia, and the Radiological Society of America. A secondary contribution was that it enabled many of us to learn the basics, and in my case more than that because I already had a strong background in health services research, and to do that research in a policy-relevant manner. A lot of health services research that is done is of very little value in developing policy, guiding policy, or guiding action in general. The analog of policy in the private sector is not legislation, regulation, and so forth but how you run an organization and so forth. I think those are the most important contributions of my program. For the program, in general, I think roughly the same things apply. My impression is that the other programs had a lot more junior-level, inexperienced people, and what they turned out were people who were less likely to be able to, at least in the short turn, contribute to policy and more likely to end up in lower-level positions or academic positions. Since they are younger and less experienced you would need to look at longer trajectories. If you look 10 years out you might find that by then they have moved into more senior positions.

2. *What was the most innovative or unique aspect of your particular program design and implementation?*

Our program was a combination of workshops, which were not just lectures but workshops and seminars that gave us background material, methods, and other knowledge, again, in a context of application. Then the second part of our program was working on real projects, and I thought that, in contrast to my experience in graduate school, for example, these workshops and seminars were more effective than traditional graduate education( I did economics at the Massachusetts Institute of Technology). Most important were the projects. I was fortunate enough to be involved in four and a half really wonderful projects through RAND during the year I was there. They were real projects, such as helping the U.S. Department of Health and Human Services (DHHS) understand what academic medical centers were going through and how to make policy that related to graduate medical education, research and training, and so forth that was appropriate for the nation's goals but that also took into account what academic medical centers could do and were doing. Another one was on the implications of alternative ways to pay physicians on quality and cost of care, and that led to my position with the Congress. A third on the National Institutes of Health decision-making process dealt with evaluations of existing practices and technology, which is a difficult issue. There were others. The projects were just absolutely wonderful.

*Can you speculate how many of your classmates or people from the classes before or after you went on to get jobs as a result of these work projects?*

My class, so to speak, was three people. One of my classmates modified his professional course to be more involved in policy, the costs of care, and manpower policy in radiology, for example, reimbursement and other regulatory policies for radiological services. The program certainly influenced his career. This person went from a faculty positions and I think assistant chairman to chairman of a department, so he moved up. Whether he would have gotten the same job anyway, I don't know. However, it is clear that it influenced what he does in that job. My other classmate did change his direction and he is now working for the Kaiser Family Foundation, I believe. He has become more involved in policy than he was in the past. For me it is absolutely clear that my career has changed. I went from a fairly typical faculty position at The University of Iowa College of Medicine to deputy director of the Physician Payment Review Commission (PPRC) for Congress. My subsequent positions were then driven out of that. As I focused on internal policy and administrative positions in private organizations and academic medical centers, I am very much involved in changing the way these places work. My expectation is that I will end up more clearly back in the policy world in a clearer public or quasipublic policy role. Right now, in my opinion there is not much going on in health policy that is really going to happen. But, there will be. There is a lot of private health policy changes that I am involved in. That just happens to be the way health policy is changing.

3.  *What was it about the curriculum that contributed or did not contribute to the program's success?*

Going back to what I said before, the seminars and workshops with their mixture of principles, methods and applications were good, and the projects were wonderful. I thought it was a really good curriculum.

*Who was in the seminars with you?*

There were my two other classmates and then some of the other graduate students at RAND and UCLA (University of California, Los Angeles) that were more like the people in the other Pew programs (less experienced and so forth). So it ranged from some with just the three midcareer people to seminars with four to eight other people. They were all taught by the full-time faculty at RAND and UCLA.

4.  *How, if at all, was the Pew approach different from the traditional teaching approach?*

I haven't really been in a traditional program, but my guess is that Pew is more about application and use and is more targeted at experience through those projects. I'm comparing it, in a sense, to my economics work.

5a. *How has your professional life changed as a result of the Pew program? What value has Pew training added to your life?*

5b. *Has your career trajectory changed as a result of your time spent in the Pew program? If yes, how?*

It completely changed the direction I was going in. It gave me tremendous opportunities that are still playing out and will play out from the rest of my career. It has been just incredibly valuable to me, because even though I had a background in economics and I was viewed within the college of medicine and within the context of academic medicine as pretty well informed about policy things, if you will, I was clearly not capable of making a major contribution in either policy or health services research that is policy relevant. I just didn't have the critical mass of understanding that you need to do that. When I finished the 1 year at RAND, I did have that. The other thing that was very valuable, and these are intertwined, was the opportunity to get to know a lot of people around the country who were doing that kind of thing at RAND, Brandeis, Harvard or in places like the Congressional Budget Office and DHHS in Washington. That is very much tied into the projects and the applied stuff. That has been wonderful.

*Has that network continued?*

Yes. Of course, some of the people turn over and some you lose track of, but there are many people I keep in touch with and talk with regularly about what is going on in policy and so forth.

6.   *If you did not complete the program do you plan to? If yes, why? If no, why?*

Not applicable.

7.   *What is the Pew "legacy" in terms of:*

a)   *health policy?*

I assume it's what people did or will do with the training. When we are talking about the younger people we have to keep in mind that it may take longer to see what they will contribute.

b)   *education?*

I think there is a real dearth of understanding in medical education of the health care systems and health care policy and so forth, and I've gotten involved with some of that at Case Western and here at Hopkins. But I know there have been others from my program and the other Pew programs that have made huge contributions to education.

*What about how the Pew training has changed, if at all, the method for training health policy makers?*

It has, but it's not the only way. There are obviously many paths by which people end up contributing to health policy. I thought the particular program I went through, the midcareer program, and the way it was designed at RAND was a really effective one, and it was able to be accomplished in only 1 year. I looked at Phil Lee's program, that was a 2-year program at UCSF at the time, and it was between those two. His was a more conventional program, certainly a very good one, but it was very attractive to me that the RAND/UCLA program was 1 year and that it was just packed with experience. I just think there is no way as effective as these projects to learn about policy, how to do policy in a high-quality way, and to be involved in it with people who are the best in the world.

c)   *your future?*

The program completely changed my future.

8.   *Are there any important issues that this interview does not address? If so, please feel free to add comments and/or concerns.*

I was angry and disappointed and thought it was a huge mistake for the Pew program to quit funding my particular version of the Pew Health Policy Program in midstream. I have no idea why they did that. I don't know who did it. Perhaps if somebody could explain to me why I would see the logic, but I thought it was really a huge mistake. It seemed to me the most innovative program, and I say that without really fully knowing the rest of them. The RAND program just seemed richest in real experience. Of course, I have a strong bias. I would just really like to know how the decision to end the RAND programs were made.

Paul Ginsburg at the Center for Studying Health Policy Change was one of the lead people at the CBO, then he spent a year at RAND, and it happened to be the same year I was there. Then he went back to Washington and became executive director of the PPRC, and I was his deputy. He is still in Washington. He is a prototypical RAND person. He is a good economist, a superb researcher and thinker, and one of the leading people who could use his academic knowledge to make sound policy.

Telephone Interview with Doctoral Alumnus
Jonathan Howland
Tuesday July 16, 1996, 1:30 p.m.

1.   *Based on your experience and familiarity with the fellows and the pro-
     grams, what did the program really accomplish? What are the most
     important contributions?*

There are definitely some people who went off into
health policy and are doing great things, so the program
kind of seeded the field in that way. There are a bunch of us
who went into academia and other things, but that too sup-
plements the field. What the program did for a lot of people
was to give them an opportunity to get their doctorate under
circumstances that if it were not for the program, they would
not have been able to have done so. There were two things
that the program did. The first was that it bestowed a certain
amount of prestige, so it was seen as a career enhancer, and
the other thing it did was to provide some funds. So, for
example, in my case I had just finished my MPH, and I was
in a sense retreating from a previous profession, and I probably would not have been able to get my PhD without the
program. So, from my own perspective what the program
did was to help us get our doctorate, which was critical to
our careers.

The Pew program was supposed to take people out of
their careers in health policy, tune them up, give them some
skills, and put them back wiser and more skilled. The extent
to which it did that I don't really know.

Certainly, one important contribution that it made in a
generic sense was that it created a prestigious fellowship for
health policy, which in and of itself said something about the
importance of health policy as a discipline and that having a
doctorate in health policy was a desirable thing. That was
important. Some of us did some research that may have been
useful. I think the issues that may have been important in
health policy 13 years ago have changed so much that we
certainly got a grounding and were able to understand what
was happening, but the extent to which fellows have gone on
and sort of changed the spin of health policy in this country,
I don't know.

2.   *What was the most innovative or unique aspect of your particular pro-
     gram design and implementation?*

I was at Boston University (BU) and I thought it was
great that we could essentially design our own curriculum
and decide what tools we wanted to get. One of the reasons

I thought that was so great was that the program enabled me to study epidemiology, which is what I wanted to do, and I was free from taking a whole lot of required courses and able to pursue the courses that were really of interest to me. That was really nice. The other thing that was really nice was that I was able to go through the program in 23 months. I did my course and my dissertation at the same time. There are very few programs that would have allowed me to do that. It was a fast-track program. Now there are good sides and bad sides to that because there were people who went through and should not have gotten the doctorate. But for others, this structure really allowed them to get through in a way that fit with their lives. Very few other programs would have afforded them that opportunity, certainly, very few programs with the kind of prestige that the Pew fellowship brought with it.

*Could you talk a bit about the integration between the BU and Brandeis program?*

I think it worked pretty well. We felt fairly cohesive as a group. For some people I didn't know what program they were in. The Pew fellows' identity was so transcendent. We felt like Pew fellows, and that had a higher profile than what school we were at. People like Steve Crane were incredibly helpful across the board for all fellows as an advocate, counselor, a mentor. On the other hand, we learned a tremendous amount from people like Stanley Wallack about health policy. I just think that it worked very well. I was very sorry that BU withdrew from the program.

*What effect did the tightly structured Brandeis curriculum have, in comparison to the more loosely structured BU program?*

The Brandeis students certainly talked about and envied our freedom. On the other hand, there were people who went through the BU program who didn't learn any methodology, who came out of the program not knowing what a regression equation was. That, to me, was really shocking. So, in a way, even though I enjoyed the freedom of being able to do what I wanted, what I wanted out of the program was skill acquisition, and so what BU did was to give me the degrees of freedom to load up on biostatistics courses. And those are the skills that I market right now. What other of my colleagues at BU did was to avoid some of the more rigorous methodological courses, and I think they came out with a shorter skill set and it showed up in their dissertation. If we did this again, I would like to see some sort of mechanism in place that would ensure that people got the necessary skills, yet still be left alone to do it. Otherwise, I would say that it is too risky and that there should be a curriculum that has a minimum skill set requirement that everyone must take. I'm sort of conservative educationally.

When I took over for Steve I inherited a bunch of my classmates as students. It was very interesting because I saw many of my peers struggle with the skills that they should have mastered. So overall I think there was some envy from the Brandeis students over the freedom that we had, and I enjoyed that freedom, but there were some students who didn't make the best choices and would have benefited from being told that they were not leaving the program without understanding what multivariate regression is.

When you have a midcareer program like this, you get two groups of people. You get one group that says, "Thank God for this window of opportunity to learn some stuff," and then you get another group of people who shook off the system for some reason like they weren't too embedded in it. The latter group came in thinking that they knew it all and they left thinking that they knew it all, but they didn't learn anything in between.

3. *What was it about the curriculum that contributed or did not contribute to the program's success? Could you also speak a bit about the dissertation process? What was it about the curriculum and/or program that enabled you to get through as quickly as you did. Was it a what, or was it a who?*

First of all, the fact that you didn't have to collect your own data and could use an existing data set helped a lot. I did my dissertation using the Framingham Data Set, which was just a beautiful data set. It was well groomed, and the school was crawling with people who knew the variables and how stuff was collected. It was an incredibly supportive environment, and that really made a huge difference. The other thing was that I think I found out in April that I had been accepted into the program, and I started looking for data sets then. I knew I was going to have to do a dissertation, and I finally ended up with a dissertation topic in December of my first year. But I had been working on it since April. So, I say that I did it in 23 months, but the fact of the matter is I gave myself a long lead time. Once I knew what I was going to do I got right to work on it. Now that was my case. A whole bunch of people just went aground on the dissertation topic, and they still haven't done it.

*Were there structures built into the curriculum that helped to guide students, like dissertation seminars?*

No, I don't think we ever had a dissertation seminar. Steve Crane was a great counselor. Steve and I spent inordinate amounts of time with some people to help with their dissertation and got, what I think, was really high-quality mentoring, yet some still never got it. I don't know how to change this.

*What about the curriculum contributed or did not contribute to the success of the program?*

Well I think, certainly at the BU side, there should have been some minimal requirements or simple learning objectives: fellows will leave with this basic skill set. People were not served well by not having those learning objectives spelled out and enforced. But for me it was a breeze because I was doing my dissertation as I was picking my courses: harmony of the spheres.

4. *How, if at all, was the Pew approach different from the traditional teaching approach?*

It's hard for me to say, not having done other doctoral programs. In other doctoral programs there is more of an adversarial relationship between the doctoral candidate and the faculty. You may have your mentor, but as a whole the department's view is that you have to prove that you are worthy of our bestowing this doctorate from our department. There is this kind of onus on individuals to prove themselves. In the Pew program the faculty had a real stake in people getting through; a high attrition rate was not a good thing. There are two sides to this: on one hand you had a very user-friendly faculty; on the other hand it allowed some people to be irresponsible in terms of the course selection, the amount of work that they did, and what learning they did. So, I guess the simplest answer to the question is that the faculty were stakeholders in the success of the program. I think that is different from other places.

*You alluded to something earlier that perhaps you could expand upon. You said that there was a strong identification with being a Pew fellow. Do you think that makes the program different than a traditional doctoral programs? And, how do you think that affects the legacy of the program?*

It had good and bad effects. In one sense it generated a sense of privilege, and rather than being graceful the Pew fellows were demanding, were often obnoxious, and had an incredible sense of specialness that often manifested itself. That comes with the prestige of the program, plus the whole way in which the Pew fellows were pumped up not only by the faculty but also by the foundation. We needed more discipline and we needed to be reminded that we were really very fortunate to have what had been bestowed upon us, and that made us responsible to behave in a gracious manner. I felt as if, because of the nature of the program and because everybody had such a big stake in our succeeding, that there was no one to come along and tell us to shape up. Once you've been through the selection process and you've been given that $10,000, attrition really isn't an option. Every failure is a failure of the program. Conversely, in a traditional PhD program, the whole process is set up for people to fail. The fact that the students had that sort of unspoken edge over the program, the fact that once they were in it was not in the program's best interest for them to leave, gave a kind of tolerance that I think bred an attitude that was not great.

**5a.** *How has your professional life changed as a result of the Pew program? What value has Pew training added to your life?*

**5b.** *Has your career trajectory changed as a result of your time spent in the Pew program? If yes, how?*

Before I started the program I was getting my MPH, and I intended on getting out and getting a job with the Department of Public Health (DPH) and I saw myself as a sort of midlevel bureaucrat. I was kind of hoping to get a job down by the regional office. Today I am celebrating the receipt of my full professorship. So, the Pew program determined the difference between what I had predicted for myself and what happened. I would have gotten a job with the DPH and I would never have gotten my doctorate. It would have been too tough. I would have been too involved and too committed, and I would never have gotten out. The program gave me the opportunity to get the education and set of skills that I just hadn't gotten before. I thought I had lost the opportunity. It was absolutely pivotal for my life and one which I feel extremely grateful for. So when I seem harsh toward the program, sometimes I don't mean to be harsh toward the foundation or the program. They both served me very well. It's just that there are some people I feel didn't get as much out of it as I did or as they could have. In a way, for something that was so good and so important for me, I kind of am always trying to figure out why that couldn't have been for everybody and whose fault that was.

6.   *If you did not complete the program do you plan to? If yes, why? If no,*
     *why? Let me rephrase this question: Can you speculate about the people*
     *who did not finish the program in terms of what value the Pew train-*
     *ing had on their career trajectories, and were there people, do you*
     *think, who came in with no intentions of completing the program?*

I think there may have been a few people like that. I can
tell you that I think that is really despicable, because the
foundation was paying your tuition and giving you a stipend
in exchange for something, and to not take that deal seriously from the word go seems to me unethical. There are
people to this day who have blown off their dissertation, but
they don't see it in that light. They see it completely from
their personal point of view, not from the perspective of a
program that invested in them to do something.

*Is it a recruitment issue?*

I don't know. I run a fellowship program now, and it's
really hard to pick who is going to make it and who is not.
But, I don't think anyone ever spelled it out for the Pew students. They never said, "If you are going to take this money
you have an obligation to follow through." I don't know
whether that would have changed the numbers overall. But I
think there are people who didn't get their doctorates yet who
don't feel at all as if they have failed or haven't fulfilled a
responsibility. Also, I think the people who didn't finish were
probably the same people who were least aggressive about
picking courses that would increase their skill set. I think what
they got out of it was 2 years of sabbatical. I'm sure they
learned some stuff, but nothing like what they could have
learned if they had come in with an aggressive program of skill
acquisition and if they had done their dissertation.

7.   *What is the Pew "legacy" in terms of:*

a)   *health policy?*

In a way it's a little premature. I think we ought to reask
this question in 20 years and see what happened to us. In a
way it's a question that seems to me most appropriately
addressed to the foundation. It's actually always something
I've always wanted to ask to the foundation: "what did you
want and did you get what you wanted?" Or even, "Do you
know what you got?" They would send evaluators around to
see what a wonderful program it as, and the first time I took
this very seriously. I think I was just out of the program a few
years, and I had very strong feelings about what the program

should be, but they weren't negative, just strong. I'd read these reports and they all seemed to be all happy-faced to me.

One of the things that the Pew program really did for a lot of people, even if they didn't get their dissertation, was to add a certain amount of cachet to their resumes.

b)    *education and training?*

I don't know whether anything about the program is so unique or so either bad or good as to leave a lasting impression on the educational landscape. There are a lot of fellowship programs. It is interesting that there are certain times in history when there is a demand for people trained in a certain area, and a foundation can come in and sort of create a cadre of those people. I think that is an interesting kind of concept. I am sure that it has happened in the past, and I am sure that it will happen in the future. Sometimes it's the federal government. When I was going to college years ago there was a whole group of people who were subsidized to study Russian or Soviet Affairs. A lot of times the marketplace will do it. I graduated with city planning as my undergraduate at a time when Lyndon Johnson was President and there was the great society, so the marketplace was creating these people. Whether or not the Robert Wood Johnson fellows or the Pew fellows will be seen as seeding the field and changing the spin of health policy, I just don't know.

c)    *your future? You've spoken about this already. Is there anything else you'd like to add?*

I will always be grateful. I know I learned to think about health policy in some ways that I just hadn't before. That information will be one of the filters that is part of the way I look at things for the rest of my career.

8.    *Is there anything else you'd like to add from the perspective of a program director?*

I started a fellowship here that takes return Peace Corps people and places them for 2 years as residents of public housing. During that time they get their MPH and they are also AmeriCorps volunteers, so they have to do good work. When I was starting this program I was very enthusiastic about it conceptually, and still am for that matter. We were forming the program and set up a lot of things to make the group of fellows feel privileged, entitled, and special because they were going to live a hard life. Throughout that whole process of early design I kept thinking that we had to be very careful that this doesn't translate into the kinds of sense of entitlement that the Pew program got into, at least at BU and Brandeis. That can get pathological and become unhealthy not only for the program but for the fellow as well. I guess that's one of the things I learned from being both a fellow and filling in for Steve for a while.

Other lessons: In recruitment you need to screen for motivation and completion and, secondly, you have to make it clear that there is an expectation that comes with being accepted to the program that you will finish your doctorate. Of course, things do happen. A lot of people don't finish doctoral programs. But in this case they were getting paid to do it.

In terms of degree requirements, I mentioned before I think a minimum skill set should be defined, and it should be skill oriented and enforced.

In terms of integration with other students and the university, we've spoken at length about it. It's a conundrum. On one hand you want the fellows to be special and to have a sense of pride in their accomplishment at having been accepted to the program, on the other hand you don't want then to go around feeling entitled. Those other students who are trying to prove themselves, these students were supported by the faculty because getting them through was one of the performance measures for the program.

If I were to give advice to another university I would tell them some of the characteristics I would look for in my recruitment screen beyond just how you did in your previous courses. I'd really look at commitment and motivation level. I would establish an independent advisery board to keep an eye on the program. That would allow the faculty people and the administrators to say that they were tempted to go native with the students. It would instill a quality control mechanism. We got in binds sometimes with students and their dissertations because on one hand we clearly had an interest in getting people through; on the other hand we were clearly letting a few people through whose work just was not up to the quality that it should have been. It was not good for us to be conflicted in that way.

I think if I were the Pew Charitable Trusts I would have taken a very close look at the infrastructure of the university, I would try to identify the level of commitment to the program, and I would ask for some prospective plan for institutionalization. I don't think this was the case at BU; rather a lot of the supporting people left.

Telephone Interview with Kate Korman
Wednesday July 3, 1996, 1 p.m.

1.   *Based on your experience and familiarity with the fellows and the programs, what did the program really accomplish? What are the most important contributions?*

The program created a national focus on health policy training which was buttressed by the six institutions in four demographically diverse cities. Each institution brought its particular strengths to the whole of the program and chose fellows whose similar aims were to study health policy. The richness of the program lay in the multitude of choices that these institutions offered. In a sense, program directors recruited fellows for all institutions: if an applicant called the RAND/UCLA (University of California, Los Angeles) office but was looking for a program which allowed him/her to remain at home and employed, the applicant was referred to the Michigan program. Another example: RAND/UCLA offered a midcareer, year-long residential study, but inquiries often came from individuals who had just finished a PhD program or medical residency, so they might be referred to UCSF (University of California, San Francisco) which had established a postdoctoral offering. It was my understanding from people like Steve Crane (Boston University [BU]), David Perlman (Michigan), and Ted Benjamin (UCSF) that they too referred fellows to us or other more appropriate programs.

The most important contributions may be the richness of the health policy community today, which boasts 250 additional minds responsible for health policy decision making in a wide variety of venues: local, state, and national governments; private foundations and institutions; universities; and research institutes. The ripple effect of this knowledge and expertise is found in the lives and future endeavors of those whom past fellows influence. Whether it be a change in policy at the local level or the influence of a teacher for a student to pursue a change in career in health policy, the ramifications are far reaching.

2.   *How and why did your specific program develop? To what extent will your program continue now that Pew funding has ceased?*

Al Williams can answer this better than I since he was involved from the very beginning, whereas I was hired after Pew funded RAND and UCLA. My understanding, however, is that there already existed loose ties between the UCLA Department of Medicine, UCLA School of Public Health, and RAND.

Those ties were individual faculty at UCLA who also had appointments in the RAND health sciences program. It must have seemed a natural progression to create programs which formally built on the strengths of each institution. RAND already had the RAND Graduate School of Policy Studies, which offered just a PhD, but no real emphasis on health (although individual students had done their research in health), and UCLA had programs in health services, community health, and epidemiology but no stated emphasis on policy. In addition, the Robert Wood Johnson Clinical Scholars program existed at UCLA, but faculty there were hungry for policy-relevant study for these scholars. From time to time senior scholars from other institutions had come to RAND or UCLA, but no formal program existed for them. Given this background the two programs were developed for the RAND/UCLA Center for Health Policy Study: (1) a residential doctoral program in health policy with students pursuing their degrees either at the UCLA School of Public Health or RAND Graduate School and (2) a residential midcareer program for scholars to steep themselves in health policy for 9 months to a year.

The residential doctoral program continues both at UCLA and at the RAND Graduate School since the courses created for the Pew program are fully vetted at both institutions. However, without outside funding the midcareer program is no longer viable.

*Is there any advice that you could give to the programs that are currently being defunded? Is it only funds or is it something more?*

I think particularly in the midcareer program you need fellowship monies to come. The curriculum that still exists is for health policy workshops, and they cover a broad range. There are four different courses, and they still exist. The midcareer fellows took these four courses along with others, but they were geared toward people who were not getting a degree to give them the fundamentals.

Midcareer people were leaving their professions for 9 to 12 months. They took a deep-pocket dip, and so the fellowship grant enabled them to come and to take an accelerated and specific course of study. When the money went, that was it for the midcareer program. It just wasn't possible to maintain it. We would need to pay the faculty separately (the courses were already developed) and we really needed the set-aside.

3. *What was the need in the health policy community when your program started, and how have those needs changed? To what extent has the Pew program met the changing needs?*

Al Williams can better answer this question. I wasn't in health until 1982.

4. *What was it about your curriculum that contributed or did not contribute to your program's success?*

I think the curriculum was the key to the program's success. It was developed by a cadre of scholars from RAND and UCLA with vital insights and contributions from Allyson Davies who was finishing her PhD in health services at UCLA while working full-time at RAND as a health policy analyst. (She once said to me that she helped create the program she wished she had when she started her studies.) She was a major contributor and actually the associate director in the beginning. Not only did the doctoral students and midcareer fellows take the course work but RWJ Clinical Scholars, nonPew doctoral students at UCLA, and postdoctoral fellows from other departments also contributed to the success and necessity for continuation of the course work even after Pew funding dried up.

I don't think there was anything about the curriculum that didn't contribute or was a problem. We had people eager to teach, and we had experts to come and do specific seminars, for instance, on Medicare. Seminars were often team taught, and people looked forward to them. I think the only possible problem may have been in how often we offered a course. In the beginning we offered the courses every year so that the midcareer fellows would have an opportunity to take them; however, we stopped that later on. We offered one each quarter, and then every other year we offered a fourth one.

*So, it was nothing really unique to Pew; rather, it was logistical?*

Yes.

5. *What was the most innovative or unique aspects of:*

a) *your program design?*

The program overall or of the set of Pew programs?

*RAND*

Okay. I think it was the crossfertilization of UCLA and RAND. I think its a unique situation where you have a think tank where you have the research ongoing and at UCLA were the teaching is such a fertile ground and has so many students available to complement the program.

b) *methods of implementation?*

A formal agreement was created between RAND and UCLA which had not existed before. There had been this loose connection of faculty, people like Bob Brook and Bob Kane who were actually faculty members at UCLA. They also had appointments at RAND, and they were the groundbreakers. They helped to make this very difficult process happen. They are very different institutions.

c) *educational process?*

Doctoral and midcareer fellows were required to align themselves with a research project or projects immediately upon entering the program. We designated this on-the-job training, and a requirement for doctoral students was 16 to 20 hours a week. This effort produced familiarity with research methods and processes "in the lab" to apply what was being learned in the classroom. As a result, our students progressed rapidly toward the degree, where in the case of midcareer fellows, they often had a publication as a result of work done while in the program.

> *At the November meeting, someone from RAND mentioned this concept of "work projects." Could you speak a bit more to that?*

There weren't formal grades given; however, I would keep tabs of how the fellows were doing in their research project area. We had periodic reports from the team leaders, and in a way they were graded if they were not pulling their weight; they would be nicely asked to look for something else to do. It didn't happen very often, but every once in a while it would. They learned pretty quickly that they couldn't get by without really producing. I made them accountable, as did the project directors. In the very beginning we didn't have this paper accountability.

The research projects were pretty much held with the same importance as the courses, because it was the project work that was supposed to lead to a dissertation. It was a unique opportunity for them, but some of them didn't take these projects quite so seriously. Some didn't realize that at the end there was a real product that was expected.

6. *What were the biggest challenges or barriers to overcome in terms of:*

a) *your program design?*

The biggest challenge seemed to be not to include the "whole world" of health policy in the curriculum. Initially, the curriculum was pretty enthusiastic, far-reaching, even overreaching. One course which was just too much was eliminated after 2 years. The students couldn't learn everything. This was challenging, because as parts of courses or whole courses were cut out or restructured, some faculty found that their roles changed. However, the program design was much too ambitious in the beginning.

*It seems like that would be a real tension in any interdisciplinary program.*

It is. We would also have seminars from time to time and invite researchers or policy people to come and speak, and so sometimes the fellows would get a flavor for different kinds of things that had been removed from the original curriculum. That was our way to touch the whole world.

b)    *methods of implementation?*

Getting the bureaucracies at RAND and UCLA to accept cross-registration of course work was challenging. It seems simple-minded, but it was actually quite challenging. That went on for at least 3 years, and part of the problem was that we had 15 doctoral student and three midcareer fellows (by the third year). At least 10 of those were taking these workshops, and so UCLA didn't understand that if it was going to be a UCLA course, why couldn't just anybody sign up for it? So we had to deal with these kinds of very political issues. But it all worked out.

c)    *educational process?*

I think the biggest challenge was getting students involved right away in ongoing research at the two institutions. We had a potluck, get acquainted session just for the new Pew people, and we had, of course, the Pew people who were already in place, but we also invited a lot of faculty, and they got up and gave a little speech about what kinds of research they were doing. We did that beginning the third year, and it really worked well. It really gave the students a taste. I spent a lot of time taking students around and introducing them to the faculty and explaining the research projects. We arranged lunches for them to talk to the individuals. Some were intimidated, others were great, and yet others would get involved in too many projects. It was sometimes hard to get people to settle down. Students seemed to work better and better as time went on. Students really got right in there. They also knew their funding was for 3 years. You know there is an end to the funding, and if nothing else, that should give you a nice clear incentive.

7.  *What lessons were learned about the educational process in terms of:*

    a)  *recruitment?*

There is a variety of needs that exist in the potential student population: postdoctoral, doctoral (both residential and non residential), midcareer. No one program can fulfill all these requirements. I think that made requirement efforts really wonderful for the people. For example, Steve Crane, Ted Benjamin, and I had a booth at the American Public Health Association annual meetings for several years, and we always placed it right next to the Michigan booth because that is where David Perlman was and we had this national program with all these offerings. It was wonderful. This was one of the things that was really interesting. We were, as directors, very eager to have really good students in our program, but if they didn't fit the mold, we were very free to advise them on what the other programs were offering and put them in touch with the other people. Recruitment was a dream. It was great.

    b)  *degree requirements?*

When implementing a new program within an existing institution, the fellowship requirements must at least meet the needs of the degree grantor, and additional requirements toward that degree may discourage some potential fellows. We put that burden on our students with our curriculum. We required four additional courses. Eventually, both UCLA and RAND accepted one of our courses as a substitute for something that was a requirement, but the other three were really additional. Programs have very little leeway in allowing you electives. There is so much required. Some were discouraged by that, but not too many. It was a burden that most students were willing to bear.

    c)  *curriculum and content?*

These areas were the great selling points of the RAND/UCLA program, it was unique to require OJT with the classroom study, and potential fellows relished the idea of the meshing of these two areas. That was a real bonus that we didn't even know we had.

    d)  *integration of fellows with other students, the university and the program?*

In the beginning there was some antipathy toward fellows who had lucrative fellowships and seemingly did not have to "work" while going to school. However, this faded over time as nonfellows and faculty began to realize that these were serious, hardworking individuals who had been legitimately honored for their previous scholarship and work. They worked just as hard in the classroom and on their research projects for their dissertations as others. Midcareer fellows were just wonderful. Here were people who came out of senior positions and we were in essence taking them back to the classroom, and they became humble very quickly. It was real interesting. There was a lot of cross-fertilization between the doctoral students and the midcareer students. They often traded notes and gained understanding from each other. It was really nice. We really didn't have any snobs in our group, at least not that I knew of. There may have been experiences that I didn't hear about.

*You also had open seminars that probably made a big difference, right?*

Yes. They did make a big difference.

e)    *relationship between faculty and students?*

Over time very strong bonds were created between faculty and students, since the students were not just faces in the classroom but integral members of research teams with faculty team leaders. That was really great, particularly at RAND. People who are doing research at RAND usually aren't doing just one project. They are usually involved in several and so they might be the leader of the research project in one area and they might be the co-principal investigator on another, or they might just being giving input as a statistician on another. And so they played various roles, and thus, the students were able to see them in different roles, and this was very good. There was a lot of camaraderie, and our faculty showed up for every award ceremony or whatever. Every year we gave a certificate for the midcareer fellows, and the faculty always showed up. There was lots of support.

f)    *completion rates (where applicable)?*

We talked about this already. Al Williams will have to speak more specifically to this issues. I no longer have access to this information. My sense is that the doctoral program has a nearly 90 percent completion rate and the midcareer program had no dropouts, which is essentially a 100 percent completion rate. It was a huge success the midcareer program. We even had people who came on their own nickel in the second funding. We funded three, but their were several years when we had four and one year when we had five, which was too many. These were people who said they really wanted to do this, and they didn't care if there was no more Pew money.

8. *To what extent do you think the program is beneficial for those who do not finish?*

The students that I remember who did not finish actually completed the course work and some research but did not finish the dissertation, which I believe is fairly common. People very rarely do 1 year and then say that's it. They usually make it to the dissertation stage. At least two of the individuals are in key positions to influence health policy. Al Williams will have to speak to the others. However, these two individuals have revealed to me recently that their experience in the RAND/UCLA program reinforced their work ethic (due to the combined on-the-job training and classroom study experience) and exposed them to a variety of health policy issues so that they have better understandings of the work they are engaged in today. I think that speaks well. One person actually applied for the midcareer program and the PhD program and then chose the PhD program. He did not complete the dissertation, but he made a conscious decision not to finish; it wasn't just that he drifted off. He got an amazing job offer and went with it. So, I don't think it hurt him in his career not to have the PhD, but I think it's obvious from the way he talks that those 2 years were really important to him.

9. *How can we measure success for those programs where completion rates do not apply (e.g., postdoctoral programs)?*

This is an unusual question. If you mean where no degree is granted, that is one issue, but the postdocs and management fellows at UCSF and the midcareer fellows at RAND/UCLA completed their programs by participation for the duration of the fellowship. However, as a measurement of success, one need only look at where those individuals are today: how they have become engaged in health policy decision making as their careers have progressed.

10. *How does the Pew program approach differ from the traditional fellowship approach? How have the major outcomes differed?*

Perhaps the greatest difference is the variety within the "set" of programs from residential to nonresidential doctoral programs, to midcareer and postdoctoral study at six institutions which offer varied research focuses: social policy, health services research, health policy management. I don't know how the outcomes have differed. One way may be that people in the clinical scholars program become clinical faculty; people who are Kellogg fellows sort of stay where they are but then go off to Turkey and China and different places, but as I see it Kellogg fellows sort of stay in the career they were in, and I think the Health Policy Fellowship Program offered more opportunities for people to either change career or really advance in their career more quickly.

11. *If you were going to give advice to another university attempting to initiate a similar program, what would you say?*

Get strong commitments from faculty and the administration because not everything works the first time around. Be flexible. Get the best students. Recruitment is key.

12. *What is the Pew program "legacy" in terms of:*

a) *health policy?*

Former fellows are involved in health policy decision making at all levels, federal, state, and local, as well as in health policy research at universities and public- and private-sector research firms. I really think that is the legacy. What they bring to those areas: they are smarter, they are better informed, and they have a broader viewm and this is true of all the programs, not just RAND.

b) *education and training?*

Former fellows have faculty positions in universities throughout the country, and they are training new health policy analysts based on the Pew training that they themselves received. Additionally, faculty from the six programs have moved from institution to institution and replicated parts of or the whole Health Policy Fellowship Program curriculum and study methods to their new institutions. A prime example is Joe Newhouse at Harvard, who took the RAND program in its entirety, tweaked it some, and put it into place at Harvard. That is seeding the field.

c) *your institution?*

It is my understanding that the RAND Graduate School and UCLA continue to train health policy students using the program set in place by Pew funding.

13. *Are there important issues you feel that this interview does not address? If so, please feel free to add comments and/or concerns.*

The pride I feel in the accomplishments not only of "my" Pew fellows but also fellows from the other programs! I think its really a wonderful feeling that I didn't know was going to happen for me. When I go to a meeting, like AHSR, and I see them receiving awards, presenting papers, leading discussions, and being on the planning committee, and then at APHA I see the same kinds of things going on. And now that I'm in Washington I see a lot of them even if they are not in Washington working. They come here, they are leading panels, and it's wonderful. And, of course, the network is phenomenal. The alumni connect with each other. People looking for jobs can just call another Pew fellow, even if they don't personally know them, and more often than not that common bond sets the stage. The whole thing happens. It's grand. Former fellows are very proud to say that they were Pew fellows. Pew ought to be very happy about that. How do you quantify that? You can't.

## Telephone Interview with Steve Crane
Tuesday July 23, 1996, 9 a.m.

1. *Based on your experience and familiarity with the fellows and the programs, what did the Pew program really accomplish? What are the
most important contributions?*

The most important contribution has been to create a
network of people who continue to interact and who continue to have important positions in the policy system, both
public and private policy. These people understand and
know each other and are able to get things done. The policy system does not work through formal authority channels
but most often through informal channels, and it's not what
you know but who you know that counts; the networking
was really important. Secondly, I think that the Pew program
got some people involved in health policy from perspectives
that would not otherwise have been present. This relates a
lot to what the Boston University (BU)/Brandeis program
specifically intended to do. One of the core concepts for the
program was to create a shortened, highly focused program
that would reduce the time and cost barriers so that people
who were already actively engaged in health care concerns
could come back and get that doctoral education and go out
and be effective. More than just getting busy people, what
we wanted to do was to get people from nontraditional sectors like business to come in and to begin to create a different type of cadre of people who could span both public- and
private-sector concerns. At the time that this program was
started there was an awakening of the notion that in fact if
change was going to occur (and we had no sense that it was
going to occur as rapidly or as dramatically as it has), we had
to get policy issues out of the public sector and involve the
private sector. So, the whole focus, at least of the Boston
University side of the BU/Brandeis program, was to try to
create links with the business community where attempts
were already being made to control costs, improve quality,
and gain a handle on what was going on in the health care
system. I think that was a pretty significant contribution of
the program in total as well as one of the major contributions of at least the BU side of the BU/Brandeis combine.

We can also say that we identified a very bright group
of dedicated people who were trained and connected to
some of the major policy leaders in the country, and we
probably shortened the amount of time that it took them to
become effective in the system. The other great thing of the
Pew program was the many different opportunities the stu-

dents had to meet the major leaders in the field, in both the public and private sectors. Those relationships gave the program a weight of influence in the system and gave the students access to those foci that they could use to influence policy more quickly.

2. *How and why did your specific program develop? To what extent will your program continue now that Pew funding has ceased?*

In terms of how our specific program developed, as a result of the competition and as a result of the institute at BU being selected to work with Brandeis, the notion there was really to see if the business community could be involved in this in some way. The particular center at BU that was involved was the Center for Industry and Health Care. A very important part of the history of our program and I think the history of the Pew program is the fact that there were really three programs at BU/Brandeis: the doctoral program, which we always talk about; and the Pew Corporate Fellows program at BU that brought together major industry leaders involved in health care issues to Boston twice a year and created a network in the business community, the results of which are still being seen today in terms of the corporate coalitions that have been created and the analyses that continue to be done on health outcomes. I think these things are attributable to the types of discussions that took place not just at BU. I think we were a catalyst for a lot of that. It is a very important part of our total program. Likewise, Bruce Spitz's Community Program at Brandeis was very important. The notion was that we needed to create change not just at the intellectual level but at the institutional level as well. Bruce's efforts to try to get communities to move and to link together business and the public sector was highly innovative and was a precursor to the coalitions of today and the more population-based research being employed today. That was a very important part of the stimulus, particularly from the BU side.

With respect to the continuation of the program, the program has ceased at BU, and it ceased not too long after I left. The major problem at BU was lack of university institutional support. There was a lot of support at the Center for Industry and Health Care for the program, but what we were trying to do was very difficult. We wanted to create a doctoral program that would get you in and out within 2 years through a challenging process. We wanted to give students a great degree of flexibility in the courses they chose so that they would waste the least amount of time taking courses that someone thought were important but weren't directly relevant. We wanted to take in students who already had an advanced degree and substantial experience and didn't have to learn what they wanted to do with their lives. We tried to identify and choose people who knew exactly what they wanted to do and who could find what they wanted here at BU, and in that way get them in and out very quickly. We ran up against some big problems in terms of typical university structure: first, where to house this program. Happily, BU had the University Professors Program that allowed for a much more loose set of courses. The problem there was that this program was designed specifically for nonpolicy science types. The program was more in the literature and arts area, so they had a hard time understanding health policy because it wasn't a specific discipline, and they had an even harder time understanding the practical orientation and the need for these people to get out quickly. As Sol Levine, the academic director of the program, put it, the philosophy was that students ought to be able to "wallow" and pursue interests that they wanted to gain the knowledge that they need for a doctoral experience. I certainly subscribed to that in my own doctoral program, but that is not what this program was about. That is not what these students were about. There was a real culture clash between the academic directors of the program where we put the students and the students themselves. That took a lot of work.

Another aspect was that BU wasn't committed in a financial way because there was no school, there was no program, there was no department, and there was no faculty. We borrowed from everyone to put it together. Without that hard, fast focus of a strong department, the program was almost invisible to the university.

Thirdly, the students were nontraditional university types. They weren't planning academic careers; they were planning careers in business and public service. They were interested not so much in peer review but in having an impact on the policy system. I think the university, the traditional academic system, looks somewhat askance at these students at BU. I think the situation was different at Brandeis, where you had a well-established academic center and well-established academics taking all the students under their wing and providing protection. That was very hard in the medical center, and probably the greatest failure of our program was not to get Dick Egdahl more invested in what was going on. But, his interest was much more on the Corporate Fellows Program. He made a great contribution there, and

Sol [Levine] and I, and later Jon Howland, I think, made a very significant contribution on the doctoral side.

*Prior to the Pew program had there been in place a corporate program on which your structure was modeled? Are there now any programs that perhaps drew upon the success of the BU program?*

The BU Corporate Fellows program still existed at BU until at least this past year or so. It has transformed itself in various ways, and Dick Egdahl has retired, so I'm not sure of its current status. Certainly at BU that tradition carried on for years after the formal ending of the Pew grant to BU. What happened at other places I really don't know. We certainly promoted this program to Pew. But Pew didn't really promote the program any further than listening to our reports, and because perhaps the centerpiece of the program became the doctoral program, nothing much was done with the Corporate Fellows program. I think it was a lost opportunity. It's ironic because one of the things that Pew really liked in the original proposal was this notion of doing something with the corporate sector, these groups of people who could benefit from the knowledge of health policy research but who generally had little access to it, and likewise to give access inside corporate knowledge to the academics. I think there were some lost opportunities there. I think a lot was accomplished and a lot of networking was done through BU, but being a fairly aggressive person on these things, I think not as much was done as might have been.

*How do you think the connection with Brandeis contributed to or hindered the success of the BU program?*

My impression of the BU/Brandeis relationship is nothing but positive. I think we worked very well together. The students had access to courses at Brandeis, but I think the greater problem was the Brandeis students who wanted to take more courses at BU but Brandeis said no. From our curriculum's perspective, we wanted our students to have any of the courses they wanted, whether it was at BU or Brandeis. We were able to negotiate this successfully. Brandeis, with its much more structured curriculum, only allowed students to take one or two courses, if that, outside of Brandeis. I think more of the frustration was on the Brandeis side rather than on the BU side. I think the BU students really appreciated the flexibility that we gave them. It was little bit difficult because they would come into the program and sort of have to find their own way, but once they did they appreciated the chance to do what they wanted to do.

We provided as much advice and guidance as we could; we forced them to take more statistics and research methods classes than they probably wanted to take. They certainly were not bereft of intellectual guidance. As the program progressed we helped students to develop a social science core (sociology, economics, and political science) so that they had a base from which to work, but the whole concept of this program was interdisciplinary. Ironically, the model that we used was Diana Chapman Walsh's. She completed the University Professors Program and then worked very closely with Dick Egdahl. Diana's role in all of this is very important. Interestingly, Allyson Ross Davies, who got the RAND/UCLA program going, was a very close friend of Diana's and modeled some of what was done at RAND and UCLA on what was done at BU with the University Professor Program. Allyson left the program fairly early, and so that legacy was lost. There is a lot of interconnectedness here in terms of the start and operation of the program.

*Some people mentioned the tension between having the flexible curriculum and getting the needed skills. Can you speak a bit to that?*

There definitely was a tension there. The program wasn't as assertive with the students in saying you must take this and this. We weren't sure what the "musts" should be. As we went along in the program and we saw what students did, we saw then what we needed to do. Toward the end we probably had a much better sense than in the beginning of what we needed to do in terms of requirements. We were learning. Certainly for some students, the lack of our knowledge early on may have created some gaps.

Secondly, we knew that some of our students had gaps. We told them that they had gaps and we told them what they had to do and for whatever reasons some chose not to follow our recommendations. From our perspective they ended up with gaps; however, I'm not sure whether from their perspective they ended up with gaps. That is a faculty issue. Faculty often want to create students in their own image. Yes, there are tensions, but what we broke out of were the traditional doctoral program of 5 years of suffering and 4 years of writing.

3.  *What was the need in the health policy community when your program started, and how have those needs changed? To what extent has the Pew program meet the changing needs?*

I answered that in part by saying that there was a real need for two fundamental things to happen. The first is an interdisciplinary approach. We wanted to get away from the strict departmental lines. The Robert Wood Johnson Scholars program that exists now at Brandeis was really inspired by the Pew program and the emphasis on interdisciplinary training. They have taken a slightly different track by taking people out of disciplines to put them together, and so interdisciplinary is defined as having representatives from each of the different disciplines in the same room. Our approach to being interdisciplinary was that each of these disciplines had to be represented in each student. We felt that the problems in the system were not unique and discipline oriented; they weren't just purely economical or purely political. To have effective people we needed to have people who had true interdisciplinary training. That was point number one. That is why the university program was so wonderful. We were able to allow the students to focus just on the interdisciplinary stuff.

The second need that existed in the system was for the public, private, and not-for-profit sectors to work more closely together. A lot of programs produced people just for the public sector or just for the academic sector, but rarely just for the private sector. What we wanted to do was to have someone who had not only the vocabulary but also the knowledge to cross-walk academics, public service, the private sector, and the nonprofit sector. That is why we tried at BU at least to pull from each of those sectors and to put these people in the same room and to give them the perspectives they needed to go out and in true interdisciplinary style solve some of these very complicated problems.

I think those needs still exist, and most of the academic programs are still turning out discipline-focused individuals. The Heller School at Brandeis is an exception. What we need are people who can understand problems from a multiplicity of viewpoints and who can create solutions that cut across disciplinary and sector perspectives. We are still short on people who can do that.

> *When the program started there was a real emphasis on training health policy researchers and health policy makers, and it seems that today the programs that are getting funding have changed that emphasis, at least in name, to health services researchers. Why is that? What is the difference between the two terms? Why is it that people seem to flip between the two terms?*

That is a good question. There is a real difference. Let me lay out a continuum. On one end of the continuum you have disciplinary research (economics, political science, and sociology). On the other end of the continuum you have policy-related research (defined generally as finding research-oriented solutions to practical problems). Between these two you have health services research. Health services research is, in a way, a systematic and rigorous analysis of how health care is delivered and the consequences of the delivery of health care. That borrows from disciplinary research, because it's often done based on theory. Its purpose is to contribute to a literature, and its main contribution is to help us understand how something works. Policy research, by contrast, takes all that information but then applies it and focuses more on solutions and change as opposed to understanding what has happened in the past. Health services research produces the information. You then take the health policy researchers to figure out where we want to go.

I think the reason why the program has drifted from health policy back to health services research is because health services research has a disciplinary base and traditional academic viewpoints prevail. Health services research is still more accepted than health policy research. Most universities haven't got the foggiest idea what to do with someone who wants to go to a state legislature and work on a bill; that is not considered academic. I think there are institutional forces that sucked those programs back to health services research. Furthermore, there is a tremendous community of support in health services research, and you tend to go where your friends are. Most of the policy-type programs tend not to be oriented toward health care but rather public administration, public policy, and political science, all a different set of institutions than we chose to involve in this program. The field itself is not well defined or well accepted. So, given all that ambiguity and uncertainty I'm not surprised at the shifting back. Again, the standards for the field have become publications and peer review journals. I see nothing wrong with that, but policy makers don't read peer review journals. They read editorials in the *New York Times*. To borrow a phrase from Bob Blendon, it's more important sometimes for people interested in these problems to publish an Op Ed piece in the *New York Times* than to publish an article in the *New England Journal of Medicine*. The academic institutions have slowed us down, again.

*How do you think the Pew Health Policy Programs changed this outlook, if at all. Were the programs merely a blip on the screen, or will they be readily institutionalized and replicated?*

I think the programs are a blip on the screen. I could also say that the academics won. The RAND program was always much more academically oriented than any of the other programs. It was a good program. Why the programs were cut off is another study in and of itself. The Michigan program structurally should have been as practically oriented as the BU program, and certainly the students who were at Michigan were closest to the types at BU/Brandeis. The problem with Michigan was that the people teaching the programs (and I was one of them who helped write the Pew grant) were all academics. Very few of them have set foot in the real world, and again, their goals are perfect academic publications. At BU, perhaps because of some radical notions that some of us had, we were willing to push the envelope and say that your dissertation came out and was used by policy makers; this is a triumph. Even the Pew newsletter, with all due respect to Marion Ein Lewin, counts the number of peer-reviewed publications. What message is that sending? We missed the point here. The traditional academics won, and this is not surprising. It was a huge battle, and what we were dealing with were institutions caught up in a lot of tradition. They were structure and process oriented, not outcomes oriented. So, there is a tremendous need for another Pew program, not so much to change health policy, although that is necessary too, but to begin to change academic institutions. We were, in the BU program in particular, a real threat to the academic structure, and there needs to be more of that.

4. *What was it about your curriculum that contributed or did not contribute to your program's success?*

I spoke a bit about the curriculum already, and the other important part was the weekly seminars. We would come together in what is termed now in the literature as a *learning community* or *learning conversation*. We would all try to take a problem and solve it from our different perspectives. People who were into economics would approach the problem from their perspective, and people from political science would approach it from theirs, and we would share views and learn from each other. That was just a tremendously stimulating activity that we could have made even stronger than it was. Nonetheless, it was an important part.

*What is an interdisciplinary dissertation? How can you bring someone through an interdisciplinary program and have them produce a product that can be used, as you mentioned above, by policy makers?*

To explain this, one needs to begin with the question, What is a disciplinary dissertation? A disciplinary dissertation is that you start with a problem statement which is, 10 to 12 pages to say what question you're going to address. Then your second part or chapter invariably is a literature review and theory discussion describing how you're going to approach the question. Then you do your analysis and make a contribution to the question and perhaps the theory as well. Because theory is fairly complex, you are encouraged to deal with the most narrow part of a problem or theory.

An interdisciplinary dissertation says that you begin to approach a problem not just from the perspective of one discipline but perhaps from several so that there may be two or three disciplinary frameworks that you would look toward to solve a problem. A simple example: One of the scenarios/ questions that I would ask students when I was interviewing them for the program was to assume that they were the assistant to the mayor of a city and that there is a real problem with garbage collection. Some neighborhoods aren't getting garbage picked up, it's mounting up, and all kinds of issues are arising. How would they undertake analysis of that problem? Invariably even students who come in and say they have an ecumenical view of the world will find a particular cut on that problem that they would use as their lens. They start talking about either resource allocation, cost, the politics, the sociology, or the psychology. I could tell pretty quickly what people's natural disciplinary perspective was based on how they answered that kind of question. In terms of a dissertation it would be the same thing, only in reverse. You would be posing your problem and then discussing the different aspects of that problem and how it could be enlightened by different disciplinary contributions. The other side of it was to have people who on the dissertation committee held divergent views to test, probe, prompt, and push students to think about things in more ways than just one. That was the other part of the dissertation process: having an interdisciplinary committee.

*Do you think that faculty in this type of program should be made up of economists, political scientists, and sociologists, or should these positions be filled with professionals who have the type of interdisciplinary degrees that Pew is granting?*

That is an interesting question. The kinds of people that the Pew programs were graduating are rare. Universities recruit straight disciplinary people. I, myself, am a product of an interdisciplinary background, and maybe I was using my model as much as anything. My program was essentially a health policy analysis program, and the core discipline, if you could define one, was economics with a lot of overlay of sociology, organization theory, and law. I ended up teaching politics without a graduate course in politics to my name. I wasn't a bad model. Another anecdote: When I went to Michigan in 1970 and 1971 the Institute for Public Policy Studies had just been created out of the old Institute for Public Administration. The whole purpose of that program was to be interdisciplinary. Their definition of interdisciplinary was to get a political scientist, a sociologist, and an economist to have an office beside one another. It just didn't work. Those folks never talked to one another. Eventually, they got it right, but it took a long time to do it. I would like to see good strong disciplinary people around the table, but they have got to be committed to listening and learning from each other. There are some disciplinary people who can do that, and there are others who cannot. A lot of disciplinary people only want to say "my discipline is right and the only way to go." Those are the people I don't want to have at the table. I think it takes a couple of people like myself and the Pew graduates to be able to ask the questions to bring those disciplinary perspectives out, but I don't think it should be all one or all other. But, I do believe that at a minimum there should be straight disciplinary people there.

5.  *What was the most innovative or unique aspects of:*

    a)  *your program design?*

    b)  *methods of implementation?*

    c)  *educational process?*

I've already spoken about the innovations.

6.  *What were the biggest challenges or barriers to overcome in terms of:*

    a)  *your program design?*

    b)  *methods of implementation?*

    c)  *educational process?*

The biggest challenge was how to get students started on a dissertation in the first week of their program when they haven't the foggiest idea of what a dissertation is. This has to be successful if you're going to get people turned out in 2 years. We succeeded in some cases but not in others. I think we solved the problem related to trying to figure out what to do for a dissertation, because we tried to screen people as best we could before that. We really wanted to get people who knew what they wanted to do. Fortunately or unfortunately, some people came in and wallowed until they found other things to write dissertations on. We also celebrate that. That was the toughest thing: how you formulate a question. One of the other big intellectual challenges that I found myself addressing all the time was teaching the students that they came to a doctoral program not to learn what they were to know but to learn what they did not know. That was, hopefully, one of the big contributions I made to the intellectual development of the students: to teach them that it's not what you know, it's what you don't know that is important. And, then I wanted to teach them how they knew or didn't know something, which was the application of research methods and analytical thinking. The other thing, our students averaged 12 to 14 years of experience when they came into the program. They had pretty well-established beliefs about the world. The first few seminars were always really tough because people who had worked up a particular view or perspective would come in and would express it and expect the rest of the world to believe it just because they said it and believed it. In the academic world, that is not good enough. You have to explain not only what you're saying but why you're saying it. To get students to understand that they have to leave their cherished beliefs behind or to keep only those that have some type of empirical or rigorous proof was really tough. It was tough because in traditional programs you have people who are younger, who have less experience, and who are less set in their ways. These were savvy, smart people, and once they got it, they got it and they were great, but getting them to that point was tough. We essentially said that maybe what they believe in wasn't right. I'm convinced that one of the other things this program did was to value the mature learner. We proved that there is a place in an academic institution for the mature learner. The discussions, the group, and the experiences that we had were just tremendous. That maturity factor was important. We as faculty sat around the table as much as the students, and the students who were there were as much faculty as we were. It was a true community of learners. Of course, there was a hierarchy, because at the end of the semester we were able to tell them whether they were right or wrong. One of the major problems the students had was fitting into the role of a student, putting themselves in a totally dependent, subservient role. For many this was very difficult. Many were highly accomplished people with big titles and far bigger salaries then we who were faculty. And, to come in and be talked to, lectured at, evaluated, measured, probed, etc., was a very uncomfortable experience. Some people adapted to it and others fought it. The ones who fought it had the toughest time.

7. *What lessons were learned about the educational process in terms of?*

   a) *recruitment?*

   b) *degree requirements?*

   c) *curriculum and content?*

   d) *integration of fellows with other students, the university, and the program?*

   e) *relationship between faculty and students?*

   f) *completion rates (where applicable)?*

I think the recruitment really is the critical issue. We were blessed because we worked very hard at it and because we had some very good applicants. The choices were always exceedingly difficult. I think that it has been said often that the quality of a program is presumably measured by what you contribute to a student. Actually it's very easy, because if you take a good student in you'll turn a good student out. I'm not sure we transformed many students. That would have taken a lot longer than a 2-year program.

A couple of lessons: (1) Two years probably was ambitious; 3 years is probably more realistic. But I would keep a 2- to 3-year time frame because if you start a 3-year program it will become a 4-year program. I think that was a lesson. (2) I would now give a much greater emphasis to research methods and slightly more attention to quantitative methods. I think overall we did OK there. There are two or three things that you get out of a doctoral program. One is analytic thinking, and that is where the research methods come in. We really need to do a lot more on research methods, and that means Campbell and Stanley stuff and not just statistics. Second, we need to help students develop that core disciplinary perspective, not so they become a disciplinarian but so that they have a good strong starting point from which to observe other disciplines and other problems. Third, I think we need (we should have) developed more of a core faculty for the program. There was a structural failure, and it was probably on the part of BU to ask for this. Dollars weren't available to pay faculty to become involved in this type of program. It's one thing to provide dollars for students. I think you have to buy people off in an academic setting. There are too many competing demands, and some dollars for faculty would have been very helpful as an inducement, which is sad but perfectly understandable. Fourth, I think that in the end Brandeis probably had a better approach to tying people to specific research projects so that the students didn't have to do primary data collection and they could work very well with a mentor and other researchers. People who worked on those kinds of projects did very well, and I think for a quick degree program that's what you want to do. If you want to learn how to collect data, then I think you ought to go to a traditional doctoral program and take longer to do because it takes longer to collect data. I think a lesson was learned there. I would give as much if not greater emphasis in the future to the policy seminars, to talking with one another. That community of learners is a critical part of all of this. There are some things you have to do on your own, but it's the group process that makes a big difference. Also, we thought that $10,000 was a generous stipend, and as one of my favorite students said when he came into the program early on, "You know we priced the program just right. It was too little to live on but too much to turn down." I always appreciated that phrase, and I've used it a lot, but I think we did a bit of disservice to our students by forcing otherwise senior people to live a student's life. You get what you pay for. I'd put more money into a stipend and help these students, particularly those with families. It was very hard for the people with families. It's hard enough to do a doctoral program without our making it more difficult. That's the monastic view of academics. I also think that we should have tried to bring in more people from the outside than we did. I think Marion's contributions to the program and the national meetings that we had were immense. We used to have two or three, and then we reduced it down to two and ultimately to one. I think that perhaps one of the most important things that we did was to have those joint national meetings where people from the different programs came together and met with outsiders. I knew it was an expensive process, but, boy, did that add a lot for all of us.

*Was that unique to Pew or was that something that you had heard of before?*

I think we did it more than some others, but the Robert Wood Johnson Clinical Scholars program did it, and that is something that is done because you have people you want to get together, and all the fellowship programs I've been involved with subsequently have had that as an essential part, but typically only once a year. I think that people should come together at a minimum twice a year to get to know one another and to become comfortable. The problems now are not institutionally oriented, they are not state oriented, they are nationally oriented. The problems cut across all the political boundaries. You need to have people who can take that view come together, and the more we spend time just in our own little cells sitting around with faculty from one institution, we are missing the fact that the problem is interdisciplinary, intersector, and national, not local, in scope.

*Kate Korman spoke about the joint recruitment effort all the programs had. Can you speak a bit to that?*

We pioneered that with our efforts to recruit people at the American Public Health Association's (APHA) annual meetings. We understood that each of the programs had a unique approach. What we wanted to do was to go out and try to get people who would be good for the program in general and then get them slotted or placed in the program that would be most appropriate for their interests. For the younger students, the ones more interested in a traditional academic career, RAND/UCLA (University of California, Los Angeles) was better for them. For the people who were more business oriented or problem oriented, the BU/Brandeis program was more appropriate. On the other side, the Michigan program was an on-job/on-campus program where people who couldn't get away from their work or didn't want to could get their degree. We all had something to contribute. We were competitive only in that we all wanted to be seen and do well by Pew and to stand in the best light. And that is very unique because most doctoral programs don't do that.

*Do you want to say anything else about the "set" of programs, how they complemented each other yet were very different? And how that benefited the health policy "scene/field"?*

I think one of the great strengths of the program as a whole were the individual faculty members involved. Can you imagine sitting down in a room with Phil Lee, Stu Altman, Stan Wallack, Dick Egdahl, Al Williams, Bob Brook—I could go on and list dozens of names—and be able to go up to them and talk with them, think and discuss with them for a day or two, and then go back to your institutions and do that on an ongoing basis, or if you want, call someone up in another institution: Phil Lee, Assistant Secretary for Health; Stuart Altman, Chairman of ProPAC (Prospective Payment Assessment Commission); and Joe Newhouse at Harvard, to speak with the people who are writing the articles, who are changing the world? Incredible. It was just incredible. So often doctoral students get stuck with assistant professors who are more interested in  fighting for tenure and their own existence. The Pew program on the other hand was just unbelievably rich, and the commitment that those senior people had to this group of students was extraordinary. That is something else that could be replicated by another program. There is still a strong need to get people from different institutions together. That phrase "inter" is really so important, not "intra" as doctoral programs traditionally are. They only look within themselves. This was "inter" in every respect of the word.

> *Almost without exception, every program director has mentioned that to have a successful program you need to have someone like Steve Crane. How does an institution go about finding that commitment and dedication?*

It's a flattering question, and I wish I had a good answer for it. A couple of things: Maybe one of the great contributions of BU was to have had a culture that would allow someone like myself to come in and gave me free reign to do what was necessary. I particularly appreciated the freedom and the tremendous resources that BU offered. This really made a big difference in what could be done. I do think it takes an individual or a group of individuals who believe very strongly in something to move a system, particularly one that is as rigid as an academic institution. There were lots of times when the answer came back, "No, that's not the way we do things," and we did it anyway. Perhaps because structurally I wasn't in a tenure track, my incentive was to keep the program going because that is where my pay was coming from. That may be a little bit of it, without demeaning it to that level. Certainly not having someone holding a tenure over my head made a huge difference. I think it takes someone who can see the possibilities and who works well with other people. I don't think there was anything unique about me, but it does very much help to have someone who has the vision and, number two, has the time to spend on this. There are a lot of people like that, I found them all over the place. The trouble is they were more constrained than I was in terms of their institutional setting or structure.

8. *To what extent do you think the program is beneficial for those who do not finish?*

This is a good question. I would like to think that people who didn't end up with a PhD degree still got a tremendous amount out of the program. We often said, and I don't know if this was right or not, in the end what is important is not whether or not you get a degree but what you learned. Nice idealized statement. We could say it though, because our goal was not to have someone go on and get a tenured track position in a university. If that was your goal and you don't get your PhD, then you have failed miserably. Our goal, however, was to produce highly capable people, people capable of effecting great change. I think we did that. I am sure that there is great personal frustration and disappointment at not being able to complete a dissertation. But in reality, while I'm sure that the academic program bears some responsibility for that result, a lot of responsibility remains with the individual. Either they got sucked back into their professional lives too quickly, they unfortunately couldn't create the time to do it, they refused to undertake the discipline to sitting down and organizing their lives so that it could get done, they couldn't quite get the notion of a single question to answer, they ran into tremendous problems with data, or they wanted to prove something that they couldn't prove and didn't want to do it if they couldn't prove what they wanted to prove. There are a whole variety of reasons for not finishing, and that's frustrating. But every one of those people, whether they finished or not, ended up as an equal part of the club. I don't think anyone in the program discriminates based on whether you finished or not. We revel and celebrate completion, but no one is considered a second-class citizen for not having finished. That's pretty amazing, because again, I think out focus was more on what you're going to do, not who you're going to be.

*Do you think the PhD is an appropriate degree?*

Ah, that's the big question. We ran into a lot of problems because it was a PhD as opposed to a DrPH or as opposed to a super master's degree. What was important about the level of education that we were talking about were a couple of things: (1) the emphasis on research methods and being not only a consumer of research, which you become with a master's degree, but a producer of research, which is signified by a PhD. People needed to have that knowledge whether or not they needed the degree for their careers. For some people the PhD was important because when you're out there battling in the world of health care that is so degree conscious, you really need to have the highest degree possible. So, from a marketing point of view, the PhD was really important. I think Michigan folks will feel a little badly about the DrPH because its considered to be a professional degree, which in the end is probably a more appropriate degree for this program, but it doesn't have the same cachet, doesn't give you the same entree or access to academic faculty positions, and doesn't give you the same identification when applying for research grants. So, on balance, I think the PhD has real value, signifying both the level at which you are working and your capability for independent research, and it puts you squarely in a position where you can look a doctor in the eye and not blink. Every other degree less than that is not as strong in that dimension. Whether you absolutely needed a PhD to be successful I would say it should be more competency based than degree based.

9. *How can we measure success for those programs where completion rates do not apply (e.g., postdoctoral programs)?*

First of all, I think the presumption of this question is all wrong. If you are defining success implicitly as being a degree, I don't think that is the right measure of success. I think again we are slipping back into the same academic mentality, like asking how many peer-reviewed publications do you have. I object to the question, but the answer to both a degree and a nondegree program is the same. It's not a degree, it's not a peer-reviewed publication, it's what you are contributing to the field. That is a soft measure, but one of the things that works very well in tenure review is when you take the number of references made to your work in the field. You're not measuring the quality of the work directly, but you're measuring it indirectly by how it is used. To me that is a tremendous measure. To the extent that the people we produce are in demand in the system, I think that's a measure. Even more important is the extent to which people have assumed leadership positions, and I don't mean to count titles, and are actively striving to make a difference, being innovative, and coming up with new ideas. All of that needs to be looked at to measure success. This program was all about change. It was not about training policy makers but was about training change makers. Change takes interdisciplinary people who can talk to one another. That was what this program was all about. One of the defining purposes of the Pew program, and one that set us apart from other PhD programs was that while we were striving to create people who could produce policy, our emphasis was more on creating people who could use policy. In essence we were creating change agents. Certainly at BU and Brandeis this was true. We focused on the intersection of the three worlds of the public sector, the private sector, and academia. We trained people to straddle the fence. Change comes from the interaction of these three sectors, and we knew that and we emphasized that. Focusing on that intersection effects lasting change. We are seeing this borne out today in the health care sector.

> *We have spoken about how the Pew HPFP goes against the very nature of a traditional PhD program, and one of the ways it did so was that the faculty were eager and had incentives to see that the fellows got their degree fast and got out. In traditional programs its almost a challenge for the students to prove that they deserve the degree. How do we address that issue?*

Again, that is partly faculty recruitment. You don't want to have involved in the program a faculty member who believes that no one is good enough to get the degree or that they should suffer for 10 years before getting the degree. There are a lot of those people out there. At the same time there are different kinds of students. There are students who say they want a quick degree just for the knowledge, to get in and get out and not to have their dissertation be their life's work. Those are appropriate students for a short-term program. We had some other people come into our program who said they wanted a fast track but who were real academics and who really wanted or needed to take the time. We couldn't track them into something faster. For those students it ended up being a mismatch. It is a recruitment issue on both the faculty and student sides, and I think the best approach is truth in advertising. The upside and the downside are to do some heavy-duty counseling in advance and monitoring as you go along.

10. *How does the Pew HPFP approach differ from the traditional fellowship approach? How have the major outcomes differed?*

I think we said enough about this.

11. *If you were going to give advice to another university attempting to initiate a similar program, what would you say?*

We've already discussed this.

12. *What is the Pew HPFP "legacy" in terms of:*

a) *health policy?*

I'll just use one example: John Dopkeen, a student at BU. He came from Boston City Hospital, knew the importance of incorporating the corporate sector with the government sectors and academia to understand health care policy problems. He made a tremendous contribution to the field in this way. The RAND/UCLA program did very significant work with satisfaction, the Brandeis program contributed at a more micro level, but still a very significant level, to issues of Medicaid, reimbursement, and prospective payment. Overall the Pew programs made lots of contributions on many different levels. The key there is not so much relating to a particular policy finding but rather the community of people who now contribute to ongoing change in policy.

b) *education and training?*

We have already identified a whole bunch of legacies in education and training: (1) the quick PhD that we pioneered, and we probably found as many problems as successes but we learned a lot; (2) the interdisciplinary approach; (3) the focus on change; (4) the intersector approach (the public, private, academic, and not-for-profit sectors); (5) the importance of discussion; (6) the need for emphasis on research methods and analytic thinking; and (7) the ability to take mature learners into the system and have them succeed. These are all very important contributions that we made to health policy education and training.

c) *your institution?*

I think the Center for Industry and Health Care probably is the last bit of legacy for BU. With Dick Egdahl retiring now, I'm not sure what will be left at BU. I think there is a tremendous legacy at Brandeis, but I assume you've gotten that from interviews.

The Pew legacy is really trite but true, and you've heard it before: the people who were trained. Even though we took in more mature students, some of whom are now in their 50s, there is still a huge crop of people coming along who are going to make a huge difference. I'm not sure that we've seen yet the contributions to health policy that the Pew students are going to make. It takes awhile. But as those folks come up and go through leadership positions, I think we'll see more and more. That emphasizes the important of trying to keep this group together as well as having them interact with some of the other program fellowship people who are around: those from the Johnson program and the Kellogg programs. All these people are unique. They are leaders, and they are going to make a contribution. The group effort is only going to enhance their already evolving skills.

It was a great time. It was Camelot.

The Pew Charitable Trusts really need to understand what positive feelings everyone has toward these programs. They have been very supportive. They are our colleagues in all of this. They hung with us when things were rough. They celebrated our victories. The Trusts deserve a lot of commendation for doing this and sticking with it. There are as many lessons to be learned on their side about how you deal with fellowship programs. This is a good point to make for other foundations. If this model is to be replicated, what the foundations are going to need to know about is not how it works at our end but how it works at their end. I could suggest a whole variety of lessons that I think foundations should have learned from this, and we can discuss this further at another time.

Telephone Interview with Al Williams
Monday July 8, 1996, 1 p.m.

1.   *Based on your experience and familiarity with the fellows and the pro-
     grams, what did the Pew program really accomplish? What are the
     most important contributions?*

We've produced a large number of successful PhD
grads and a smaller of number of midcareer folks who made
substantial shifts in their professional interest and orientation
to health policy. In addition, we built a strong curriculum
structure which is continued.

2.   *How and why did your specific program develop? To what extent will
     your program continue now that Pew funding has ceased?*

The program was born out of a long term relationship
between UCLA (University of California, Los Angeles) and
RAND. When Pew sent the letters way back, they sent a let-
ter to both UCLA and RAND and basically said that we
should get together and write a proposal. So that's what we
did, and that proposal was obviously successful. And, yes, it
continues in the sense that we have joint courses taught by
faculty at both the RAND Graduate School and the UCLA
School of Public Health. What doesn't continue in any consistent way is a rich fellowship. We do have fellowships, but
they are not as reliable and not as rich as they were in the
Pew days. I think we tend to get more MDs who have the
means to support themselves taking the programs. Thus, in
recent years we've produced more MDs/PhDs, some of
whom have had the RWJ Clinical Scholars support.

3.   *What was the need in the health policy community when your program
     started, and how have those needs changed? To what extent has the Pew
     program met the changing needs?*

The need was clearly expressed in terms of inadequate
numbers of broadly trained health policy people. Most of that
need and demand was in the public sector, and over time the
public sector, if it has not shrunk, has certainly not expanded,
at least on the federal side. More people are going into private activities in some degree in the state government. Our
folks tend to be quite strongly trained health policy
researchers, and there are as many positions as there were
before. We clearly have done well in meeting those needs in
the sense that our fellows have gotten good positions. But
there just aren't as many positions except in the private sector
now. There is clearly a movement toward private-sector jobs.

4. *What was it about your curriculum that contributed or did not contribute to your program's success?*

The main thing was this broad integrated policy research that was going on at RAND and, at the time, to a somewhat lesser extent at UCLA. That continues and has grown so that is a base on which to build a strong program. We also had in the RAND Graduate School a structure of policy workshops that was well suited to the kind of people we attracted. It was more collegial and less academic in terms of the culture as opposed to the content, and so I think the fellows did really well in that environment. But the strongest thing was the long-term relationship between RAND and UCLA and the substantial body of work.

5. *What was the most innovative or unique aspects of:*

a) *your program design?*

Probably what we call workshops or seminars on broad policy domains with a set of modules dealing with particular things were the most unique. For example, there is one on technology, regulation, innovation, and diffusion, and we deal with everything from the National Institutes of Health process of awarding grants to drug regulation. The one on health care financing has modules that deal with the hospital side, the physician side, and now the managed care side. That has worked well. Another thing that was unique (and one never knows just how unique one's own program is, as you only hear about the others) was that the exercises were in the form of short policy exercises: a short policy memo, a presentation, etc., all oriented toward current problems which captures the fellows.

The workshop model was a modification of part of the curriculum at the RAND Graduate School. It's oriented toward health and has become more stylized. That basic model was there, and what we tried to do was to apply it to health policy problems.

b) *methods of implementation and*

c) *educational process?*

This is a health policy emphasis grafted on two separate programs. One is a broad public policy PhD (at the RAND Graduate School), and the other is mainly a health services PhD at the UCLA School of Public Health. There is a heavy dose of required seminars that take the place of electives that existed in the program before. The fellows can cross-register at each place, but there is a common core of seminars that the folks take.

6. *What were the biggest challenges or barriers to overcome in terms of:*

   a) *your program design, b) methods of implementation, and c) educational process?*

I think that there was a short-term challenge in the form of leadership problems at UCLA for about 2 years that made things more difficult in terms of coordination and getting good people at UCLA. And there were the minor logistical problems that every program has with courses and instructors.

7. *What lessons were learned about the educational process in terms of:*

   a) *recruitment?*

We had a very low attrition rate, so I guess we did well in recruitment. We had basically two components. One was the PhD and the other was the midcareer component. I think except for some of the usual misjudging of how committed somebody is to doing something, we were pretty successful and didn't necessarily learn anything in particular. I guess we learned that we were doing things pretty well.

   *How about the midcareer program? That was a unique and innovative program. How did you go about recruiting these people?*

Basically, we sent out an announcement, and there was a fair amount of word of mouth. Over a fairly long period of time we have had tailored sabbaticals for people coming here. The midcareer program did not continue after the Pew funding ceased simply because we did not have the funding. We offer them an intensive, didactic, almost tutorial with one teacher and no more than three to five participants. That has ended, but we have continued to have people come when they come with their own money or own support from someplace. It pretty much recruited itself. We sent out formal announcement, but it was the word of mouth really.

   b) *degree requirements?*

Our fellows for the most part came in with a master's. We were looking for people who had already done work that required, in the case of the PhD students, their commitment to health, and in the case of the midcareer folks we basically took in people who had to convince us that they were committed. In most cases, the midcareer fellows had demonstrated substantial capability in a domain other than policy. We took people from a fairly broad range into the midcareer program. We have a fairly strong quantitative program. The program at UCLA is somewhat less oriented toward the quantitative. In both cases we basically looked for people who had strong backgrounds in this area.

*What about the dissertation process?*

The RAND Graduate Program has another unique feature that I didn't even mention because it has been around so long, and that is the on-the-job training component that's been there from the beginning. The fellows spend about half their time on projects. What we try to do is get them on a project that will lead toward their dissertation. It doesn't always work. That is not a requirement of the project time, but that is a component of guidance. That tends to get them started, and probably half of them tend to follow that. There are a lot of mentors around because we have a large research program, and so if it's not clicking with one person they move and eventually find someone with whom they click. It works. Obviously, some take longer than others. I could only count two that I would call dropouts (dropped out before completing the course requirements or exams) and only three who I don't think have completed the PhD.

c) *curriculum and content?*

I think it works well. The particular kind of workshop has been one that has been copied elsewhere. To some substantial degree Joe Newhouse's program at Harvard follows it. Imitation is a form of endorsement. Joe taught here until he moved there. I guess the other thing that worked better than I thought it would was that when we had the workshops we expected the midcareer fellows to take the workshops too. That turned out to be a leavening experience both ways. They learned from the more academically and methodologically oriented doctoral students, and the doctoral students learned from the real-world experience of the midcareer fellows.

d) *integration of fellows with other students, the university, and the program?*

Basically we opened up the workshops to people outside the fellowship program, and we had a fair number of takers and we still have a fair number of takers. That form of integration occurred. The RAND Graduate School program is by nature a small program, and so unless the class doesn't bond (which is very rare) there is almost forced integration. The workshops are still going. I just finished teaching a module on drug regulation. Only about half were committed health policy people from the beginning; others were taking the course because they wanted to increase their understanding of regulatory policies or the state of health technology. That is an example of integration.

There was perhaps a little bit of jealously in the early on. The Pew folks were looked at as being particularly well off and particularly free of having to worrying about getting projects. We changed that over time.

    e)    *relationship between faculty and students?*

It's by nature close. I mentioned earlier that it is more of a collegial atmosphere.

8.    *To what extent do you think the program is beneficial for those who do not finish?*

For those who drop out before completing the courses and exams I don't think much. I've lost track of one of them. Two people up front looked like risks and the program did really work for them, so I wouldn't want to take any credit for how they've done. For the three who haven't finished and are at least in theory in process, I think unequivocally for one the program very strongly affected his career and he has had a major role in the private sector. About the other two I'm a little less clear, but they are both doing health work, last I heard. I think in that sense they have been using their training. The answer is that those who get to the point of passing the general exams stay in health and do good work, yet it's not the same as a PhD. In the private sector, of course, they don't care so much.

9.    *How can we measure success for those programs where completion rates do not apply (e.g., postdoctoral programs)?*

We had essentially no one who didn't complete the midcareer program, but the question is how to measure success when completion rates do not apply. I think you simply look at their career and you have the testimonial there.

10.    *How does the Pew program approach differ from the traditional fellowship approach? How have the major outcomes differed?*

From the beginning we tried to [attract the] cream [of the crop]. We intentionally made it a rich program because we wanted to get the best students. Most programs cannot do that, and we can't do it now in the same way. The other thing was the UCLA and RAND relationship and the availability of cross-registering. For instance, the RAND Graduate School doesn't teach epidemiology but they have an epidemiology program at UCLA and a business school at UCLA. At both sides there is a lot of going back and forth across campuses. I don't think that is that common. My sense is, however, that BU and Brandeis did not integrate to the extent that we did.

I think that as a whole the Pew fellows have gone toward policy in a more focused way than people in the past. It did emphasize policy. The emphasis was different across the set of programs, but the policy side was more focused than I think is common. When Paul Ginsburg was running the Physician Payment Review Commission he hired several of our graduates and specifically noted that he preferred our graduates because while he needed people with strong analytic skills, he also needed people who had a background in the health care system and health policy. We created that mix of skills that set our fellows apart. The term management was in the title; however, we took that to mean policy management.

*Maybe you could just say a bit more about the common theme among the "set of programs?"*

I think they focused on what is a policy and what happens when you have one. That was a theme that I think existed across all programs: the declaration of a policy doesn't mean you have one. We certainly probed that, and I think it was probed at the annual meetings and at the other schools.

11. *If you were going to give advice to another university attempting to initiate a similar program, what would you say?*

I can't think of any other place, other than Joe Newhouse's at Harvard, that has concentrated their focus on getting the best people, as we did. Clearly, though trite, money helps. RAND and UCLA have been doing things together for a long time, but the impetus for sustained cooperation that was in the educational program wasn't there in the absence of funding. In particular, the existence of the Pew program brought the two programs together, particularly on the educational side. Money makes the difference. We have a unique situation here because we had existing programs and we didn't have to hire people to fill new positions. I would think it would be harder to start from scratch.

Thinking back about other programs, my sense is that Minnesota has developed a stronger policy focus over time. The program wasn't established before. The same is true with the program at Penn's Wharton School.

We were a test. The program was defunded and it's continuing. I don't think it would continue in the absence of funding if not for the strong research ties between the two institutions. The people who teach jointly for the most part are people who are also involved in joint research. My guess is that that is an uncommon situation. We clearly have a legacy of continuing joint courses between the two institutions and a fair amount of movement back and forth.

12. *What is the Pew HPFP "legacy" in terms of a) health policy, b) education and training, and c) your institution?*

The legacy is a continued collaboration between the two institutions; there is also the legacy of continuing collaboration with former Pew fellows. Many of the fellows go through a transition period after they complete their degree. They continue to consult on the projects they were involved in for a while after.

13. *Are there important issues you feel this interview does not address? If so, please feel free to add comments and/or concerns.*

There is a criticism. Pew became a pretty bumpy place, at least toward the end of our relationship, especially in the health area. The turnover has been great.

Is it reasonable for a foundation to start a program with the idea at the beginning that somehow it will become self-sufficient? I think we have done pretty well, but I don't think the premise for that is strongly based in history. I am sure that were it not for the strong research program here, it would not have continued. The current health program at RAND is about $16 million, and that provides a base for supporting students to some degree, but that is getting harder and harder to do with budgets getting cut, etc. It is very hard to maintain a program in the absence of a strong research base and strong research funding.

Kate and I will try to dig up some statistics and any other information you may find helpful to represent the RAND/UCLA program.

**Telephone Interview with Midcareer Alumna
Kathleen Eyre**
Monday July 8, 1996, 11 a.m.

**1a.** *Based on your experience and familiarity with the Pew program, what did the program really accomplish? What are the most important contributions?*

I did the midcareer program, that unusual 1-year fellowship that brought professionals into the health policy realm. I would have to say that the greatest accomplishment was introducing a paradigm or a way of thinking to existing professionals. We all came out of professional positions. I had a physician and another lawyer in my class. So, we came in with our own professional set of skills and analytic tools, and what we were introduced to for the first time was a rigorous policy analysis paradigm and way of thinking, the kinds of questions to ask, and the different disciplines that influence policy (it's very varied, obviously).I in our brief year we were exposed to all kinds of different academic settings and disciplines. The greatest accomplishment, therefore, for the midcareer fellows was the introduction of a paradigm, of an analytic set of tools that was an overlay to an existing set of professional skills and that was extremely useful in going forward. Other kinds of things would be that professionals were introduced into the academic world, giving us an understanding how academics think and work, and also vice versa, exposing academics to other professionals in terms of "in the real world we would think this way." There was probably pretty positive cross-fertilization both ways. Then, of course, as you hear from everybody the great network that was developed. I just can't underscore that enough. It's been such a huge advantage for me in the policy world, particularly since I've been back in Washington, just to call people up and say "what about doing this project," and there is a lot of good examples of that which I'll talk about later.

In terms of the overall accomplishments, the Pew programs as a set of programs set up a curriculum for the training of health policy analysts and professionals. It really established a model for training in a lot of different settings that will continue in those particular settings and in many others, I'm sure.

**2.** *What was the most innovative or unique aspect of your program design and implementation?*

It was the opportunity of stepping out of a successful professional career for a year. It's really unusual to be able to do that. The timing, the setting, the stipend, all of those things contributed to the ability of existing professionals to step out and add that layer of analytic skills to their existing policy skills without investing a huge amount of time or a huge amount of financial sacrifice. It's that incredible unusual opportunity of being able to go back to school, having intensive training in policy analysis, and taking that out into the world.

> *How did you come to make this obviously difficult decision to leave work? What brought you to the RAND program?*

I started as a federal health care antitrust prosecutor. That was my first job out of law school: competition issues for the U.S. Department of Justice, hospital mergers, and physician boycotts. I did some policy-related work, commented on federal regulations and Health Care Financing Administration policies, and the like and really enjoyed that, but decided I wanted to be exposed to the private sector so I went to the law firm, which had its own rewards, but what I really missed from my prior experience was the policy stuff. The decisions we were making then were going to influence an entire industry and the big picture, global movement of the world thing. I really missed those, and I didn't find those desires satisfied in the private sector. So, I left private practice, a very lucrative career, to do my Pew fellowship. However, being able to add that layer of very specific policy analytic skills and move my career in that direction was just tremendous. It was a tremendous opportunity, and I feel very privileged to have had that opportunity. It really made a big difference in my career path.

3. *What was it about the curriculum that contributed or did not contribute to the program's success?*

Just the basics. Having the opportunity to understand the economic paradigm and the sociological and behavioral sciences. Getting exposed to the social science ways of thinking were the greatest contributions of the curriculum. We also had very specific sets of policy analysis courses, and we had quality of care with Bob Brook and all these absolutely fabulous introductory courses to health policy issues. Then we were able to take that a step further with project work. I think Arlene Leibowitz's class was probably the best that we had in the curriculum. It was competition, regulation, and the notion of understanding markets in an economic point of view and she was just terrific. That was the most enlightening class of the entire spectrum. And then applying those introductory skills to specific sets of projects and being able to work on projects. I worked on a big MEWA (multiple employer welfare arrangements) project and small employer insurance options project. I worked on some tax-exempt hospital issues. It was very fun to have the ability to apply the sets of skills that we gained into specific projects. I think those were successes in the curriculum.

I think the thing that we missed in my program was that we didn't do a lot of general discussions on the major health policy issues. We didn't have a roundtable on reform, for example. Those were all touched upon, of course, in the course work that we took, but we didn't have a regular, organized, high-level discussion on, for instance, health care reform, which was the hot topic at that time (1989-1990). I missed that. I know that this type of thing happened at other campuses. I know UCSF (University of California, San Francisco) has a regular brown bag session on different topics of fairly global interest. We just didn't have opportunities to take cuts at the big picture. That's the major criticism that I would have of the midcareer program. I don't know if it was because of the time constraints. I think some of it was that, but some of it was that the focus was on giving you your basic skills. That was the most important part of the program. I think being able to put that in context would have been useful as well. Maybe it was a general philosophy of the institution. RAND isn't as liberal leaning as some of the other campuses. It was more concerned about the nuts and bolts of research and getting answers to important research questions. Some of that is just the nature of RAND. They do like to really be careful of any perception that they lean one way or another politically. They work for many different nonprofit clients, and so maybe there was an intentional effort to avoid any overt political discussion.

4. *How was the Pew approach different from the traditional teaching approach?*

The difference was the integration of the different social sciences and the specific focus on handling problems with a health policy framework. It's hard to understand what exactly "the Pew approach" means. I knew what my program was. I guess it is an interdisciplinary approach across the board, a rigorous exercise in disciplined thinking.

5a. *How has your professional life changed as a result of the Pew program? What value has Pew training added to your life?*

5b. *Has your career trajectory changed as a result of your time spent in the Pew program? If yes, how?*

It was a complete change for me, I got out of the law entirely. I left the program, consulted at RAND for a year, and then became director of health policy and advocacy for Blue Cross of California, so I worked on the private side in a health plan to help them understand policy issues and develop their own positions. That was really fun. I worked for Leonard Schaffer, who continues to be very interested in the national policy scene and a very thoughtful and controversial commentator on health markets and changes. I wouldn't have gotten the job, nor would I have been ready for the job without having had the policy training. It was really fabulous and wild. I directly link that switch in my career path to being able to do the midcareer program for the year. It was terrific. I then left (about 2 and a half years ago) to come to this institute which is a small nonprofit funded by 10 plans and have focused on managed care best practices. Obviously, it is a very hot topic: how do you integrate public programs into managed care settings, quality issues, and all those important issues? Again, this move was a direct result of the ability to have had the policy training. I can't say enough about how great it was for me. It allowed me to make a major career shift, and I am very happy with the decision that I made. The law was just too narrow, too contentious, and not aimed at thinking and solving the bigger picture issues. The work I do now, I feel, is contributing to society much more directly than the legal work I ever did. People feel differently.

*Can your speculate about your fellow classmates?*

Yes, I know the two folks in my cohort; Grant Bagley is now at the Health Care Financing Administration, he is an OB-GYN, a lawyer, and more. He is with the bureau of policy development working on things like coverage decision making, how you pay for particular procedures. He is most definitely using his Pew experience. He was at the Food and Drug Administration before that, so he is definitely using his policy spin. Lucy Eisenberg was my other classmate. I have not been in touch with her; however, as I understand it she went back to the law firm she had come from. I presume she is using her policy skills in her health practice, but I don't know for sure. I know all the PhDs I went to school with are doing incredible, fun, and interesting things.

*How was the interaction between the midcareer fellows and the doctoral students?*

It was very good, very healthy. Of course, they had much more strenuous courses, and dealing with the first year of a doctoral program is always hard, but the interaction was very often and very good. We worked together in courses and on projects. Part of the benefit of the program was for us to be able to be working with professional students like them.

6.  *If you did not complete the program do you plan to? If yes, why? If no, why?*

Not applicable.

7.  *What is the Pew "legacy" in terms of:*

a)  *health policy?*

A cadre of incredible well-trained people now exists. They are out there doing it in a lot of different sectors, both private and public sectors. It's an amorphous thing. You've got well-trained people working in the field in a variety of settings making changes. That's a huge legacy. Furthermore, they are talking to each other, which is part of the legacy, having developed that network.

b)  *education?*

The development of an established curriculum that I presume will be disseminated and used all over, again is invaluable. It is a terrific investment for the foundation folks.

c)  *your future?*

I'm going to continue in the policy world. It may not be in this same position. I'm going to be moving to California in the fall. My husband has a job at Berkeley, so I'll be making some changes, but I will continue to do policy-related work. I will always be grateful for the training, the exposure, the connection, the network, and the exposure to people at RAND. It has been invaluable and will continue to be invaluable for me. I can't say enough positive things about how great the program was. It has had real, genuine, important effects. I'd like to thank the Pew Charitable Trusts for creating the program and including me as a participant.

8.  *Are there any important issues that this interview does not address? If so, please feel free to add comments and/or concerns.*

Some of this is selective memory, of course, but overall I had really positive feelings. There were some criticisms at the time, the major one being that lack of the big picture that I already discussed.

Other than that I think this interview does a great job at getting at the issues. I'm thrilled that you called. We did feel slighted at the last couple of meetings, and I understand that the information just wasn't there, but in terms of presentation, we need some acknowledgment because its produced some really fine researchers who, in fact, in some respects are probably better trained than those from some of the other programs on the quantitative side.

**Telephone Interview with Doctoral Alumnus Leighton Ku**
Tuesday July 9, 1996, 10 a.m.

1a. *Based on your experience and familiarity with the Pew program, what did the program really accomplish? What are the most important contributions?*

I'm not sure I can differentiate between the contributions and the accomplishments. However, on a personal level, it helped me to get my PhD, which changed my career orientation. In addition, it put me in contact with a network of people who also were involved in health policy issues. At a broader level, I think that the important contributions or accomplishments of the program were that it helped establish health policy as an area of study, which had not been much studied at the point when the program began, and certainly took it out of somewhat, the traditional areas in which health policy was usually associated with, which was either as an adjunct to hospital administration or health economics. The Pew program brought health policy out from there.

There have been great changes in other health policy programs, and I think part of that is a result of what the Pew programs accomplished.

*Can you name any particular programs?*

There are certainly many more health policy programs than there used to be. For example Harvard has one, and Hopkins now has a fairly large and well-established health policy program. I don't think Hopkins had much of one all that long ago. So, here you have two of the biggest, most prestigious programs around, neither of which got any direct funding from Pew for their health policy programs yet, nonetheless, I think in part modeled some of Pew's activities. I remember back in November at the networking dinner that Kate Korman mentioned that Joe Newhouse took the Pew program to Harvard with him. The other place where Pew may have had an influence (and I'm not sure exactly what they are doing now) is at Berkeley. Helen Schauffler was a Pew fellow and is now one of the health policy professors at the School of Public Health. My impression has been that she sort of carried over some of what she studied.

*Can you speak a bit to the overall accomplishments of the Pew programs as a network or set of programs?*

The most direct benefit was that they trained a relatively large cadre of researchers and then, for the UCSF (University of California, San Francisco) program, program administrators who were able to do a continuing amount of work in health policy at the state and local levels and at the federal level at a time in which the issue suddenly became much more nationally prominent. I think there was definitely an element of fortuitous timing there.

2. *What was the most innovative or unique aspect of your program design and implementation?*

The most unique aspect of the Boston University (BU)/Brandeis program was the attempt to have a very accelerated program that provided a fair amount of program flexibility. I think the other thing that made it unique was, shall we not say a structural aspect, but it was something that was brought at the personal level, and that was that a lot of the faculty treated students really as friends and as peers. I think that was actually quite important in the program. I think that is one of the things that happened, certainly at our program and at the Michigan program, which may have been related to the fact that a lot of the students were older students who had experience in the field.

*What can you say about the integration of BU and Brandeis?*

Basically it worked fairly well, insofar as it really let students access facilities, faculty, and such at either institution. For example, I was normally at BU, but in fact, the dissertation that I did was mostly with someone who was at Brandeis. And that is just really unheard of. It was not a perfect marriage. But, in general, it worked about as well at it could have. Right now it's Brandeis only. As much as anything else what happened was that the people at BU left for greener pastures. In some respects the institution was there but the people were not. The real difference between BU and Brandeis was that BU had fewer requirements than Brandeis did and BU had the disadvantage that, whereas at Brandeis you were fully part of the Heller School and so had a place to function from, at BU you weren't part of the School of Public Health or the School of Management, you were part of this University Professors Program. So on one hand you had the flexibility to go anywhere, so some people did stuff with the School of Management, others did things with the Public Health School, and others did things that related to neither. This made it a bit more difficult because you felt like you didn't have a place to sit. You didn't really belong to a particular institution or a larger entity.

3. *What was it about the curriculum that contributed or did not contribute to the program's success?*

I have mixed feelings about the curriculum. On one hand the freedom of the curriculum was one of the things that the students liked a lot; on the other hand I think that the BU/Brandeis program didn't give people a good enough methodological training. It was not rigorous enough in methods.

*What can you say about the dissertation process?*

The process for me was relatively painless. I had a topic that worked fairly well and a dissertation committee that was nice, compliant, and responsive. They would read my things and generally not take me to task too badly. It went well for me.

*Were there structures built into the curriculum that kept the process going or at least helped to keep it at that fast pace?*

There were definitely efforts to try to start it up. The major problem was that the hardest thing is to find the topic, find the niche, and find some way to deal with that, and then different students have different strategies on how they build their committees. I prefer to find my own project and then pick a committee that will give me support in the areas that I need and not give me a lot of hassles. Other students think they have to pick out the most prestigious names and the biggest experts in a given area to help guide them. That had its virtues too.

4. *How, if at all, was the Pew approach different from the traditional teaching approach?*

The Pew approach was somewhat different because there was a given set of classes and a slightly different program philosophy. I'm not sure when all was said and done that there was a massive approach difference, but maybe there was something that was a little different: My impression was that at Brandeis, perhaps there was somewhat more of an emphasis to think that either I'm a political scientist, an economist, or a sociologist, whereas at BU there was not an emphasis to identify with one or another social science discipline.

5a. *How has your professional life changed as a result of the Pew program? What value has Pew training added to your life?*

5b. *Has your career trajectory changed as a result of your time spent in the Pew program? If yes, how?*

It certainly changed my professional life somewhat. I was doing policy work and policy research in the federal government beforehand. On the other hand, the area that I was working in, food and nutrition and welfare policy, was fairly different from what I do now, so it permitted me to shift areas into a somewhat broader area and get some extra training. That was very useful and very helpful to me.

6. *If you did not complete the program do you plan to? If yes, why? If no, why? Obviously you completed the program. Do you have any ideas how valuable the program was for those who did not complete?*

There are two things. The first is that they all got some additional training, regardless of whether or not they finished. I think the other thing is that a fairly high proportion of those who did not complete the program (meaning that they did not get their PhD) still harbor a hope that at some point they will complete it. I know this because when I periodically talk to some of the people who didn't complete the program in the first 2 years, they say that they still plan on getting around to the dissertation any day now. At the least they harbor some hope of completing it. I think that in any PhD program there are those who after the first few years don't complete the program, and then there is a small percentage of the noncompleters who then do finally complete it.

*Would you guess that an accelerated program produced more or fewer completers?*

I think that it produced a fair number of completers in the time frame. It may well be that one of the things that happened, because of the emphasis on a quick time frame, is that if you didn't complete the program within the first few years, then you sort of had to go out and find a real job and perhaps move away from the Boston area, and then there was a greater likelihood that you wouldn't complete it. There is a different philosophy than that perhaps at Michigan, where you knew you were in it for the long haul and you didn't feel the same pressure to complete the program quickly. I will say that my recollection from the statistics that you showed in Washington was that I think fellows at BU/Brandeis had among the lowest completion rates. However, by the time I completed the program, BU/Brandeis had lots of completers and Michigan had maybe two. It was an issue of different timing.

7. *What is the Pew "legacy" in terms of:*

a) *health policy?*

It would be difficult to say that there is a clear and unique Pew legacy in terms of health policy. Actually, just recently I saw the video of *Mr. Holland's Opus.* Remember at the end when the people say, "Gee, Mr. Holland, you didn't do your opus, but we are your opus." That's sort of what the Pew legacy is. Is there a grand work or something that Pew can say is their legacy? I'm not sure that there is something sitting out there brassy and shiny, but there are lots of people that it affected both from the students' perspective and I think also from the program directors' and faculty's perspective. It encouraged faculty to do teaching and furthered them as well.

b) *education?*

One of the things that Pew did was that it helped make more formal the idea that health policy was an area of interest, and it is slowly gaining in acceptance. I do a lot of work for the Association of Health Policy and Management, and the health policy group there seems to keep getting a bit stronger and bigger. Still, that was well reflected in the journal, but partly they are correct because there are lots of health journals but there are not that many management and welfare policy journals so they want to emphasize that. I still wish I'd see a few more health articles in the journal though.

c) *your future?*

I'm still doing the sorts of things that I studied. It had a long-term effect on my past and I assume it will affect my future in the same way.

*At the November meeting you made reference to the fact that you are no longer in government and yet you have more influence on policy in your current position than before. The context of this statement was that we were talking about what Pew wanted to produce. Can you speak a bit to that?*

Partly it is because when you're in government, at least when I was in government, and for what I did dealing with the program, I was sort of the major policy and budget analyst for a long time, but you are always sort of fitting in and just trying to keep up with a broader administrative agenda for the Administration and/or for Congress. You can shape things, but you're shaping things within that context. If you're on the outside doing policy research, then you can try to shape the agenda somewhat. Whereas when you're working in the government, the way the government is set up it's very hierarchical. Basically speaking, most government people work in relative anonymity, and information goes up the administrative hierarchy and then occasionally goes across into other policy circles, whereas if you're on the outside at a place like the Urban Institute, you can deal on lots of levels with policy makers in government, in the executive branch, in Congress, at state levels, and with some of the other associations. In the past few months I've given talks to the national council and state legislators, and the American Medical Association, and it is the sort of thing that would be unusual to do if I were still in the government.

8.   *Are there any important issues that this interview does not address? If so, please feel free to add comments and/or concerns.*

Not that I can think of at the moment. Is Pew at this point having any clear thoughts about what it wants to do in the future in this area?

*As far as I know they are not thinking about health policy. They did start up another program that is more clinically based.*

## Face-to-Face Interview with Doctoral Alumna Linda Simoni-Wastila
Wednesday July 3, 1996, 10 a.m.

1.  *Based on your experience and familiarity with the Pew program, what did the program really accomplish? What are the most important contributions?*

I think the best thing that the Pew program did was that it took people, mostly from different disciplines, and gave them very similar training. There were four programs and each one had different goals but essentially it developed this cohort of people who could do health services research, who could do health policy, and who could talk the language and walk the walk and put them out there all over the place. Pew developed this huge network. Not only did it help those who went through the program but it also helped shape health care and health policy. I think that's one of the most important contributions.

I can go anywhere, to any meeting, and start talking, and someone will say, "What's your background?" I'll happen to mention that I'm a Pew health policy fellow and they'll say, "Oh yeah? I was a health policy fellow too!" I think the other thing for me, on a personal level, is that I really felt nurtured through the program by the staff and faculty, particularly Steve Crane (even though he was at BU; we had the joint program then). He was a real mentor. I also got some good mentoring here, and we nurtured each other. My class was particularly tight. We nurtured each other and sort of developed a need to mentor other people. That was nice; I enjoyed that. Now I find myself in a mentoring position for students and even for some colleagues, and I am prepared. The Pew program sort of facilitated that.

Network building began in the first year. In the first year, all the first-year fellows go to Washington, D.C. You were introduced right away to the Washington scene and the hot issues of the moment, the real cutting-edge issues. If you wanted to know about health care reform you got the latest and the greatest right there. It got students really excited. And, it helped to bridge the programs, to develop that commonality and similar approach to health and health policy. The same thing was true of the annual meetings. The great thing about the Pew program is that it got people excited about the issues and exposed them to the experts, and I'm sad to see that ending. It was almost as if you too became a cutting-edge person. The conversations are incredibly intellectual yet practical at the same time. You felt like, "Wow, we can change the world!" You just don't get that a lot in typical academic programs. You know, even for me, I'm very specialized, I'm not out there doing health care reform, but I was able to apply my interests and expertise. I would love to have a weekend retreat like that every year. I know the AHCPR (Agency for Health Care Policy and Research) fellowships are happening, but I don't think they have the same sort of bringing together of people from across the country and exposing them to some of the leading minds and practitioners. That was one of the biggest benefits of the Pew program.

2. *What was the most innovative or unique aspect of your particular program design and implementation?*

The most useful and very unique aspect when I was here (the program was a joint BU/Brandeis program) was the dissertation seminar where we were exposed to the second- and third-year students. It really was a dissertation seminar. Every other week there would be a presentation of different research methods and designs. We would spend a whole 2 to 3 hours discussing internal and external validity. The issues discussed were very relevant for the dissertation proposal work. One could take the issues beyond the dissertation process per se; however, they were specific enough to apply to whatever you were working on. It was very useful. It was basic yet thorough: Epidemiology, research methods, and some biostatistics thrown in. The discussions were very cogent. What was even more useful was that we were all, the first- and second-year students, told that we had to be present. This was not something that was taken lightly. Our sessions were 2 to 3 hours; they were long and everyone participated. You didn't get credit, but everyone came. The second-year students and even some of the third-year students came and were helpful in getting us younger folks to start formalizing our ideas. At the same time we were exposed to different processes and different levels of the process. For example, we might have someone come in and say that they were defending their proposal next week and would like to have a dry run, so we'd see what a formal dissertation proposal would look like, and we were then able to provide feedback and hear feedback that was given by other students and/or professors. We had a very good idea what to expect before we actually went through the process ourselves. We even had dry runs for people who were defending their entire dissertations, so by the end of my first year, I was no longer afraid of the dissertation. It was no longer that big huge "D." It was no longer the big black hole that so many students talk about. They don't see that there are steps to it and that there is a sequential process and that it happens over time. I was able to see very clearly after 1 year what the process was, what the steps were, and what sort of things I should consider. And these principles are not just useful for the dissertation process; they are principles that any researcher or user of research will apply throughout his or her career.

Another thing that I liked about the program at Brandeis was that every year we had a seminar series that focused on an area. Some of them were very good, and some weren't so good. We had one that Stan Wallack did on health care financing that was extremely tedious, I guess, but we were exposed to the latest economics in health care in terms of financing and reimbursement and it was excellent, very in-depth. It provided us with an evaluation of the literature. There was another seminar on people's dissertations that were made into books. They were all related to health care. We were thus able to discuss these issues and at the same time examine other people's research. Our focus was mostly qualitative, which is important because I think most research programs don't have enough qualitative courses. One year we had one just on AIDS, which was fantastic. Jonathan Mann came and spoke to us.

Overall, the dissertation seminars were the best. We really learned from each other and developed connections that still exist today. I still call on people, and vice versa. Going through the process together bonded us personally and professionally.

3. *What was it about the curriculum that contributed or did not contribute to the program's success?*

From the Brandeis side—and it's not a fault of the Pew program, rather, it is a fault of the Heller School—most of the curriculum offered at the Heller School is just not rigorous enough. We had to go off campus to get more economics, econometrics, or statistics. Bill Crown was great. When you get into the Pew program you've already come from a background that's pretty rigorous, like the Agency for Health Care Policy and Research (AHCPR), and so for the most part we really didn't need all this introductory stuff that you get here. That's my one complaint. Part of it may have been that I was younger than most people, and the program was really geared toward people who had been out of school for awhile. I came out of a fantastic master's program and was very well prepared. So indirectly, the Heller School curriculum did not do much to increase the Pew program's success. (I should note that The Heller School has since addressed this concern by overhauling its PhD program curriculum.)

4. *How, if at all, was the Pew approach different from the traditional teaching approach?*

It was different by the fact that there were smaller seminars, more one on one. There was a lot more mentoring. There was a lot of collegiality between faculty and students in my master's program, which is really unusual for a master's program. So, I thought that would continue in my PhD program. I dreamed of working alongside some great experts and solving the problems of the world. Yet, when I came here I thought this was the most closed-door place I had ever been. At first I thought it was just this place, but then I talked with my friends at Harvard and Johns Hopkins and they said it was the same everywhere. But, the Pew program helped immensely in that area. Some key faculty were available and eager to mentor the Pew fellows. We had ready access. It was built in. We had Stan Wallack, Steve Crane, Jon Chilingerian later, and many others, mostly BU people, which is interesting. Having that available, as well as a really good group of folks, made it different. But it is interesting: a lot of other students resented that; they hated the Pew fellows. Part of it may have been that the seminars were closed off to non-Pew fellows. And so during my last semester we opened it up but only one other person came. But one of the best things about the seminars was that they were so small. There was a real sense of camaraderie. We didn't really want it to be opened up. On the other hand, it was a great opportunity, and all doctoral students should have the same opportunity. So there was a real conflict in my mind about how I felt about the setup. There was also a lot of fuss made about the Pew fellows which I didn't think was appropriate.

5a. *How has your professional life changed as a result of the Pew program? What value has Pew training added to your life?*

I don't think I would be where I am now if I had just gone through the Heller School PhD program and not specifically the Pew program. I think the Pew program just gave it that extra boost. I don't even know if I would have finished my PhD otherwise. Yes, the funding facilitated it, but the pressure and support to get done also facilitated it. I almost quit the program after 1 year. I thought I might follow another interest of mine, art, but the reason I didn't was because I kept on thinking about what Marion Ein Lewin said at the meetings, "OK, you guys, you can all get done, you can all do it." She would always talk about how important is was to finish. And, then I said to myself that I've got to get done, I've got to do this, I'm not a quitter. I'm really glad I did it. That kind of support motivated me to want to contribute. And, I'm very pleased with my position. My experience with Pew continues to motivate me. When I get the Pew newsletter and I see where everyone is and what they are doing I think, wow, that's great. It makes me want to go out there and publish more, contribute more, and do more. In that way Pew has touched me professionally. It has made me more enthusiastic about what I do, not that I wasn't before, but it has given me that extra boost. It made the Heller program, which was pretty good, excellent.

**5b.** *Has your career trajectory changed as a result of your time spent in the Pew program? If yes, how?*

When I finished my master's program I had applied for the Presidential Management Internship but didn't get it. I thought I had wanted to work in Washington. I have many friends who did that and are now "Beltway Bandits." I thought I wanted to be down there doing policy. I thought I wanted to be a policy wonk. But, the Pew program made me realize (even though it is a policy program) that I was not a policy wonk. It didn't make me dislike policy. I actually believe that my research is policy relevant. But, it made me realize that I have a personality that doesn't fit that role. And that's just fine. Yet, it reiterated to me the importance of policy and to study things that have some sort of relevance to a policy, political, or social issue, to strive to deliver as much truth as possible to that particular policy area. In that regard, yes, Pew changed my career trajectory: I realized I was a research nerd. But I do research with practical applications.

**6.** *If you did not complete the program do you plan to? If yes, why? If no, why?*

I did complete the program. Just going through the course work is the easy part. All it is is foundation. The hardest part is doing the dissertation. The comprehensive exams don't pull all our knowledge together. Nothing but the dissertation can do that. That is the big challenge. People who don't finish haven't met that challenge. I feel sorry for them. I really think they've missed out on the best part of the whole program. I don't know why they haven't finished.

Maybe people think they can come in here and pull it off while keeping their full-time jobs, running a family with two kids, and all that going on. Some people can actually do all that. But, you have to really make a commitment to completing the program, and the dissertation needs to be a real priority. I teach a dissertation seminar, and I tell people this: "Don't plan on remodeling your house in the next 2 years. Try to limit everything else. Focus on your dissertation. It's only 1, 2, maybe 3 years of your life." And people get tied up with thinking they need to have blocks of time. You don't need that. You just need a few hours a day or even an hour a day. People just don't see that. I think one of the reasons the Pew program wasn't refunded was because there was a low completion rate. I get a little angry about that. I think it's been denied to other people, this great opportunity to get exposed and get the funding, etc. Of course they still made great contacts. Unfortunately, I think some people come into this just to make the contacts and they sort of leapfrog over people.

7. *What is the Pew "legacy" in terms of:*

   a) *health policy?*

What it has really done is to put people out there who have superb training and an interesting way of attacking problems. These people are now in high-profile positions. They are able to make a real contribution to the field. I think that's real important. I also think that below that there is a level of people, like myself, who are more background people, who do the research. And I think we are real important too, because what we are doing is building a foundation of knowledge that has practical applications, and I hope is done as objectively as possible and as rigorously as possible. But, there are definitely two layers. Policy isn't just those people working for Rockefeller or Kennedy or the bureaucrats in the U.S. Department of Health and Human Services. It's also about the people who do the background work. Pew has done an excellent job of supplying these kinds of people.

   b) *education?*

There are two levels here as well. I do some education too. I think it's real important that I return the mentoring that I received, and I think a lot of people came out with that attitude. There are now incredible role models out there for people who are starting out. There is a high profile of Pew people, and that is a real legacy. To have those type of role models out there and for them to be visible.

It seems to me that the Pew programs provided some consistency to the whole arena of health policy in terms of the quality and expertise of people that may not have been there before. That was achieved through the educational mission and policy focus.

What Pew had also done was to make sure that programs like those at Brandeis, UCLA, and UCSF have the programs even without funding. They all have a real strong interest in continuing programs like this through other funding sources, like AHCPR. They all continue to build this health policy area, broadly speaking. Pew really enabled a few programs to develop educational programs in health policy and gave people fantastic skills. And they are now ongoing. It was like seed money. It's really important. Everyone else can't find jobs, but this is one area where there will always be jobs. Health policy keeps on growing. Pew fostered that, and that's the legacy.

*c)* *your future?*

Pew gave me a head start. It allowed me to evolve my ideas in a less pressured environment. I didn't have to worry about where my next paycheck was coming from. I didn't have to worry about not having colleagues and peers to support me and mentor me. It gave me a real boost. I'm really happy for that. I'm grateful for that. I know a lot of graduate students who feel like they are in perpetual alienation. Pew prevented that from happening to me.

8. *Are there any important issues that this interview does not address? If so, please feel free to add comments and/or concerns.*

We have to address the gaps that will now exist without Pew funding. For instance, if AHCPR does go under or if other foundations fail to kick in, hopefully, Pew will reconsider this sort of program, again, but maybe in a different way or with different institutions. We need to always be thinking about training health policy professionals at the pre- and postdoctoral levels. We need to keep an eye on the field and seeing where and what the gaps are in health and medical training.

# APPENDIX B.
*Curriculum and Course Offerings*[7]

The University of Michigan curriculum consists of approximately 50 credit hours of course work. The overall goal of the curriculum is to ensure that at the completion of the program every student has a high level of literacy in the concepts and methods that are basic to health policy analysis and research. Because of the nonresidential nature of the program, in which the students come to campus once a month for 4 days, all Pew students take the same courses in lockstep fashion. All courses in the curriculum are required, and there are no electives. The curriculum is grouped into four categories: orientational and instrumental courses, statistics and methodology, core skills and concepts, and the public health core. Several dissertation-related courses are also required.

## Orientational and Instrumental Courses

Some of the instruction provided early in the program is designed to enable students to make full and efficient use of the resources and facilities available to them through the Pew program at the University of Michigan. These offerings include computer instruction.

Although there is no formal course in computers, time is set aside during the first three sessions of the program to teach students how to use key features of the university's mainframe system. This includes the electronic mail and conferencing systems that Pew students are expected to use to communicate with one another and the faculty. It also includes the university library's computerized catalog as well as relevant literature and journal databases. In addition, instruction is provided in the microcomputer statistical

[7] *Information included in this appendix comes from program narratives and interviews with program directors and faculty.*

301

package that Pew students use in their statistics and methodology courses.

Similarly, the introductory course taught at the beginning of the program aims to give students a clearer understanding of the goals and structure of the program so that as they proceed in their course work they have a solid sense of how the various components fit together. This includes an understanding of how the course work relates to the qualifying examination, which they need to take to achieve candidacy, as well as to the dissertation, and how all of these elements are intended to serve the basic goals of the program.

Another part of this introductory course consists of presentations and seminars by guest lecturers, which are intended to expose students to a broad range of approaches to the analysis of health policy issues. An important goal of this series of seminars is to illustrate how several of the individual elements covered in Pew program courses are brought together by experienced analysts and researchers in addressing specific policy questions and issues.

## Statistics and Methodology

Graduates of the Pew program at the University of Michigan are expected to have the kind of grounding in statistics and research methods that will enable them to make discerning use of the literature and to know what is required to turn out high-quality health policy research and evaluations. Since they are not being trained to be full-time researchers, the emphasis is on gaining a firm grasp of the fundamentals and of the methods and approaches most likely to be of use for health policy. This is seen as providing the necessary base for any subsequent learning of more intricate or specialized approaches that individuals may wish to pursue or for collaborating with those who have specialized knowledge about such approaches.

A series of four courses is offered in this area. Each course is meant to reinforce and build upon previously acquired knowledge. In addition, the topics covered in these four courses come up again and are expanded upon in other courses, such as epidemiology, economics, and the seminar on disease prevention and the environment.

Statistics is one of the areas in which the Pew students must pass a so-called prerequisite examination at the start of the program. To pass it students must demonstrate knowledge at the level of an introductory graduate course in statistics. The biostatistics course that is given early in the program (BIOS 524) starts with a brief review of the basic material in probability theory and statistical methods that the qualifying examination covers. The biostatistics course itself concentrates on regression methods and analysis of variance and covariance. Also taught early in the program is a course that deals with research and evaluation methods (HSMP 854). These two initial courses in statistics and methods focus heavily on the nature and use of key concepts and tools. Two other courses taught in the latter part of the program, applied statistics and applied methodology, focus on the hands-on, actual application to specific health policy issues of the concepts and tools taught in the initial two courses. These two applications-oriented courses run concurrently, and their coverage of topics is coordinated as to be mutually supportive and reinforcing.

### Core Skills and Concepts

Central to the Pew program's curriculum is a set of courses, each of which deals with the concepts and frameworks from a specific discipline or area and with the application of these to the analysis of health policy issues. To ensure that these courses are taught at the appropriate doctoral level and can devote the necessary time to health policy applications rather than to teaching of basic concepts, students must demonstrate mastery of the basics in three areas: economics, political science, and organizational behavior. Similarly, the medical care organization course assumes a basic knowledge of how the U.S. health care system is structured and how it operates. Students with deficiencies in this area are provided with resources and guidance to remedy this through self-study prior to the start of the course.

### Public Health Core

The degree that Pew fellows earn from Michigan is a doctorate in public health. Like all other programs leading to a public health degree awarded by the university's School of Public Health, the Pew program must include in its curriculum certain basic public health courses. The courses in this set are the only ones that were not specifically created for the Pew program. Nonetheless, as offered in the Pew program construct, each of these courses emphasizes policy applications and implications.

### Dissertation Courses

As part of the strategies developed over time to help students in the Pew program make timely and satisfactory progress toward their dissertations, a formal dissertation seminar was established as part of the curriculum. Its purpose is to provide, systematically and concisely, information of what is known about effective ways to structure and manage the dissertation. It also serves as a forum for the discussion of generic and specific problems related to the dissertation and their solutions, as well as a forum for students to present preliminary topics to their fellow classmates, which have been proven to be useful exercises.

In addition, during the final stage of the program, each student must sign up with a faculty member of the student's choosing for an independent study course focusing on the dissertation. In the context of this course the student works with the faculty adviser to select a topic, prepare a dissertation proposal, and identify the proposed membership for the student's dissertation committee.

To help sustain the momentum toward the dissertation that these courses are expected to generate during the second year of the program, students are brought back to Ann Arbor on three separate occasions during the third year of the program. At each of these sessions students are expected to meet with their dissertation advisers. They also meet as a group at the dissertation seminar, where they report back to the group and leading faculty member on their progress, and receive feedback from them.

### Lessons Learned

Over time, some lessons were learned regarding the curriculum, over time. Leon Wyszewianski explained that at the beginning there was a division between the more didactic courses and the policy seminars. At the seminars the emphasis was on discussion and on interaction. However, what the program directors learned was that the fellows really did not want free-form seminar discussion; rather, they wanted discussion in the context of much "harder-hitting" didactic material. Other changes included increasing the depth of the methodological aspects of the curriculum. One way this was done was to require that the fellows have some minimum level of competence, as determined by an entrance examination, prior to beginning the courses. This helped the faculty gear their lectures to the middle of the class rather than to the lowest denominator. The formal dissertation seminars were also brought about through curriculum reform. As discussed at length in the main body of the report, the program learned that just because its fellows excelled in the field and at being students, these factors did not mean that they could just automatically write a dissertation on their own. Formal structures that helped the fellows move through the complex dissertation process were instituted. Leon Wyszewianski also discussed the early problems related to the multiple incompletes that were being accumulated by the fellows. The faculty were discouraged from assigning a major paper due at the end of the term; rather, pieces of a term paper were required to be handed in throughout the semester. Having frequent and smaller deliverables was found to greatly assist the fellows in completing the required course work.

## COURSE OFFERINGS AT THE UNIVERSITY OF MICHIGAN
### Course Requirements
#### Orientation and Instrumental Courses

*Computer Instruction.* Although there is no formal course in computers, time is set aside during the first three sessions of the program to teach students how to use key features of the university's mainframe computer system (including electronic mail and conferencing systems, the library's computerized catalog, and relevant literature and journal databases). Instruction is also provided in the microcomputer statistical package that Pew students use in their statistics and methodology courses.

*Introduction to Health Policy and Research.* This course gives students an understanding of the goals and structure of the Pew Doctoral Program in Health Policy and to the health policy field in general. The balance of the course is devoted to an examination of how health policy research is conducted, and a varied group of guests who are active in policy research and analysis are invited to make presentations and conduct seminars.

#### Statistics and Methodology

*Biostatistics for Clinical Researchers.* This course reviews the basic probability theory and statistical methods, including design of experiments, observational studies, point and interval estimation, and hypothesis testing. The topics for this course are simple and multiple regression analyses and analysis of variance and covariance.

*Research and Evaluation Methods in Health Policy.* This course aims to acquaint students with major analytical and methodological issues in understanding, criticizing, and designing formal research and evaluation programs in the health policy field, including the design and use of experiments and quasiexperiments; choice and operationalization of measures and hypotheses in health policy studies; randomized clinical trails and their bearing on policy; methods and limits of technology assessment; and Delphi techniques and consensus methods.

*Applied Statistics.* This course begins with a review of simple and multiple regression analyses and analysis of variance and covariance. The course itself centers on the application of these and other statistical tools to the analysis of health policy questions.

*Applied Methodology.* This course is designed to reinforce and expand upon the material covered in the Research and Evaluation Methods in Health Policy course. The course uses actual studies and data sets to provide hands-on experience in the use of methodological and design approaches to address specific policy issues and questions. The structure includes a module on survey research methods.

### Core Skills and Concepts

*Organizational Issues in Health Policy.* This course offers application of current theory and research to health policy-relevant cases in organizational design, organizational environments, boundary setting and boundary spanning, organizational conflict, and organizational change. The structure emphasizes theoretical formulations; critical analysis of current research, especially its utility for organizational policies and practices; and application of theory and research to complex case material.

*Economics of Health Policies.* This course offers an application of microeconomic concepts and methods to health care policy formulation, implementation, and evaluation. The structure emphasizes applicability of market analyses, cost-benefit and cost-effectiveness analyses, allocational and distributional considerations, and design and implementation of incentives and regulation.

*Legal Issues in Health Care Policy.* This course analyzes selected legal issues demonstrating the role of law and the

Anglo-American legal system in the implementation of health care policy. Emphasis is placed on issues of current significance including health planning, antitrust legislation, rights to access to care, the government's role in environmental and occupational health, taxation and regulation of providers, the status of allied health professionals, and the legal aspects of termination of care. Each subject is considered in the context of the political, economic, administrative, and ethical/moral values that shape the development of law.

*Issues in Medical Care Organization and Delivery.* This course offers analysis and description of selected issues, problems, and tasks in the financing, organization, and evaluation of personal health care services. Topics include social values and objectives, assessment of the need for health services, assessment of health care resources, features of system design that influence key aspects of performance, and assessing, monitoring, and enhancing the quality of care. The course emphasizes the use of concepts and frameworks in analyzing policy issues related to these topics.

*Politics in Health Care Policy.* This course focuses on the political aspects of health care policy. The emphasis is placed on the processes by which decisions are made about the allocation of key resources and the institutions and forces affecting these processes, including the president, the U.S. Congress, the bureaucracy, interest groups, the professions, and state and local governments. The course aims to show fellows how to make effective use of political science concepts and frameworks to analyze health policy issues.

*Policy Seminar in Disease Prevention and the Environment.* This course reviews concepts of disease prevention in a policy context, with consideration of prevention as a social health care strategy and of the political economy of prevention. Emphasis is placed on the application of policy analytic tools to contemporary behavioral and environmental issues of disease prevention, relying heavily on case studies and recent and ongoing research.

## Public Health Core

*Strategies and Uses of Epidemiology.* The course reviews basic epidemiology for the public health professional, with a review of the fundamental principles and concepts and application of these principles and concepts to selected examples of communicable diseases and chronic degenerative diseases. A strong emphasis is placed on the policy aspects of the examples discussed.

*Principles of Health Behavior.* This course provides an overview of psychosocial factors related to health and illness behavior and to processes of belief and behavior change in relation to health, including strategies for change at the individual, group, and community levels. Again, a strong emphasis is placed on the policy implications of the issues discussed.

*Principles of Environmental Health Sciences.* This course focuses on giving the fellows basic knowledge and skills required to assess the impacts of environmental health contaminants. The teaching format uses representative examples of environmental health problems. Environmental interactions, health effects, risk assessment, and control measures are assessed for each example.

### Dissertation

*Dissertation Seminar.* This course is intended to help the fellows structure their work on the dissertation and thereby facilitate a satisfactory and timely completion of a critical requirement for the DrPH. Strategies for structuring and managing the dissertation are presented and discussed, along with ways to deal with common problems and pitfalls.

*Dissertation Research for Precandidates.* This consists of independent study with a faculty member of the student's choosing. The goal is to select a topic, prepare a prospectus, and identify the proposed membership of the dissertation committee.

*Dissertation Research for Doctoral Students.* This consists of a series of three visits to the University of Michigan campus during the third year of the program, during which fellows meet with their dissertation advisers.

### CURRICULUM AT UCSF

The University of California at San Francisco (UCSF) Pew program curriculum consists of seminars, formal courses, faculty-fellow interaction and mentoring, research experiences, and field placement experiences in federal, state, or local government or in other policy-relevant organizations. Seminars and courses introduce fellows to a broad range of issues and a multidisciplinary understanding of the policy-making process. Courses designed to strengthen research skills are also made available. For fellows wishing to pursue a research career, participation in a multidisciplinary research team on one or more research projects is required. For fellows pursuing a career in health policy practice, field placements, mentoring, and networking become relatively more important elements. Defining and refining the curricula are complex and ongoing tasks that include formal course evaluations, a panel discussion of each health policy seminar series, and interviews with former fellows.

Each element of the UCSF program, the courses, seminars, faculty-fellow mentoring relationship, learning-by-doing model, field placement, and participation in multidisciplinary research, is geared toward the highly diverse backgrounds and range of needs of both the postdoctoral and the midcareer fellows (UCSF Lessons Learned, 1992-1993). Thus, the UCSF program curricula underwent continual revisions and reformations throughout the tenure of the Pew program. The program directors stated that one of the most valuable tools used to shape the curriculum was the input of current and former fellows. Alumni maintain contact with the faculty long after the program has been completed, and through this continued interaction the program directors learn which aspects of the program are most helpful for the fellows. The process for gathering information about the program from the fellows and alumni has been formalized over the years with the addition of written evaluations and a panel discussion of each health policy seminar series. During 1991 and 1992, the Pew program faculty, as part of the review of the program, conducted telephone interviews with former fellows to evaluate the fellows' introduction to, experience with, and continuing ties with the program and to make suggestions for improvements (Lessons Learned, 92-93). Furthermore, the Fellowship Committee includes two current faculty who were former fellows, as well as a representative of current fellows, further strengthening the input of past and present fellows. The varied teaching and training experiences of the Fellowship Committee members have stimulated curriculum development. Each member brings the best aspects of his or her training to bear on the curriculum. Members also made suggestions based on what they thought was missing from their own training. In addition, the committee members who teach program courses are willing to experiment with novel teaching methods.

In 1991 and 1992, a more structured core curriculum was implemented. This curriculum was required for all full-time fellows and was recommended for part-time fellows. Program seminars are organized into four general topics: introduction to health policy, methodology for health policy research, health policy processes, and health policy issues. The Health Policy Seminar, Writing Seminar, and Journal Club are held weekly throughout the year (11 months), and all fellows attend and participate in the seminars. In addition, a research methods course is required of all physicians and others with limited research training. A rich roster of other courses is offered to fellows, with timely information on available courses and advice on which courses would best fill educational needs being provided. For fellows with particular interests in health policy and the elderly, the Department of Social and Behavioral Sciences of the School of Nursing offers special courses.

Institute seminars and courses have proven to be important in achieving three overall training objectives: proving an educational experience for the fellows addressing both policy issues and research applied to policy, offering fellows the opportunity to interact with researchers and policy makers from a variety of settings, and providing an excellent means to create a social support system for the fellows and to assist in their socialization into the world of public policy.

Assistance in career planning and placement is also provided. Initially, this assistance was provided on an informal basis, but it is provided in a more formalized structure as the program has evolved. The faculty systematically distribute descriptions of job openings to fellows, discuss job seeking with them beginning in the first year of the fellowship, and provide fellows with general information on preparing a curriculum vitae, interviewing, and other aspects of job hunting. Career counseling is made a specific responsibility of the fellow's mentor, and progress is reviewed periodically by the faculty fellowship committee.

## Lessons Learned

Hal Luft discussed the ongoing tension over how much curriculum structure was too much and how much was too little. He explained that it was in fact the Pew Charitable Trusts that encouraged UCSF to add more structure in terms of the seminars and courses offered. Hal Luft stated that although the Health Policy Seminar had always been successful, making it more formal by structuring internal sequences increased its effectiveness. Nonetheless, Hal Luft stated that the program was continually being further structured; for instance, the mentoring relationships were standardized with formal guidelines (included in Appendix C). This process was instituted to ensure that the fellows were as productive as possible.

Carroll Estes underscored the importance of requiring certain courses at specific times during the program. She stated that the directors learned over time that is was very important to be explicit and to have some details and firm requirements such as the Writing Seminar and the Pew Dissertation Seminar. Participation in these seminars is required unconditionally, as with the methods courses. The faculty wanted to ensure that all fellows emerged from the program with skills in the art and science of proposal writing. On the other hand, Carroll Estes discussed the importance of having some flexibility for other aspects within the curriculum, for instance, allowing the fellows to explore new avenues and areas that they are interested in.

## COURSE OFFERINGS AT UCSF
### Core Seminar Requirements

*Health Policy Seminar (eight quarters).* The health policy seminar introduces fellows from disparate backgrounds to a broad range of health policy topics. The seminar focuses on policy questions and how research may help answer those questions. It includes a series of four to six seminars on a specific theme (such as AIDS, women's health, or private sector reform perspectives) to give fellows a chance to immerse themselves in a topic and see how researchers or policy makers from different disciplines approach the same topic.

Fellows in the UCSF postdoctoral program typically come into the program with most of the specific skills they will need for their careers. What the Pew program aims to teach these fellows is how to apply those skills to the questions that policy makers need to answer. Therefore, the core health policy seminar focuses on policy questions and how research may help answer those questions. These seminars are often held in an informal fashion, with faculty members raising various questions about topics and attempting to elicit discussion. All fellows and all key faculty take part in the weekly seminars. Exposure to faculty thinking and insights regarding the seminars strengthens the educational component of the seminar series for the fellows.

*The Art and Science of Health Services Research (one quarter).* The emphasis of this course is on how to approach a research problem, how to plan a project, how to develop a proposal, and how to manage a project. It addresses the nuts and bolts of identifying data sources, checking and cleaning data, developing budgets, identifying publishable findings, and being alert to the ethical issues inherent in policy-oriented research.

This course was created so that fellows would receive some formal training in such areas as how grants are reviewed, how to develop a time line, how to estimate a budget, and how to target papers to appropriate journals. Courses in quantitative methods typically deal with the theory of statistics and the appropriate applications of various tests, but not how to determine if the data have errors or even how to locate specific types of data.

*The Writing Seminar (eight quarters).* This seminar was created so that fellows would have a forum in which to sharpen their communication skills. The goals of the writing seminar include recognizing good research design and analysis and how to acquire the habits and practices that make for good scientific papers on relevant subjects; communicating with policy makers; being taught the skills of constructive review, that is, how to assess critically the work of others; being taught the absolute necessity for receiving and using criticism from colleagues; being taught the realities and subtleties of scientific and lay publication and the skills of constructive review; involving fellows in vigorous and informed debate with other fellows and faculty; inculcating the idea that there are important ethical principles throughout this process; and showing that open exchange of ideas and criticism is the best way to achieve good science and the best insurance against error and fraud.

This seminar addresses the fact that although fellows are expected to publish papers, they have very little experience doing so. They receive balanced criticism, both supportive and critical, with constructive criticism focusing on how to improve the paper. This is supplemented with a combination of written comments handed in by the fellow classmates, along with an oral discussion. Faculty input is important in keeping comments balanced and helpful. Faculty also submit papers for the fellows to review, thereby demonstrating that they too write things in need of improvement and that the fellows are not aspiring to the impossible. Special seminars are held prior to national meetings to allow fellows to practice their presentations and receive feedback.

*The Journal Club (four quarters)*. The goals of this course are similar to those of the Writing Seminar. Fellows are expected to learn to communicate effectively, critique the design and analysis in the published manuscripts reviewed during the sessions, understand the realities of the publication process, and evaluate the ethics of publication. In addition, fellows are expected to understand the policy relevance and implications of the papers discussed. The discussions concentrate on two areas: scientific merit and policy implications.

*Research Methods (one quarter)*. The components of a research program are systematically examined through the workshop format with both didactic and small-group sessions. Topics include the research question, selection of study subjects, measurement of study variables, study designs, sample size calculations, ethical considerations and consent forms, pretests and pilot studies, and National Institutes of Health (NIH grant proposal requirements. At the end of the course, participants prepare and defend a complete study proposal.

Proposals begun during this course by Pew fellows have developed into federally funded research projects. This course is valuable even for fellows not planning a research career because it can enhance their understanding of research and allow them to use findings effectively in the practice of health policy.

*Perspectives on Public Policy (one quarter)*. This course offers a systematic overview of health policy in modern U.S. government. The course examines major trends in the U.S. health care system since 1945 as a context for examining two broad policy issues: (1) the changing role of the public sector, including an analysis of market and regulatory approaches to reform, and (2) the role of federal versus state and local governments in health care reform. Discussion of this second policy issue includes case studies of federal, state, and local government efforts at cost-containment. In addition, the course provides an overview of the policy process, with special attention to policy formulation and implementation within the federal system. Fellows are required to analyze selected policy reform issues and develop a paper examining the policy process in one substantive area.

*Translating Research into Policy (one quarter, alternate years)*. This course identifies areas of research that are particularly relevant to health policy, examines barriers to the translation of research into policy, and discusses strategies for the effective translation of research into policy. The class discusses the use of research from a variety of disciplines, including basic sciences, health services research, economics, and epidemiology. Faculty use a tutorial, case-study approach for this course, with sessions on the use of research to shape policy related to specific topics, such as lead poisoning, physician supply and distribution, and environmental tobacco smoke. Each class consists of a presentation by the fellows of a case study that they developed following consultation with faculty.

*Health Policy Leadership (one quarter, alternate years).* This course includes discussions of communication, consensus building, networking, negotiation, mediation, conflict resolution, and conflict prevention. In the future this course may require fellows to work (intern) in policy environments where real problems must be solved.

*Optional Course Work.* Fellows are provided with several opportunities to take elective course work at both UCSF and the University of California at Berkeley, enabling them to structure a program that meets their individual training needs. Fellows are attracted to the Pew program at UCSF in part because of the program's ability to tailor fellowships to meet individual needs.

The UCSF curriculum also places heavy emphasis on the faculty-fellow interaction and mentoring relationship. This is discussed in detail in the main body of the report. Likewise, the importance of field placements in training effective researchers and practitioners is a vital component of the curriculum and is discussed further in the report.

## CURRICULUM AT RAND/UCLA

The design of the curriculum of the doctoral program of RAND and the University of California at Los Angeles (UCLA) recognized that health policy analysis could and should be taught at different levels, depending on the specific backgrounds of individuals in the training program. Those individuals already engaged in the development of public policy may need to expand their knowledge of policy issues and to refine the skills that enable them to contribute to and use the results of policy analytic studies. Clinicians and other health care providers may seek to understand the effects that their clinical decisions have, beyond the individual patient, on the distribution and use of health care resources. Cognizant of these issues, the RAND/UCLA Center for Health Policy Study created a series of modules differing in the level, intensity, and disciplinary mix of the academic component. All modules provided considerable exposure to substantive issues of health care organization, delivery systems, personnel, financing, and regulation. Students pursued quantitative and technical skills at different levels of understanding while participating together in the substantive workshops. Differences among students attracted to the various modules are important to the success of any health policy training program because they underscore the interdisciplinary and multilevel nature of the health policy process.

The RAND/UCLA Center incorporated the resources from the RAND Health Science Program, the RAND Graduate School of Policy Studies, the UCLA School of Public Health, and the UCLA School of Medicine. Faculty, research, and course work were drawn from each institution, creating a complete health policy training environment.

## Doctoral Programs

The doctoral programs provided students with the analytical expertise and close understanding of the health services system and its relationship to patient consumers that is necessary to formulate and evaluate alternative health policies and policy management strategies.

Doctoral training combined a firm grounding in quantitative and analytical methods with study and applied work on substantive problems of the health care system. Two approaches were taken to achieve this goal: (1) The RAND school's basic curriculum trained students with the primary emphasis on the use and application of policy analytic techniques, but with a substantive specialization in health policy topics; (2) the UCLA School of Public Health's basic curriculum trained students with the primary emphasis on the substantive issues in the public health field with specialization in policy analysis methods and their applications.

In addition to the individual institutional program curriculum, doctoral students were required to take a core set of health policy workshops and apply their classroom study to ongoing or self-initiated health policy research projects.

## Midcareer Program

The purpose of the midcareer intensive study was to improve the ability of those already (or potentially) involved in the health policy process and to contribute to and use the results of health services research and policy analysis, but it did not intend for program participants to perform such analyses or studies themselves.

The program was designed to provide an understanding of the basic concepts of economics, statistics, and behavioral sciences as they apply to health policy. Therefore, the students were required to take a set of courses created specifically for this program, including Economics in Health Policy, Statistics, and Social Sciences in Health Policy, on top of the core health policy workshops mentioned above.

### Health Policy Workshops

As mentioned earlier, all students of health policy at the predoctoral, postdoctoral, or midcareer level enroll in this series of workshops. The workshops remained substantially unchanged during the latter half of the program.

### Lessons Learned

Several amendments within the curriculum were made over the 10-year period; however, the focus remained constant: quantitative and analytic training combined with a series of substantive workshops spanning the broad topical spectrum of health policy and health services. The quantitative and analytic course work remained unchanged. Topical areas in the health policy workshops were dependent on faculty availability, so changes were made. In particular, the Special Populations workshop became more focused on the underinsured and uninsured over time.

Initially, a requirement of the doctoral program was a summer practicum that was designed to familiarize students with the organization and practice of medicine through a series of seminars, tours of facilities, and direct observations of clinical encounters. At the UCLA Center for Health Science students spent 3 weeks rotating from the ambulatory medical ward to the end-stage renal disease ward to the medical surgical ward. Students were assigned to a physician each week of the rotation. Student and physician/instructor evaluations over a 4-year period determined that this form of study should be optional rather than required. The varied backgrounds of individual students pointed to a high degree of preprogram experience and exposure to academic medicine, which made such a practicum redundant in most cases.

Kate Korman explained that curriculum development

at RAND/UCLA was unique in that it incorporated the ideas and suggestions from former fellows, creating a program that many of the developers stated they wished they had gone through themselves. The biggest challenge, as discussed in the main body of the report, was not to include the whole world of health policy in the curriculum. Kate Korman explained that early on the curriculum was perhaps too enthusiastic, "even overreaching." Some restructuring of the courses and eliminating a few courses took care of this logistical problem early on.

One interesting lesson learned by the program directors was that a structure they had put in place from the start, the on-the-job (OJT) training component, turned out to be one of the greatest selling points of the program. It was extremely innovative and subsequently extremely successful to require OJT with classroom study, and the fellows relished in the idea of meshing their newly acquired skills with applied projects in the field. Furthermore, requiring that the fellows be evaluated on their performance in the field made the whole experience that much more valuable. In many cases these field projects turned into dissertation projects or, for the midcareer fellows, publications.

## COURSE OFFERINGS AT RAND/UCLA
### Health Policy Workshops
#### Development, Diffusion, and Regulation of Medical Technology

*Diffusion of Innovation.* The federal government is concerned with the efficient diffusion of medical technology for two reasons. First, the government promotes the development of new technology through its investment in research. Second, as a major payer for health care services, the government pays for these innovations as new technologies become "accepted practice." There is no consensus, however, about the role that government should play in influencing the diffusion of new technologies. (Texts: reprints pertinent to topic.)

*Technology Assessment.* Government and private payers are becoming increasingly involved in assessing the efficacy and appropriateness of new medical technologies. The most difficult judgments involve how to weigh the costs and benefits of new technologies. (Texts: reprints pertinent to topic.)

*Biomedical Research Policy.* The federal government is the primary supporter of biomedical research, which is an important source of new medical technology. NIH is widely regarded as the most efficient and effective pool of the federal government's scientific enterprise. However, the biomedical research community has successfully resisted most efforts at scientific evaluation of NIH programs, and skeptics believe that NIH's reputation is based primarily on dogma. (Texts: reprints pertinent to topic.)

*Drug and Device Regulation.* In the United States there is a long-standing tradition of regulating the market for pharmaceuticals. Regulation in this area therefore often serves as a prototype for regulation of other markets for medical technology. The Food and Drug Administration is criticized simultaneously for being too lax in approving new drugs and devices and for withholding approval of valuable therapies. (Texts: Grabowski, *Drug Regulation and Innovation,* and reprints pertinent to topic.)

*Objectives of Health Policy:* Good Health and Good Care (Texts: Donabedian, *Explorations in Quality Assessment and Monitoring,* vol. I, II, and III, and reprints pertinent to topics)

*Health Status Outcomes.* Issues of Definition/Measurement (1) methods to assess and evaluate quality of life measures and (2) selected survey of instruments of measurement.

*Patient Satisfaction.* Indicator of outcomes and predictor of health-related behavior. Methods to measure patient satisfaction with ambulatory and hospital care.

*Quality of Care.* Assessment and assurance. Introduction to quality assessment, measurement of the appropriateness of medical care, quality assurance principles, and the Professional Review Organization program.

*The Relationship of Microprocess to Outcome.* (1) clinical use of health status measures and assessing the quality of long term care in long-term-care facilities, (2) overview of severity of illness measures used to adjust for outcomes in the hospital setting as well as description of modern techniques for developing detailed process of care criteria mainly for hospitalized patients, and (3) introduction to the principles of continuos quality improvement.

*Health Care Financing, Competition, and Regulation* (Texts: Reprints pertinent to topics)

*Insurance and the Demand for Care.* Issues in insurance, including the effect of insurance on demand for medical care, the demand for insurance, and the uninsured.

*Competition (in the Fee-for-Service System) and Health Maintenance Organizations (HMOs).* Competition and alternatives to fee-for-service medicine, including analyses of the competitiveness of the physician market, advertising in health, and HMOs.

*Medicare Program and Global Budgeting.* Payment schemes in medical care, including analysis of the hospital market, nursing home regulation, and prospective payment.

*Special Populations: Access to Health Care for Low-Income Populations* (Texts: Reprints pertinent to topics)
Poverty and health care policy in historical perspective; theoretical frameworks for studying and understanding access; programs and institutions for the poor: (1) public health care and (2) Medicaid; health insurance coverage (private health care coverage and the uninsured: how many, who, why are they increasing and consequences); public policy and access to care for the low-income uninsured population (targeted programs and policies, including mandating coverage by employers; universal approaches such as state and national proposals); children (advocacy for child health); the homeless population; and congressional and state legislative actions and perspectives.

## The Midcareer Core
*Quantitative Methods.* Quantitative methods is taught by using a combination of case studies, lectures, and hands-on analysis of data by computer. The course covers a range of topics in data analysis, statistics, and applied probability. Students learn to organize data, do exploratory data analyses, and fit statistical models (including regression, contingency tables, and distribution-free models) to multivariate data. Statistical topics covered include design, inference (confidence intervals, tests, standard errors, etc.), and statistical decision analysis. Students learn fundamental concepts in statistical inference, decision analysis, and some applied models. Course topics are illustrated with examples drawn primarily from the health policy field. Students learn to be good critics of quantitative studies, as well as learn how to conduct their own analyses. (Texts: Freedman/Pisani/Purves, *Statistics;* Bailer and Mosteller,

*Medical Uses of Statistics;* Huff, *How to Lie with Statistics;* and Ryan/Joiner/Ryan *Minitab* statistical software.)

*Economics in Health Policy Analysis.* The first half of the course reviews the aspects of price theory and welfare economics that are most pertinent to health services research and policy analysis. The review illustrates how economics apply these concepts and tools to problems of demand for medical care, insurance, and supply of physicians and services. The second half of the course focuses on selected concepts and tools of policy analysis in an attempt to understand the economic rationale for government actions in the health arena. These concepts include population models, cost-benefit analysis, discounting, and decision analysis. In this section, the course also addresses the issues of the value of lifesaving and the value of research. In both parts of the course, students work through a number of simple problems designed to illustrate the economic theories and methods under consideration. (Texts: Mansfield, *Microeconomics: Theory and Applications,* and various reprints of health policy articles).

*Social Sciences in Health Policy Analysis.* This course examines the contributions of behavioral and social science concepts and methods to health policy analysis. The instructors identify and explain applied theories of individual and social behavior and critically review examples of actual applications to health policy analysis. As a rule, several sessions are devoted to each broad theoretical or methodological domain. Examples include attitudes and behavior, attribution, social inference, mass communication, behavioral analysis of incentives, environment and behavior, psychological measurement, and diffusion of innovation. (Texts: health policy and health services research reprints pertinent to topic.)

## CURRICULUM AT BRANDEIS

Brandeis University recognized in the late 1980s and early 1990s that the field of health policy was rapidly expanding. Those areas developing most extensively were identification of social problems in health care and the changing nature of delivery systems. The Pew program at Brandeis responded to these changing trends with the creation of a curriculum that trained students with the ability to successfully draw upon a broad range of disciplines and conduct action-oriented policy research. As the curriculum became more multidisciplinary, the requirements for health specialization became much more specific (Raskin et al., 1992).

During the first phase of the program, Brandeis and Boston University (BU) had a joint program. The interdisciplinary core curriculum was initially developed by Sol Levine, a sociologist, and Stan Wallack, an economist. The four specially designed Pew courses were Health Financing, taught by Stan Wallack; Health Politics and Organization, taught by Deborah Stone; Health Sociology, taught by Sol Levine; and Health Care Utilization and Illness, taught by Dick Egdahl. A fifth course, the Pew Dissertation Seminar, was added to introduce students to how to conduct research. Initially, the dissertation seminar was led by Sol Levine and Stan Wallack. The goal was to bring Pew students from both universities together to begin thinking about their dissertation. Early on, Steve Crane became involved in teaching the seminar, and he focused on teaching students how to define a research problem and conduct the investigation that would lead to completing a dissertation within the 2-year time frame.

During the second phase of the program, the focus of the curriculum shifted from acute medical care services and cost-containment to encompass a broader array of policy issues related to the most underserved and vulnerable populations. The program was moved completely to the Institute for Health Policy at the Heller School at Brandeis. Nonetheless, Brandeis maintained its ties with BU's professional schools of medicine, public health, law, and management.

The curriculum during the second phase required students to take 14 courses, including 3 social science theory courses and 3 or more courses in research methods. The health specialization at the Heller School, which became required for all doctoral students interested in health policy, consisted of four required courses: Issues in National Health Policy, taught by Stanley Wallack and Stuart Altman; Health Economics, taught by Christine Bishop; Health Care Organization and Politics, taught by Deborah Stone; and Social, Ethical and Legal Issues in Health Policy, taught by George Annas and other BU faculty. These four courses have been modified since the program began to reflect changes in reimbursement and organization of health care delivery, new technology, an interest in healthier lifestyles, and policy changes that have shifted decision making from the federal level to state and local authorities. Students specializing in health policy are also required to take at least one of the courses in either the health policy core or the special populations core and to attend the Seminar in Health Policy Research led by Jon Chilingerian, codirector of the Brandeis Pew program.

The Heller School offers a PhD in social welfare policy. The school has a strong commitment to providing broad interdisciplinary training in economics, political science, sociology, and research methods. As part of the effort to integrate the core curriculum of the Heller School and to have the full resources of the Health Policy Institute available to students specializing in health policy, a Pew Curriculum Planning Committee was created. The committee included the dean and four faculty members from the Heller School plus the director of the Institute for Health Policy and four senior researchers from the institute. At the same time, the Heller School was also seeing a dramatic increase in the number of other doctoral students seeking to specialize in health policy. To help accommodate the growth in the number of students specializing in health policy, the Institute for Health Policy created an Institute Fellows program beginning in the 1992–1993 academic year and selected four fellows whose course requirements and activities paralleled those of the Pew fellows. In contrast to the Pew fellows, however, Institute fellows were required to work 1 day a week at the institute in exchange for an annual stipend.

From the outset, the content of the core curriculum was interdisciplinary. The doctoral program at the Heller School consists of course work in the basic social sciences, statistics and research methods, policy analysis, economics, and advanced work in substantive policy areas. Substantive areas are organized around the school's research centers and institutes.

Pew fellows have studied and conducted research (including their dissertations) in a wide variety of health policy areas such as cost-containment, technology, rural health delivery, and emergency care. Some students have explored emerging issues such as violence, AIDS, substance abuse, disability, and the influence of gender on professional behavior. Students are required to attend a dissertation seminar that provides in-depth exposure to the processes of conducting research. The goal has been to bring students together to begin thinking about their dissertations. Students are taught how to define the research problem and conduct the investigation, leading to completion of a dissertation within the 2-year time frame.

### Lessons Learned

Operating an accelerated doctoral program alongside a more traditional model was difficult at Brandeis, however, the Pew program turned out to be a catalyst for educational reform and change. On the basis of the experience of the Pew program, adjustments and reforms were made to the policies, procedures, and curriculum of the traditional educational program. Four problems had to be resolved: initial faculty concerns about the quality of an accelerated program, the need to change educational policy and curriculum rules, requiring an early dissertation seminar, and balancing a loose versus tight curriculum structure.

At the outset of the Pew program, some Heller School faculty challenged the concept of a doctoral program that was trying to produce high-quality, academically oriented students in only 2 or 3 years. The outcomes of the Pew experience allayed these fears. The faculty found that some of the best and brightest students in the program were Pew fellows, and some of the best dissertations were completed by Pew fellows in less than 3 years. Although 2 years was indeed fast, the faculty learned that there was no correlation between taking 5 more years and producing better scholars.

A second problem was the inertia in educational polices and procedures that evolved around a traditional educational model. In the early years, the Pew fellows found that to complete the degree in 2 years, educational policies had to become more flexible. For example, there was a requirement that all doctoral students had to pass general examinations in January of their second year. Only after passing all exams could fellows defend their dissertation proposal. Several Pew fellows felt that waiting until that time to take the exams was an obstacle to finishing the program in 2 years. Students therefore requested to take the exams in the spring of their first year so that they could hold a dissertation proposal hearing in the fall of their second year. The faculty reexamined the policy and chose to allow some Pew fellows and other doctoral students to take their exams earlier, accommodating those on a faster track.

A third problem was when should a doctoral program ask students to think about finding a dissertation topic? The Pew program required four dissertation seminars starting in the first semester of study. The seminars provided an opportunity to inculcate the goal of finishing in 2 years. On the first day of the fall seminar, the first-year doctoral students were told to think about their research interests and to winnow a list of dissertation topics. The seminar became the opportunity for Pew fellows to develop, negotiate, and formalize the idea of a 2- or 3-year target for completion. Furthermore, the seminar allowed the fellows to interact with a psychological support group that had the same educational objectives. Other doctoral students at Brandeis were not encouraged to join such a seminar until their third year, which often added 2 or 3 years onto their programs. The Pew program faculty learned that setting difficult and specific goals, such as finishing a dissertation in 3 years, may lead to higher performance. Although many Pew fellows took more than 3 years to finish, the average Pew fellow finished much faster than other Heller School doctoral students.

Finally, the educational philosophy of Brandeis's social policy doctoral program posed a problem for the Pew fellows. The traditional doctoral program allowed students to design a highly individualized plan of study, which often took 6 or 7 years to complete. The program had evolved to maximize student's freedom to chose courses—hence, a more a loosely structured curriculum. For example, the core curriculum consisted of three perspective courses in sociology, economics, and political science, three courses in research methods, and a minimum of eight free electives. Some doctoral students never took any statistics courses, opting for research methods, qualitative methods, and evaluation research.

The idea of graduating students in 2 to 3 years without a more stringent set of requirements made no sense for an accelerated program. Many Pew fellows found that the looser structure added time (in years) to their program. During each reapplication for Pew funding the Brandeis Pew curriculum increased its required courses, added more milestones, and worked toward a more structured curriculum and a better-integrated learning sequence. Complaints from other Heller School doctoral students who preferred the structure of the Pew curriculum resulted in the Heller School reforming its doctoral education and requiring an early dissertation seminar.

In conclusion, four lessons regarding curriculum structure were learned. First, an accelerated doctoral program can produce highly qualified PhDs. Second, to accommodate an accelerated program, flexibility with respect to rules is required. Third, requiring students to think about a dissertation in the first semester may be challenging, but many students will rise to the occasion. Finally, an innovative doctoral program funded by a foundation could have a lasting impact on a school by becoming a catalyst for change.

## COURSE OFFERINGS AT BRANDEIS UNIVERSITY
### Social Science Core Courses

*Economics Perspectives on Social Policy.* This course has three broad objectives: (1) to introduce the economist's way of thinking; (2) to introduce alternative modes of analysis, including Marxian; and (3) to illustrate how economic analysis can be useful in analyzing areas of social behavior and policy. The course introduces basic concepts from microeconomics like the market mechanism, economic models of choice, and efficiency. It considers how alternative systems solve economic problems. It offers illustrations of how the economic concepts can be used in policy analysis.

*Political Perspectives on Social Policy.* This course is about politics, policy analysis, and political argument. Part I is an introduction to the concepts of power, conflict, and interest in political science. Part II examines the broad goals of social policy, such as equality or security, to understand their substantive meanings and how these ideals become strategic weapons in the conduct of political disputes. Part III examines how institutions and rules of politics shape the context and effectiveness of policy.

*Sociological Perspectives on Social Policy.* This core course selectively reviews the insights that various sociological theories and methods can bring to social policy analysis. The course features theories in sociology that are particularly relevant to the practical goals of social welfare. In addition, the course considers four key elements of society and how they change: culture, institutions, collectives and roles. Major alternative theories, research traditions, and social policies associated with them are discussed.

### Required Health Policy Courses

*Issues in National Health Policy.* This seminar examines and critically analyzes the health care system in the United States, emphasizing the major issues and trends that have made it the subject of intense public concern and governmental interest. In particular, the course will concentrate on the activities of the federal government: what problems it has attempted to confront, how it has attempted to solve these problems, how successful it has been; and what types of activities are likely in the future.

*Health Economics.* The objective of this course is to introduce students to an economic approach to analyzing resource allocation in the health care sector. The course will teach students to use economic models of demand, production, and markets for goods and services to analyze the key resource allocation questions in health care: Who receives health care?, How is health care production carried out and at what cost?, and What kind of care and how much care are produced? The course will apply economic models to questions of utilization and supply, encompassing issues of cost, efficiency, and accessibility of care. The incentives and behaviors of consumers and producers of health care will be considered by using these models.

*Health Care Organization and Politics.* This seminar examines some of the major structural and cultural features of U.S. health policy. It focuses on four elements of health care that make it politically distinctive: labor organized around a concept of professionalism; a "product" consisting of human caring for sick people, yet driven by technological devices; financing through insurance rather than direct capitalization; and distribution through complex organizations.

*Social, Ethical, and Legal Issues in Health Care.* This course presents contemporary issues of social justice and social choice as they arise in the U.S. health care delivery system. The course also highlights the ethical and legal problems that originate from the development of new medical technology and the rights of patients. Students are taught to think analytically about important social problems from legal and ethical perspectives.

*Seminar in Health Policy Research.* This seminar was designed to introduce students to investigative tools and methodological approaches that would aid conceptual thinking during various stages of the research process. The seminar assists students in identifying research topics for their dissertations by the end of the first year of the program and provides psychological support for the challenging 2-year learning sequence.

### Health Policy Core

*Financing and Payment of Health Care.* This seminar will examine health insurance and payment practices to health care providers, the problems with the current methods, and possible modifications. Because reimbursement policies vary widely by provider type, the course will focus only on physician services, hospital care, and prepaid plans. Also, the increasing problems of the private market in providing insurance protection and the possible universal health financing solutions will be discussed.

*Management of Health Care Organizations.* This course introduces PhD and master's students to some management theories, analytic concepts, tools, and hands-on approaches to managing health care organizations. By the end of the course, students will understand how to research or participate in strategic management activities as well as general management situations; moreover, students will learn how to use some of the important analytic tools used by health care managers.

### Statistics and Research Methods

*Statistics.* This course is designed to provide students with a working knowledge of descriptive statistics, the logic of statistical inference, the concept of standard error, confidence limits, hypothesis, analysis of variance, correlation, and simple regression analysis. Problem sets using SPSS will be integrated with classroom presentations.

*Research Methods.* This course covers basic issues in research design beginning with an overview of conceptions of knowledge, theory design, the development of empirical research models, and basic strategies for developing knowledge through research. The research strategies reviewed include survey research, experimental designs, field observational methods, and evaluation research. Issues of sampling and measurement are emphasized. In addition to course content, class time is devoted to discussing the practical aspects of designing a research project. Each student is required to develop his or her own research design during the course.

*Regression Analysis.* This is an applications-oriented course covering multiple regression, as well as an introduction to logit analysis and simultaneous equation methods. The course is designed to teach students how to select appropriate statistical techniques for particular applications and how to interpret the results that are obtained.

*Econometrics.* This course is designed to provide students with an in-depth understanding of discrete choice techniques such as logit, probit, and tobit models. This is an applications-oriented course. Students will learn how to select the appropriate statistical techniques for particular applications, how to estimate these models using the Time Series Processor statistical package, and how to interpret results.

*Factor Analysis and Multivariate Design.* Students are introduced to multivariate methods. Assignments include the completion and report of a multivariate analysis using computer techniques.

*Causal Modeling.* Models based on theoretical knowledge of the causal links between variables representing a social or economic system may be tested against empirical data using various computer algorithms such as LISREL modeling.

*Other Courses.* Also offered are the courses Qualitative Research, Survey Research, Evaluation Research, Applied Research, and Social Forecasting Methodology

## Special Populations and Social Policy[2]

*Race/Ethnicity, Gender and Health Care.* This course explores how race/ethnicity and gender are factors in health care policies and programs in the United States. Evidence for race/ethnicity and gender differences in health care needs, utilization, and outcomes are presented for different age groups. The importance of these differences is discussed in terms of alternate concepts of justice for health care. A broad range of theoretical perspectives on the causes of race/ethnicity and gender effects on health care are reviewed. Diversity and health research opportunities and methods are described. Implications of inequitable access by race/ethnicity and gender for health care practice and policies are examined.

*Research and Policy Issues in Mental Retardation and Developmental Disabilities.* This seminar focuses on the major policy changes during the past two decades involving both educational services and treatment programs for children and adults with disabilities. In addition to investigating these changes on the basis of reviews of court decisions, legislation, and historical accounts, selected topics will be analyzed in detail by using research reports. Students will become familiar with the current research literature on these topics and will be able to critically evaluate research findings and methods in the field.

[2] *Only representative examples of courses in this area are described.*

*Long-Term Care Policies and Planning.* One of the most important health policy issues facing the nation in the 1990s is how to finance long-term care to chronically ill and disabled people. This course will acquaint students with current information on the size and characteristics of the population at risk, the nature of service delivery systems, and methods of financing and managing existing services. The primary focus will be on aged individuals, but other populations with disabilities will be considered. The performance of the current system will be evaluated against several policy objectives, and major unresolved issues will be identified. The underlying issues of values and ethics will be raised throughout the course.

# APPENDIX C.

## UCSF Fellow-Mentor Arrangements

The development of strong preceptorial relationships is a key aspect of the Pew Health Policy Program (PHPP). The goals of such a relationship are for the fellow to (1) gain specific research skills and (2) make the transition from being a student to being an independent researcher. This is often a difficult process that requires a clear understanding of the goals and expectations for both fellows and faculty.

### RESEARCH SKILLS

Health policy research is an applied field that draws upon a wide range of disciplines and methodologies including anthropology, decision analysis, economics, epidemiology, political science, and sociology. It is generally the case, however, that regardless or how well trained a fellow may be in his or her discipline, there is much to be learned about how to apply those skills to health policy questions. For example, a fellow with a background in economics and a dissertation in health economics will, in general, still have much to learn about applying the tools of economics to real-world data to arrive at conclusions that will be useful from a policy perspective. A fellow may want to gain experience with the methods and techniques used in a new field relevant to his or her chosen career path. For example, a sociologist interested in health behaviors and infectious diseases may want to learn about the methods used by epidemiologists. In cases like this, basic terminology and methods are often best learned through some formal course work, with no expectation that the fellow will become truly competent in the new field. Rather, the goal for Pew fellows is to learn how to ask the right questions of the appropriate experts and how to apply the knowledge in new situations.

For fellows with clinical backgrounds, the appropriate research goals are somewhat different. It normally takes a PhD trainee at least five years to gain the necessary theoretical and methodological skills required to be a competent researcher and then another 2 years of postdoctoral training to know how to apply those skills to health services research problems. Thus, one cannot expect a clinician to do all this in a 2-year postdoctoral fellowship. However, someone with a clinical background can learn how to become a collaborator with other formally trained health policy researchers. This requires both learning the basic terminology and methods and, more importantly, developing an appreciation of how people in a specific field (e.g., economics or sociology) address a problem, pose questions, and undertake the research. Although some of this knowledge can be acquired through introductory courses, one of the most effective methods is collaboration with skilled investigators on specific projects.

## BECOMING AN INDEPENDENT RESEARCHER

Although one can acquire specific research skills in various ways, ranging from course work to learning by doing, becoming an independent researcher is a process that requires active involvement of the fellow and the support of the faculty. The academic and policy researcher needs to understand a set of activities, including formulating problems, developing research proposals and writing grants, investigating specific research questions, interpreting findings, preparing papers for publication, understanding the publication review process, and presenting results at professional meetings. Although a fellow might be able to do all this in a 2-year period, it is not likely to happen without careful consideration of the fellow's roles in specific research projects. Given the time frames involved in grant writing and research, it is impossible for a fellow to follow a project from its inception to completion within a 2-year period. However, it is possible for the fellow to experience the various elements through involvement in multiple projects. The following is an example of this:

■ Upon arrival, the fellow identifies a preceptor with an ongoing research project that has the potential for some independent investigations. The fellow can then become a member of the project team and observe the principal investigator (PI) managing the main study, leading the analysis, and writing up the findings. The greatest problems faced by fellows often involve knowing how to write up results and determining when papers are ready for submission.  Observing the PI in the process is a key aspect of the learning experience.

▪      In the normal course of events, most large projects generate potential subsidiary studies that can use the data of the main project but that are not integral aspects of the project.  The fellow can help develop these ideas, undertake the analysis, write up the results, and be first author on this subsidiary project.  Since the PI typically has intimate knowledge of the data and analytic issues, it should be relatively easy to involve him or her as a collaborator.  However, the goal of the fellowship is to let the fellow acquire experience, which means letting him or her take responsibility and the credit for this piece of work.  The subsidiary project requires careful design, in that it should be doable within a relatively short period of time so that the fellow can write one or more papers based on it for submission before the end of the fellowship period.  Given the normal delays, the project should be doable within a year, which would imply submitting papers by early winter of the fellow's second year.

▪      Learning how to design a project and write a grant are two additional goals of the fellowship.  Again, it is probably best to follow a "see one, do one" pattern.  This means that the fellow should work with an experienced faculty member who is developing a proposal for submission.  This will allow the fellow to see how an idea is developed, honed, and structured to fit within the constraints of the granting agency.  Learning how to develop budgets and work plans is a key part of this experience. Although the fellow should be a part of the process, the fellow's lack of experience means that the PI or a senior research associate will have the primary responsibility for designing and writing the proposal.

▪      It is one thing to work on someone else's proposal and quite another to write one's own.  The fellow should also have the experience of developing a proposal for a small project on which he or she would be the major researcher.  University and agency guidelines typically do not allow fellows to be PIs; however, a senior faculty member will often be willing to be the PI for a small percentage of time, with most of the work to be done by the fellow.  In the ideal situation, the fellow would be able to transfer the grant to his or her new institution after completing the fellowship.

## FELLOW-PRECEPTOR RELATIONSHIPS
Although the preceptorial model has many advantages, its highly decentralized structure requires careful monitoring to

be sure that specific pairings are working well for both faculty member and the fellow. The preceptorship model has certain potential points of friction. Teaching research skills on a one-to-one basis can be time-consuming and frustrating for the faculty, especially since there is no course credit given for such instruction and the program has no funds available for faculty support. On the other hand, fellows may feel that they are receiving too little guidance and are asked to do too much "scut work." Careful delineation of fellow-preceptor relationships can avoid many of these problems. This involves well-defined expectations for both fellows and faculty.

During the interview process faculty will attempt to identify potential preceptors and projects for each applicant. If it is impossible to identify a faculty member on either campus who could serve as a preceptor, acceptance of the fellow would be unwise. Situations can change, however, between the time of interview and arrival in the Bay Area. Thus, during the first 2 months after joining the program, the fellow will be expected to meet with at least six faculty members to discuss potential areas of mutual interest that may result in either major or minor preceptorial relationships.

Preceptorial relationships should be beneficial for both the faculty and the fellow. The faculty member is offering both hands-on training and an introduction to the real world of health policy research. In addition, the faculty member can usually provide access to the data and computer resources of a large project as well as space and membership in a larger working group. Affiliation with a project may also lead to the presentation of results at professional meetings, with travel costs covered by the project. In turn, the fellow is offering enthusiastic assistance in carrying out the main project and undertaking supplementary projects, with salary support covered by the fellowship.

The primary goal of the preceptorships is educational, and this goal is sometimes best met by involvement with more than one preceptor. Usually this is accomplished by having a major involvement with one project and smaller commitments with one or more other projects. Multiple affiliations are encouraged because they allow more experience with both a wider variety of disciplines and faculty with different styles. Involvement in multiple professional networks is also a major advantage. On the other hand, multiple involvements may lead to conflicting demands on a fellow's time. If this becomes a problem, or if any other problems arise with a preceptorial relationship, the fellow or faculty member may raise the issue with any member of the Executive Committee of the fellowship program.

## SUMMARY

As outlined above, it is expected that each fellow will become involved in one or more research projects, publish one or more papers based on a subsidiary project for which he or she takes primary responsibility and is first author, be a coauthor on one or more papers that are part of a large project, collaborate on a faculty member's grant proposal, and design and submit his or her own proposal. Fellows who have recently completed a dissertation will also be expected to prepare for publication articles or a book from that work. Fellows with a clinical background may focus part of their time on specific methods courses. In addition, all fellows will attend core writing and policy seminars and the journal club.

After a general orientation meeting with the faculty, the fellow will begin the program with a series of meetings with faculty members on both campuses to identify potential research projects and preceptorial relationships. Although it is certainly possible that new opportunities will develop over time and relationships will be renegotiated, at the end of the fellow's second month he or she will prepare a memorandum outlining the projects on which he or she will be working and the expected products. Thereafter, fellows will prepare a progress report on their activities every 3 months. Preceptors will provide an evaluation of the fellow every 6 months. The Executive Committee will provide semiannual feedback to the fellows on their progress and continued eligibility for support.

## QUESTIONS TO ASK OF A MENTOR

1. Who are the powerful and important people in the department, the institution, and the discipline worldwide? Who has their ear?

2. How do you write a successful grant application? Where should you apply?

3. How do people in the field find out about, get nominated for, and win awards and prizes.

4. What are the leading journals in the field? How should coauthorships be handled?

5. What scientific organizations are the most important to join? What conferences are the ones to attend? Who can help a person get on the program?

6. What is the best way of getting feedback on a manuscript? To whom should drafts be circulated?

7. What are appropriate and accepted ways to raise different kinds of concerns, issues, and problems (e.g., verbally or by memo) and with whom?

8. What are the department's formal and informal criteria for promotion and tenure? Who can clarify these criteria? How does one build a promotion packet? Who can influence these decisions?

9. What departmental and institutional decisions that might affect positions in the department are pending? Who can influence these decisions?

10. How can I attract graduate students and postdoctoral fellows to work with me?

## BENEFITS OF MENTORING FOR THE PROTÉGÉ

Protégés can gain a host of benefits from a single mentor and can also form more limited relationships that address specific needs for skills or information. These include:

1. individual recognition and encouragement;

2. honest criticism and informal feedback;

3. advice on how to balance teaching, research, and other responsibilities and how to set professional priorities;

4. knowledge of the informal rules for advancement as well as political and substantive pitfalls to be avoided;

5. information on how to "behave" in a variety of professional settings;

6. appropriate ways of making contact with authorities in a discipline;

7. skills for showcasing one's own work;

8. an understanding of how to build a circle of friends and contacts both within and outside one's institution; and

9. a perspective on long-term career planning.

## WHAT TO LOOK FOR IN MENTORS

What a newcomer looks for in mentors depends on the novice's particular needs in a given field; here are some questions to consider:

1. What is the mentor's own achievement in key areas?

2. Does the mentor know what is excellent in a given area and set high standards for him or herself?

3. Is the mentor someone who believes wholeheartedly in your abilities?

4. What has happened to this person's former protégés in terms of positions, grants, publications, etc.? Are there significant differences between what has happened to male and female protégés? To minority and nonminority protégés?

5. What is the mentor's relationship to various groups and networks in the department, school, and discipline on campus?

6. Is the mentor not only good at giving advice and direction but also able to understand your own views about your needs and goals?

7. If he or she is unable to provide you with the information, skills, and knowledge you need, will the mentor help you find someone who can?

8. Are you comfortable interacting with this individual?

## HOW TO GET TO KNOW POTENTIAL MENTORS

Individuals can do more than merely wait for a senior person to notice their achievements and choose them. By actively seeking mentors, you can make yourself more visible as a potential protégé:

1. Introduce yourself and make the first contact in relation to a professional subject.

2. Begin to ask for help regarding the strengths and weaknesses in your work.

3. Take the initiative in putting the relationship on a more collegial basis if it seems appropriate.

4. Ask a colleague to mention you or your work to a potential mentor.

5. Volunteer to serve on a task force, committee, or project on which your potential mentor is also a mentor.

6. Invite your potential mentor to be a guest lecturer in your class.

## PRACTICAL SUGGESTIONS FOR A SUCCESSFUL MENTORING RELATIONSHIP FOR THE PROTÉGÉ

1. Set up regular lunch meetings on a monthly basis. Come prepared to discuss specific agenda items on a pre-arranged basis. This agenda may span a year and would function like a curriculum in regard to the relationship. As much as possible, adhere to the schedule agreed upon.

2. Seek the mentor's assistance and sponsorship for the identification of special research projects, committee, or other university-related tasks.

3. Share examples of your own written documents (e.g., letters, reports, manuscripts, grant submissions, and curriculum vitae with your mentor and solicit comments for improvement.

4. Ask your mentor to provide you with insights on the structure of the university and the roles and personalities

of university officials and the types of work that they perform. When feasible, indicate a willingness to attend meetings or lunch so that you can meet and observe some of these people. Ask to be introduced to people you might not otherwise meet.

5. Ask your mentor to introduce you to other scientists whose work you would like to know better. Have your mentor set up the interviews or visits for you.

6. Ask your mentor for advice on obtaining departmental support and resources for specific projects.

7. Ask your mentor to identify faculty who have excellent reputations in teaching, how to effectively teach particular materials, and how to be assigned to teach courses in your preferred area of interest.

# APPENDIX D.

## *Examples of Career Trajectories*

nformation in this index comes from the Directories of Pew Health Policy Fellows and Alumni published by the National Academy of Sciences. The information regarding title before the Pew Program was retrieved from the directory that was published during the year that the fellow started the program and represents the position that the fellow held immediately before entering the program. The information regarding title after the Pew Program represents the current title held by the alumni, and this information was retrieved from the 1996 Pew Directory. Positions held between the time of completion of the program and 1996 are not provided. For each category at least one to a maximum of three examples of career trajectories are provided. The numbers in parentheses represent the total number of fellows whose career trajectories followed the stated pattern. Career trajectories for those fellows who remained in the same field are not shown, although their titles and/or status may have changed.

## ACADEMIA — GOVERNMENT (4)

| *Title Before Pew Program* | *Title After Pew Program* |
|---|---|
| Associate Director, Division of Public Health, University of Massachusetts–Amherst | Deputy Director, Office of Statewide Health Planning and Development, Sacramento, CA |
| Research Assistant, University of California, San Francisco | Scientist, Air Policy Branch, Environmental Protection Agency, Washington, DC |
| Deputy Director of the Supportive Services Program for Older Persons, Heller School, Brandeis University, Waltham, MA | Project Leader, Office of Evaluation and Inspections, Office of the Inspector General, U.S. Department of Health and Human Services |

## ACADEMIA — RESEARCH (7)

| Title Before Pew Program | Title After Pew Program |
|---|---|
| Lecturer, Department of Sociology, University of Miami, Coral Gables, Florida | Research Scientist, New England Research Institutes, Watertown, MA |
| Lecturer, Children's Hospital and Medical Center, Seattle, WA | Biostatistician, Clinical Quality Management Department, Harvard Pilgrim Health Care, Brookline, MA |
| Associate Professor of Sociology, California State University, Los Angeles | RAND, Santa Monica, CA |

## ACADEMIA — CONSULTING (4)

| Title Before Pew Program | Title After Pew Program |
|---|---|
| Senior Research Associate, Heller School, Brandeis University, Waltham, MA | Project Manager, The MEDSTAT Group, Cambridge, MA |
| Instructor of Sociology, Yale University, New Haven, CT | Consultant, Interactive Technologies in Health Care, San Francisco, CA |
| Project Director, Institute for Health and Aging and Adjunct Professor, Social and Behavioral Science, University of California, San Francisco | Vice President and Health of California Office, The Lewin Group, Sausalito, CA |

## ACADEMIA — HEALTH CARE MANAGEMENT (5)

| Title Before Pew Program | Title After Pew Program |
|---|---|
| Assistant Professor of Pathology, College of Medicine, University of Iowa | Vice President for Performance Improvement, The Johns Hopkins Hospital, Baltimore, MD |
| Project Manager, Multi-Hospital Study of Variations in Medical Practice and Clinical Outcomes, University of California, Los Angeles | Associate Chief, Evaluation and Decision Support Service, Sepulveda VA Medical Center, Sepulveda, CA |
| Coordinator of Educational Programs, Heller Graduate School, Brandeis University, Waltham, MA | Research Coordinator, Department of Occupational Therapy, Rush-Presbyterian–St. Luke's Medical Center, Chicago, IL |

## ACADEMIA — PROFESSIONAL ASSOCIATIONS (0)

## ACADEMIA — OTHER (1)

| Title Before Pew Program | Title After Pew Program |
|---|---|
| Research Associate, Division of Population and Family Health, School of Public Health, UCLA | Founding Partner, 2 Cow HERD, Internet Service Provider, Venice, CA |

## RESEARCH — ACADEMIA (3)

| *Title Before Pew Program* | *Title After Pew Program* |
|---|---|
| Research Scientist, Aerospace Medical Research, Douglas Aircraft Company, Santa Monica, CA | Associate Professor of Surgery, Division of Emergency Medicine, Emergency Department, University of Texas–Southwestern Medical Center |
| Research Assistant, RAND, Santa Monica, CA | Research Associate, Institute for Health Promotion and Disease Prevention, University of Southern California School of Medicine |
| Research Assistant, RAND, Santa Monica, CA | Center for Health Administration Studies, University of Chicago |

## RESEARCH — GOVERNMENT (3)

| *Title Before Pew Program* | *Title After Pew Program* |
|---|---|
| Research Assistant, RAND, Santa Monica, CA | Director, Medicare Part A Analysis, Office of Legislative and Intergovernmental Affairs, Health Care Financing Administration, Washington, DC |
| Research Assistant, RAND, Santa Monica, CA | National Expert, European Commission, Directorate of Public Health and Safety at Work, Office of Public Health Analysis, Policy and Program Coordination, Development and Evaluation, Luxembourg |
| Research Associate, RAND, Santa Monica, CA | Senior Analyst, Prospective Payment Review Commission, Washington, DC |

## RESEARCH — CONSULTING (0)

## RESEARCH — HEALTH CARE MANAGEMENT (2)

| *Title Before Pew Program* | *Title After Pew Program* |
|---|---|
| Director of Research, Arizona Long Term Care Gerontology Center, AZ | Pew Health Policy Program, San Francisco General Hospital, San Francisco, CA |
| Research Associate, RAND, Santa Monica, CA | Vice President, Client Services/ UMWA Health and Retirement Funds, First Health Services, Coraopolis, PA |

## RESEARCH — PROFESSIONAL ASSOCIATIONS (0)

## RESEARCH — OTHER (0)

## HEALTH CARE MANAGEMENT — ACADEMIA (8)

| Title Before Pew Program | Title After Pew Program |
| --- | --- |
| Executive Vice President, Massachusetts Eye and Ear Infirmary, Boston, MA | Assistant Professor, Clark University, Worcester, MA |
| Manager of Health Care Cost Containment, Johnson and Johnson, New Brunswick, NJ | Senior Research Associate, Institute for Circumpolar Health Studies, University of Alaska |
| Hospital Administrator, Westworld Community Health Care | Project Manager, Department of Health Services Management and Policy, University of Michigan |

## HEALTH CARE MANAGEMENT — RESEARCH (5)

| Title Before Pew Program | Title After Pew Program |
| --- | --- |
| Director of Research, California Association of Public Hospitals | Director, Quality Measurement and Analysis, Department of Quality, Kaiser Foundation Health Plan, Oakland, CA |
| Research Director, Multicultural AIDS Coalition, Boston, MA | Senior Research Analyst, COSMOS Corporation, Rockville, MD |
| Senior Planner, New York City Health and Hospitals Corporation, NYC | Senior Policy Analyst, Health Department of Public Policy, Community Service Society of New York |

## HEALTH CARE MANAGEMENT — GOVERNMENT (6)

| Title Before Pew Program | Title After Pew Program |
| --- | --- |
| Project Coordinator, US Corporation for Health Management | Acting Deputy Director, Health Policy and Planning Division, Office of Statewide Health Planning and Development, Sacramento, CA |
| Medical Director, Alaska Native Hospital, Kotzebue, AK | State Epidemiologist, Director of Epidemiology and Prevention Branch, Division of Public Health, Georgia Department of Human Resources |
| Interim Medical Director, West Berkeley Community Health Center, Berkeley, CA | Medical Officer, National Center on Drug Abuse, National Institutes of Health, Rockville, MD |

## HEALTH CARE MANAGEMENT — CONSULTING (8)

| Title Before Pew Program | Title After Pew Program |
| --- | --- |
| Manager of Program Development and Planning, Dallas Region, Kaiser Permanente, Dallas, TX | Consultant, Comparative Medical Outcomes Research and Evaluation, Golden, CO |
| Risk Manager, New York City Health and Hospitals Corporation | Senior Manager, The Lewin Group, Fairfax, VA |
| Executive Director, AIDS Action Council | Health Policy Consultant |

## HEALTH CARE MANAGEMENT — PROFESSIONAL ASSOCIATIONS (1)

| Title Before Pew Program | Title After Pew Program |
| --- | --- |
| Staffing Coordinator, Stanford Hospital, Stanford, CA | Washington Health Foundation |

## HEALTH CARE MANAGEMENT — OTHER (1)

| *Title Before Pew Program* | *Title After Pew Program* |
|---|---|
| Associate Director, Department of Medicine, Cedars-Sinai Medical Center, Los Angeles, CA | Physician, Cedars-Sinai Medical Center, Los Angeles, CA |

## GOVERNMENT — ACADEMIA (12)

| *Title Before Pew Program* | *Title After Pew Program* |
|---|---|
| Program Analyst, Office of the Inspector General, U.S. Department of Health and Human Services | Tufts School of Nutrition, Cambridge, MA |
| Regional Coordinator, Center for Health Promotion and Environmental Disease Prevention, Massachusetts Department of Public Health | Associate Professor of Health Policy, Director, Joint Program in Public Policy and Public Health, School of Public Health, University of California, Berkeley |
| Coordinator, Protocol for Comparison of CT and MRI, National Cancer Institute, NIH | Assistant Professor, School of Nursing, Indiana State University |

## GOVERNMENT — RESEARCH (10)

| *Title Before Pew Program* | *Title After Pew Program* |
|---|---|
| Deputy Director for Special Projects, Policy and Budget Coordination, Governor's Office, SC | Research Director, Sarah Shuptrine and Associates and Research Director, Columbia, SC |
| Policy Analyst, Legislative and Budget Analysis Branch, Office of Analysis and Evaluation, Food and Nutrition Service, U.S. Department of Agriculture | Senior Research Associate, The Urban Institute, Washington, DC |
| Special Assistant to the Director/Senior Research Analyst, Office of Research and Demonstration, Health Care Financing Administration | Economist, Abt Associates, Bethesda, MD |

## GOVERNMENT — HEALTH CARE MANAGEMENT (6)

| *Title Before Pew Program* | *Title After Pew Program* |
|---|---|
| Director, Indigent Health Care Project, Texas Department of Human Services | President, Children's Hospital Association of Texas, Austin |
| Project Director, Bureau of Ambulatory Care Reimbursement, NY State Department of Health | Director, HIV Special Needs Plan, The Partnership/Village Center for Care, New York |
| Deputy Director, Office of Policy Analysis, National Institute of Alcohol Abuse and Alcoholism, U.S. Department of Health and Human Services | Vice President, Public Policy and Counsel to the President, Managed Care and Employee Benefit Operations, The Travelers Companies, Hartford, CT |

## GOVERNMENT — CONSULTING (4)

| *Title Before Pew Program* | *Title After Pew Program* |
|---|---|
| Director, Bureau of Long Term Care, Massachusetts Rate Setting Commission, Boston | Program Manager, The MEDSTAT Group, Cambridge, MA |
| Chief, Evaluation Branch, Office of Program Development, Bureau of Maternal and Child Health Resource Development, U.S. Department of Health and Human Services | Health Planning and Policy Consultant |
| Research Associate, Health Services Research and Development, Veterans Administration, UT | Senior Scientist, Health and Human Development Programs, Education Development Center, MA |

## GOVERNMENT — PROFESSIONAL ASSOCIATIONS (1)

| *Title Before Pew Program* | *Title After Pew Program* |
|---|---|
| Nurse Practitioner, Multnomah County Health Department, Portland, OR | Health Policy Analyst, Oregon Nurses Association |

## GOVERNMENT — OTHER (0)

## CONSULTING — ACADEMIA (4)

| *Title Before Pew Program* | *Title After Pew Program* |
|---|---|
| Senior Consultant, MEDSTAT Systems, Inc., Boston, MA | Research Associate, Institute for Health Policy, Heller Graduate School, Brandeis University, Waltham, MA |
| Consultant, Center for Social Science Computation and Research, University of Washington | Research Assistant Professor, Department of Psychosocial and Community Health, School of Nursing, University of Washington, Seattle, WA |
| Senior Consultant, National Health Mothers, Healthy Babies Coalition, Washington, DC | Clinical Core Faculty, Department of Health Psychology, California School of Professional Psychology, Los Angeles Campus, CA |

## CONSULTING — RESEARCH (3)

| *Title Before Pew Program* | *Title After Pew Program* |
|---|---|
| Health Policy Consultant | Senior Project Manager, Jobs for the Future, Boston, MA |
| Senior Consultant, MEDSTAT Systems, Inc., Cambridge, MA | Director of Research, Pacific Business Group on Health, Los Angeles, CA |
| Resident Consultant, School of Public Health, University of California, Los Angeles | RAND, Santa Monica, CA |

## CONSULTING — HEALTH CARE MANAGEMENT (0)

## CONSULTING — GOVERNMENT (0)

## CONSULTING — PROFESSIONAL ASSOCIATIONS (0)

| *Title Before Pew Program* | *Title After Pew Program* |
|---|---|
| Financing Specialist, On Lok Senior Health Services, San Francisco, CA | Executive Director, National PACE Association |

## CONSULTING — OTHER (2)

| *Title Before Pew Program* | *Title After Pew Program* |
|---|---|
| Senior Associate, Lewin ICF, Inc., Fairfax, VA | Attorney, Proskauer, Rose, Goetz & Mendelsohn, Washington, DC |

## OTHER — ACADEMIA (11)

| *Title Before Pew Program* | *Title After Pew Program* |
|---|---|
| Executive Director, Managing Attorney and Clinical Social Worker, The Hawkins Center of Law and Services for the Disabled, Richmond, CA | Assistant Professor, School of Social Welfare, UCLA School of Public Policy and Social Research, Los Angeles, CA |
| Associate Attorney, Fordham & Starrett and Sullivan & Worcester | Associate Professor of Law and Public Policy, School of Public and Environmental Affairs, Indiana University, Bloomington |
| Medical Practitioner, Mission Neighborhood Health Center | Associate Professor, Departments of Family and Community Medicine and Epidemiology and Biostatistics, Institute for Health Policy Studies, University of California, San Francisco |

## OTHER — RESEARCH (1)

| *Title Before Pew Program* | *Title After Pew Program* |
|---|---|
| Physician, Neighborhood Health Centers, Boston, MA | Senior Research Scientist, John Snow, Inc., Boston, MA |

## OTHER — GOVERNMENT (3)

| *Title Before Pew Program* | *Title After Pew Program* |
|---|---|
| Staff Attorney, ABLE, Inc., Boston, MA | Assistant Attorney General, State of Tennessee, Office of the Attorney General, Nashville |
| Dentist, Clinical Practice | California Epidemiologic Investigation Service Resident, Office of Dental Health, Alameda County Health Care Services, Oakland |
| Assistant Director of Public Affairs, American Trucking Association | Health Policy Analyst, Program Evaluation and Methodology Division, U.S. General Accounting Office, Washington, DC |

## OTHER — CONSULTING (2)

| Title Before Pew Program | Title After Pew Program |
| --- | --- |
| Staff Attorney, Youth Law Center, San Francisco | Consultant, National Center for Youth Law, CA |
| Psychotherapist | Research Consultant, American Academy of Physician Assistants, Washington, DC |

## OTHER — HEALTH CARE MANAGEMENT (6)

| Title Before Pew Program | Title After Pew Program |
| --- | --- |
| Attorney, Sidely & Austin, Washington, DC | Senior Director of Policy and Research, National Institute for Health Care Management |
| Physician | Director, Alternative Medicine and Complementary Therapies, St. Elizabeth's Medical Center, Brighton, MA |
| Emergency Physician | Physician Director for National Accounts, Kaiser Permanente Medical Care Program, Oakland, CA |

## OTHER — PROFESSIONAL ASSOCIATIONS (1)

| Title Before Pew Program | Title After Pew Program |
| --- | --- |
| Associate Editor, *Health Care Reporter*, Times Journal Company | Director, Community Programs, Milton S. Eisenhower Foundation, Washington, DC |